Dedication

To the many colleagues, students, and friends who assisted in making this book possible—every contribution is important. This book is also dedicated to Helen.

Heather R. Hall

I am most appreciative of our contributors and stakeholders who create healthcare environments that translate best practices for improvement. Thank you for your tireless efforts, commitment, and relentlessness to safe, quality care for those we are privileged to partner with in innovation and sustained improvement.

Linda A. Roussel

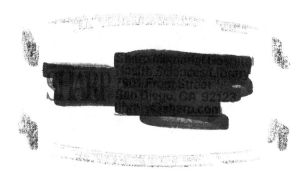

Contents

Contributors

Handan Boztepe, PhD, RN
Assistant Professor
Hacettepe University Faculty of Health Sciences
Child Health and Illness Nursing Department
Ankara, Turkey

Ellen B. Buckner, PhD, RN, CNE
Professor
University of South Alabama
Mobile, Alabama

Clista Clanton, MSLS
Education and Clinical Librarian Coordinator/Circulation Coordinator
University of South Alabama
Mobile, Alabama

Valorie Dearmon, DNP, RN, NEA-BC
Associate Professor and Chair, Maternal Child Nursing Department
University of South Alabama
Mobile, Alabama

Gordana Dermody, MSN, RN, CNL
Clinical Assistant Professor
Washington State University
Spokane, Washington

Sharon M. Fruh, PhD, RN, FNP-BC
Professor
University of South Alabama
Mobile, Alabama

Mary E. Geary, PhD, RN
Consultant
Pensacola, Florida

J. Carolyn Graff, PhD, RN, FAAIDD
Professor and Director, PhD in Nursing Science Program
University of Tennessee Health Science Center
Memphis, Tennessee

James L. Harris, PhD, APRN-BC, MBA, CNL, FAAN
Professor
University of South Alabama
Mobile, Alabama

Duygu Hiçdurmaz, PhD, RN
Assistant Professor
Hacettepe University Faculty of Health Sciences
Psychiatric Nursing Department
Ankara, Turkey

Kenda Jezek, PhD, RN
Professor and Dean
Oral Roberts University
Tulsa, Oklahoma

Carolynn T. Jones, DNP, MSPH, RN
Assistant Professor
Ohio State University
Columbus, Ohio

Trey Lemley, MSLS, JD, AHIP
Information Services and Scholarly Communications Librarian
University of South Alabama Biomedical Library
Mobile, Alabama

Robin Lennon-Dearing, PhD, MSW
Assistant Professor of Social Work
University of Memphis
Memphis, Tennessee

Sara C. Majors, DNP, RNC, NNP-BC, PNP-BC
Clinical Professor of Nursing
Berry College
Mount Berry, Georgia

Anne Miller, PhD, RN
Associate Professor
Vanderbilt University
Nashville, Tennessee

Madhuri S. Mulekar, PhD
Professor and Chair, Department of Mathematics and Statistics
University of South Alabama
Mobile, Alabama

Susan L. Neely-Barnes, PhD, MSW
Associate Professor of Social Work
University of Memphis
Memphis, Tennessee

Shea Polancich, PhD, RN
Assistant Professor/Assistant Dean
University of Alabama Medical Center/School of Nursing
Birmingham, Alabama

Elizabeth S. Pratt, DNP, RN, ACNS-BC
Nurse Scientist and Clinical Nurse Specialist
Acute Medicine and Surgery
Barnes-Jewish Hospital
St. Louis, Missouri

Patricia L. Thomas, PhD, RN, FACHE, NEA-BC, ACNS-BC, CNL
Vice President, Home Care Services
Trinity Health
Farmington Hills, Michigan

▪ Exemplar Contributors:

Erica Arnold, MSN, RN, CNL
Care Coordinator, Heart Failure Clinic
University of Alabama at Birmingham Medical Center
Birmingham, Alabama

Debra Berger, DNP, JD, RN, CRNP
Faculty
Loyola University Nursing
New Orleans, Louisiana

Mary Callens, DNP, RN, CRNP
University of Alabama at Birmingham Medical Center
Birmingham, Alabama

Shannon DeLuca, MSN, AGACNP-BC
University of Alabama at Birmingham Medical Center
Birmingham, Alabama

Susan J. Garpiel, RN, MSN, C-EFM,
Director of Perinatal Clinical Practice
Trinity Health
Farmington Hills, Michigan

David James, DNP, RN, CNS
Center for Nursing Excellence
University of Alabama at Birmingham Medical Center
Birmingham, Alabama

Clare Krntz, MSN, RN, CRNP
Instructor
University of Alabama at Birmingham School of Nursing
Birmingham, Alabama

Quinton Ming, DNP, RN
Case Manager
University of Alabama at Birmingham Medical Center
Birmingham, Alabama

Dana Mitchell, DNP, ACNP-BC
Heart Failure Clinic
University of Alabama at Birmingham Medical Center
Birmingham, Alabama

Sallie Shipman, EdD, MSN, RN, CNL
Instructor
University of Alabama at Birmingham School of Nursing
Birmingham, Alabama

Maria Shirey, PhD, RN, NEA-BC, ANEF, FACHE, FAAN
Department Chair, Acute Care
University of Alabama at Birmingham School of Nursing
Birmingham, Alabama

Donna Stevens, DNP, RN, CRNP
University of Alabama at Birmingham Medical Center
Birmingham, Alabama

Debra M. Swanzy, DNP, RN
Assistant Professor
University of South Alabama College of Nursing
Mobile, Alabama

Lenora Wade, DNP, RN, CRNP
University of Alabama at Birmingham Medical Center
Birmingham, Alabama

Connie White-Williams, PhD, RN, NE-BC, FAAN
Director
Center for Nursing Excellence
University of Alabama at Birmingham Medical Center
Birmingham, Alabama

Foreword

The rapid unfolding of new knowledge in contemporary nursing and the other disciplines that impact nursing, specifically medicine and other healthcare professions, is both a blessing and burden to our large community of clinicians, practitioners, educators, executives, and all others involved in nursing in some capacity. We are blessed by being part of a "living discipline" that is on the cutting-edge of developing, implementing, and evaluating new health information that can directly and indirectly the lives and communities of people across the globe. For this reason, during the Great Recession of 2007–2009, data indicate that industries with the largest volume of employment growth were internet-related, hospitals and health care, health, wellness and fitness, oil and energy, internet technology, and renewables (Nicholson, 2012). In addition, as reported in the *New York Times* in 2014, the largest middle-wage industries with the greatest growth potential were overwhelmingly in health care (Ashkenas & Parlapiano, 2014). These indicators point to nursing being thoroughly part of the growing knowledge economy, resulting in very high growth in our BSN, master's, and DNP programs (American Association of Colleges of Nursing [AACN], 2015).

But we are also burdened by the difficulties of managing this rapid knowledge expansion, and bedside nurses are specifically challenged by the realities of all the data they are required to report and outcomes they are accountable for that are tracked and measured on every shift. We are also challenged to come out of our comfortable nursing silos and be more visible members and leaders on today's modern interdisciplinary and interprofessional healthcare teams. Hall and Roussel's second edition of their book, *Evidence-Based Practice: An Integrative Approach to Research, Administration, and Practice*, is a significant contribution to professional, advanced, and doctoral advanced nursing practice because its editors and contributors seek to better navigate this sometimes contradictory world of the critical appraisal of research findings that is essential to any nursing practice. Individuals or patients can now go on the Internet to investigate their illnesses or conditions and easily be overwhelmed by what various websites indicate they should or should not eat, for example. It is the nurse's role, as health educators at all levels, to synthesize this information and, based on an evaluation of the best evidence, including using the new Joanna Briggs Institute Levels of Evidence (2014), share their professional assessments. In this new data-driven world even competent managers and leaders are expected to make decisions based on evidence. Thus, the scholarship of administrative practice, an emphasis in Part II of this book, is an important contribution. Good management and leadership (and good teaching!) require mastery of specific advanced content, and the idea that an excellent clinical nurse can instantly become an excellent manager or teacher should have been dispelled by now. Today's successful administrator, really no matter the discipline, must not only have expertise in improvement and healthcare safety science, but also keen interpersonal skills and the ability to persuade others while mastering the art of listening.

The third section of this text focuses on the scholarship of clinical practice. This is certainly one of the more challenging topics with which to generate consensus. Everyone knows what clinical practice looks like. But what is the "scholarship" of clinical practice? This text suggests that it is evidence that is disseminated in some professional manner. The question that remains is how are professional, advanced, and doctoral advanced practice nurses educated and mentored to disseminate their knowledge that might enhance care and improve the health of aggregate populations. It is accepted that the PhD-prepared nurse in most settings is supposed to publish research. But DNP-prepared nurses have been sent very confusing messages, likely during their education, about what constitutes their role in the relationship to the generation of evidence. Although some attest that the PhD should generate evidence and the DNP not generate but instead evaluate and translate evidence into practice, this view is an oversimplification and not practical or even helpful to the discipline. It is almost impossible to draw finite distinctions among mathematical, basic, applied, clinical, and translational science, even in nursing science. The generation of "practice evidence" ought to be the chief domain of the DNP student and graduate (Dreher, 2015), where the generation, implementation, and evaluation of evidence is constructed along collaborative healthcare disciplinary guidelines that are understood by all.

Hall and Roussel also revisit the use of theoretical and conceptual models that can guide clinical practice. This is an excellent, often neglected perspective that is emphasized in this new book. My own School of Nursing has used a human-caring, holistic model of care that has guided our curriculum at the baccalaureate and masters (and soon doctoral) levels for several decades. In a time in which our experience with knowledge management (just look at the size of current undergraduate nursing texts!) and the acquisition of specific clinical skills has perhaps marginalized to some degree our focus on the interpersonal and ethical aspects of nursing care in baccalaureate and master's nursing education (I note the reduction at least in the prominence on the emphasis of ethics in the revised 2011 AACN's *Essentials of Master's Education in Nursing*), this text revisits the inherent value of guiding principles that should be overt, not covert or mostly invisible, in any mission statement or degree learning outcomes. In my own time as Dean, I have encouraged the faculty to be more explicit in our mission and framework in our various curricula. Moreover, it has been satisfying to our health agency partners that we emphasize core elements of our human-caring, holistic framework that they indeed later see when they hire our graduates.

Nursing remains a vibrant profession and the focus on healthy eating, exercise, integrative health, and other self-care activities must be driven by evidence and science that our nursing profession can determine advances health and wellness and improves palliative and end-of-life care. The recent emergence and use of big data in nursing prominently discussed at the closing plenary at the 2016 AACN Doctoral Conference in Naples, Florida will be an important challenge to us as a profession (Corwin et al., 2016). The healthcare sector is increasingly requiring that we better defend what we do and be fully accountable for our direct nursing-sensitive outcomes in particular. I am reminded that I recently wrote that even with the move to more evidence-based and practice-based nursing practice that we be cautious to avoid any "consequential reductionist effect on nursing care delivery . . . [that may] . . . possibly interfere with or oversimplify the uniqueness of every single nurse-individual/family interaction" (Dreher, 2015, p. 4). It is evident that Hall and Roussel have navigated this balance of evidence and contemporary nursing practice, especially as interdisciplinary healthcare teams benefit from the visibility and active participation of the highly educated nurse.

H. Michael Dreher, PhD, RN, FAAN
Dean and Professor
The College of New Rochelle

SOURCES

American Association of Colleges of Nursing. (2011). *The essentials of master's education in nursing.* Retrieved from http://www.aacn.nche.edu/education-resources/MastersEssentials11.pdf

American Association of Colleges of Nursing. (2015). *2015 annual report: Leading excellence and innovation in academic nursing.* Retrieved from http://www.aacn.nche.edu/publications/AnnualReport15 .pdf

Ashkenas, J., & Parlapiano, A. (2014, June 6). How the recession reshaped the economy, in 255 charts. *The New York Times.com: The UpShot.*

Corwin, E. J., Delaney, C. W., McCarthy, A. M., McDaniel, A. M., Pechacek, J. M., & Weaver, M. T. (2016). *Closing program session: Enhancing nursing science and improving patient care: PhD-DNP collaborative studies.* American Association of Colleges of Nursing, 2016 Doctoral Education Conference, Naples, Florida, January 21–23, 2016.

Dreher, H. M. (2015). Next steps toward practice knowledge development: An emerging epistemology in nursing. In M. D. Dahnke & H. M. Dreher's *Philosophy of science for nursing practice: Concepts and application* (2nd ed., pp. 355–391). New York, NY: Springer.

Joanna Briggs Institute Levels of Evidence and Grades of Recommendation Working Party. (2014). *New JBI levels of evidence.* Retrieved from http://joannabriggs.org/assets/docs/approach/JBI-Levels-of-evidence_2014.pdf

Nicholson, S. (2012, March 8). *LinkedIn industry trends: Winners and losers during the Great Recession.* LinkedIn.com.

Preface

We are privileged to be part of the ongoing dialogue that informs healthcare education in the 21st century. We are honored to be given continued opportunities to offer up our lived experiences in research, administration, and practice in putting together this collaborative effort shaped by our work with patients, students, stakeholders, and colleagues.

The first edition of this work began as an effort to better guide our graduate students in their understanding of the research, evidence-based practice (EBP), and quality improvement connection. We have observed students struggling with the magnitude of scientific studies and the complexity of health systems. This led to a discussion between the two of us related to the need for better models and structures to frame EBP from learning, translation, and application experiences. From ongoing feedback from our students, patients, and colleagues, we noted the disconnect between students' overall practice experience with research and the use of evidence. We, as editors, were inspired by our experience teaching doctoral students and guiding them through what was for many their first experience with EBP and quality improvement translation in health care. Gaps were identified in the foundational knowledge when graduate students entered into coursework, as evidenced by their confusion about asking the clinical question, finding the best research evidence, and synthesizing the volumes of studies, as well as their limited critical appraisal skills. Following this through, we noted difficulties with translating evidence into practice and connecting improvement and team science to the process of change and innovation. Although there is much respected literature, we wanted a book that would be user friendly and filled with great examples, tools, and reflective questions. In addition, the book needed to be relevant throughout the student's educational experience.

We believe that combining our own personal experiences and those of our contributors will be beneficial to multiple disciplines. This work has continued to evolve up to the final edits of the second edition. We live in a fast-paced health system that demands that we move forward as we reflect on our past and create our future. These experiences, along with our own search for meaning, have shaped our scholarship and professionalism. We have had a number of iterations and deep reflections, which were necessary for our own scholarship. In the spirit of these reflections and the synthesis of this work, we were able to extract the necessary components of research, administration, and practice.

The book has three components: Part I: Critical Appraisal of Research to Support Scholarship, Part II: Scholarship of Administrative Practice, and Part III: Scholarship of Clinical Practice. Each component consists of chapters that provide detailed, specific information on the targeted area. Each chapter has learning objectives, key ideas, and reflective activities. As we expanded our own understanding and application of EBP and improvement science, we included the wisdom and struggles from our international colleagues. The future of safe, quality care depends heavily on our ability to integrate our research, administrative, and clinical practices through inter-collaborative teams.

■ Acknowledgments

We would like to thank Rebecca Stephenson, Danielle Bessette, and Amanda Martin, as well as the rest of the staff at Jones & Bartlett Learning, who have been supportive throughout this process.

Finally, we would like to acknowledge each other in our work together. Writing together has provided many opportunities to engage in discussions that always (or mostly!) led to new ways of thinking and understanding our work. We have learned so much from each other and truly appreciate the power of friendship and teamwork.

Heather R. Hall, PhD, RNC, NNP-BC
Linda A. Roussel, PhD, RN, NEA-BC, CNL, FAAN

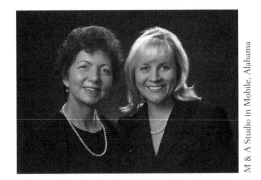

M & A Studio in Mobile, Alabama

Linda A. Roussel and Heather R. Hall

Interdisciplinary Collaboration and the Integration of Evidence-Based Practice

■ HEATHER R. HALL AND LINDA A. ROUSSEL ■

I dentified gaps in the application of research and knowledge have affected policy changes in education and practice in health care. Such gaps have proved costly in terms of patient outcomes, death notwithstanding. Freshman, Rubino, and Chassiakos (2010) described collaboration in the healthcare setting as a coming together of professionals that occurs among the healthcare team. Professionals from multiple disciplines come together to increase collaborative efforts to add value and improve communication processes. Additionally, collaboration among the healthcare team enhances understanding of system processes. The system includes a variety of disciplines responsible for the patient; integrative collaboration is a cornerstone of successful patient care (Freshman et al., 2010).

Goldman and Kahnweiler (2000) provide a classic definition of collaboration as "a mutually beneficial and well defined relationship entered into by two or more organizations to achieve common goals" (p. 435). Collaboration across professions and nations is being encouraged by higher education institutes and research and health organizations (e.g., World Health Organizations [WHO], International Council of Nurses [ICN], and Sigma Theta Tau International [STT]). These collaborations are particularly being encouraged in research and scholarly activities to identify best practices across the world (Uhrenfeldt, Lakanmaa, Flinkman, Basto, & Attree, 2014).

Uhrenfeldt et al. (2014) identified two key factors related to international scholarly collaboration that were consistent with the literature. These factors include "Facilitators" and "Barriers" that encompassed "both the individual (micro) and contextual/organizational (meso/macro) level factors" that either supported or obstructed collaboration (Uhrenfeldt et al., 2014, p. 495). In regard to Facilitators, personal attributes that assist with collaboration at the micro level include obligation, common goals, aiming to succeed and develop, and enthusiasm. Factors related to the contextual and organizational factors that are essential to collaboration at the meso and macro level include coordination, organization, networks, occasions, funding, and guidance by others. Inhibiting "Factors/Barriers" identified from the analysis included

Table 1 Literature Review Search and Results

Database	Search terms and combinations	Limitations	Hits	Included after abstract review
Medline (OVID)	(scholarly activities OR research) AND international AND collaboration AND nursing	2045–2010 Abstract/full text available English	117	5
CINAHL (EBSCO)	(scholarly activities OR research) AND international AND collaboration AND nursing	2005–2010 Abstract/full text available English	31 (one duplicate)	2
Google Scholar	Scholarly collaboration AND research AND international	2045–2010 In article title, social sciences, arts and humanities	67	
Manual data search				6
Result: papers included after abstract review				14

© 2012 John Wiley & Sons Ltd *Journal of Nursing Management,* 2014, 22, 485–498

deficiency in support and older mentors (Edwards, Webber, Mill, Kahwa, & Roelofs, 2009). Other inhibiting factors include unmet requirements for time and funding for research, workload burden, pressure, conflict in the role, inadequate resources (Uhrenfeldt et al., 2014).

A conceptual model of the "Critical Success Factors for Collaboration" comprising three key criteria attributes (Structures/Inputs, Process/Mechanisms, and Outcomes) was developed (Uhrenfeldt et al., 2014). The initial success factors to complete for collaboration are considered to be structures, contexts, and inputs. The processes are predicted as essential collaborative mechanisms and are considered core collaborative skills. The structures/contexts and processes/mechanisms are thought to be required circumstances for the accomplishment of the necessary outcomes of collaboration (see **Table 1**) (Uhrenfeldt et al., 2014, p. 496). The critical success factors for the collaboration model is initial work, with additional research required to validate the components (Uhrenfeldt et al., 2014).

A collaborative meeting would create a consensus to include knowledge and learning. Leadership is required in collaboration; however, leadership can take on a social structure among unrestricted groups. Team success can be enhanced using

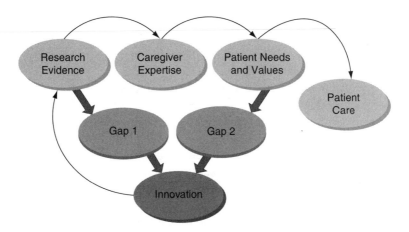

■ Gap Identification: Evidence-Based Practice and Innovation Leadership

Source: Porter-O'Grady, T., & Malloch, K. (2010). *Innovation leadership: Creating the landscape of health care.* Sudbury, MA: Jones & Bartlett.

collaborative team methods to problem-solve with the limited resources available (Straus & Layton, 2002). Porter-O'Grady and Malloch (2010) described paying attention, encouragement of feedback, and the resolution of conflict as constituting the basis of efficient collaboration. A leader of innovation will flourish in a team with professionals from multiple disciplines. The leader and members of the team will use an approach that is evidence based to recognize gaps in the literature in order to establish whether the gap is based on the needs of the patient or on published evidence (see **Figure 1**). To address complexity and novel ideas, transdisciplinary conversations must take place (Porter-O'Grady & Malloch, 2010). Members of the team should be persuaded to comment on all ideas presented. The process is considered counterproductive if members refuse to comment (Porter-O'Grady & Malloch, 2010).

Bennett and Gadlin (2011) stated that collaboration is supported by healthcare providers who come together to improve patient outcomes and simplify processes. A few of the rationales of collaborating include (a) access to skills provided by experts, (b) access to resources, and (c) multidisciplinary transformation. Many advances are brought forth secondary to collaboration. These improvements include increased funding, improved learning, and enhanced cross-training among disciplines. If healthcare providers are aware of individual jobs, the clinical pathways and protocols will be developed effortlessly (Bennett & Gadlin, 2011).

Bennett and Gadlin (2011) described productive collision as "a process by which parties who see different aspects of a problem can constructively explore their differences and search for solutions that go beyond their own limited vision of what is possible" (Slide 4). A lack of collaboration can result in the following: (a) problems without reason and definition differences; (b) future interests of many stakeholders; (c) stakeholders struggling with power difficulties; (d) lack of access to various levels of necessary information and experts; (e) difficulties distinguished by technological and scientific insecurity; (f) differences of opinions related to a problem-causing conflict; (g) unproductive work; and (h) inefficiencies in procedures to solve problems (Bennett & Gadlin, 2011).

Team members face challenges in any form of collaboration. Such problems may include: (a) decline in listening; (b) reduction of original terminology; (c) arguments related to goals and system success; (d) conflicts in conceptual frameworks; (e) rivalries related to authority, control, and credit; (f) self-esteem and/or rank intimidation; (g) failure to integrate a diverse point of view; (h) unsuccessful attempts to have differences of opinions appreciated; (i) difficulties accessing funds; and (j) problems finding publication sources (Bennett & Gadlin, 2011).

In the Institute of Medicine publication *Crossing the Quality Chasm: A New Health System for the 21st Century* (Briere, 2001), a common process to organize health care is the use of multidisciplinary teams. Much consideration has been placed on the value of such teams. For teams to be efficient, they must be maintained. Members of the team are usually educated separately, which does not include working collaboratively (Briere, 2001). Leaders take on the responsibility of developing and communicating the goals of the organization. To facilitate success, these individuals need to listen to the goals of others, give direction, develop incentives, integrate efforts for improvement, encourage environment of support, and encourage developments to facilitate success (Briere, 2001). It is important for leaders to use their own observations and thoughts related to quality improvement to provide reinforcement for team members. It is vital for leaders to understand "how units relate to each other—a form of systems thinking—and to facilitate the transfer of learning across units and practices" (Briere, 2001, p. 138).

Elwell and White (2011) noted that integrative or holistic health care is provided by the advanced practice nurse. "Nurses are educated to be holistic practitioners—attentive to the whole person, the mind, body, and spirit" (Kreitzer, Kligler, & Meeker, 2009, p. 13). Scholars included in the research component of health care may include PhD-prepared or research nurses, statisticians, or other stakeholders with common interests. Administration team members often include directors, quality improvement officers, chief officers, and managers. The translational nursing component often includes the Doctor of Nursing Practice (DNP), clinical pharmacists, nurse educators, bedside nurses, physical/occupational therapists, social workers, and other direct patient care providers. The multidisciplinary team is assembled to enable collaborative efforts that lead to evidence-based policy and quality improvement systems change. The aim of this book is to explore how each aspect—research, administration, and practice—can be integrated by multidisciplinary scholars collaborating with each other in evidence-based practice (EBP).

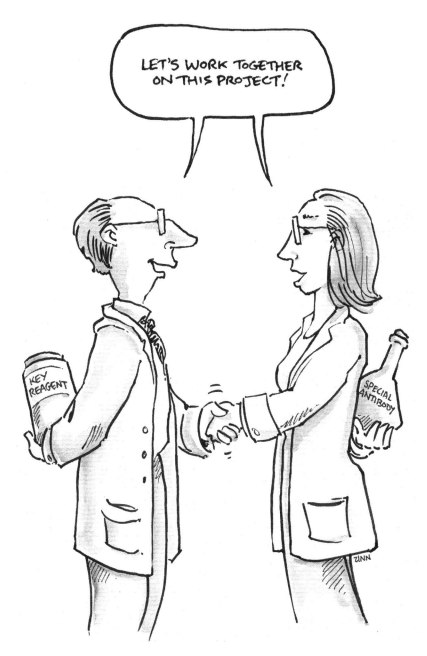

■ Collaboration or Competition?

Source: Illustration by David Zinn, © 2011, www.zinnart.com.

■ Integration and Collaboration

EBP is a part of the success of a system or organization. Polit and Beck (2012) described the emphasis of EBP as integrating the best available research evidence with other facets. The integration of research evidence needs to be included along with knowledge and clinical expertise. Important aspects of EBP and integration include the preferences and values of the patient. For example, the patient may reveal a negative perspective on a possible beneficial intervention (Polit & Beck, 2012). *Decision aids*, tools used to assist a patient in considering all available options, prove helpful so the patient can make an informed decision. Research evidence is crucial to EBP; however, the expertise of the clinician, preference of the patient, and the circumstances must be integrated into the final decision (Livesley & Howarth, 2007).

■ Scholarship

Scholarship is a process that has evolved over time. The profession level increases secondary to this evolution through involvement in generating new knowledge and participating in the exchange of ideas (Tymkow, 2011). Clinical scholarship includes applying and disseminating the evidence, which leads to a greater understanding of knowledge development (Dreher, 1999). While in the early phase of international collaboration, specific strategies for publishing should be established (Suhonen, Saarikoski, & Leino-Kilpi, 2009). The American Association of Colleges of Nursing (AACN, 2006) stated that scholarship and research are two core elements in doctoral education. Graduates from a research doctoral program are prepared with skills in research necessary to identify new knowledge in nursing (AACN, 2006). Practice experts should be well versed in "knowledge management, poised to extract information and apply it in a novel or utilitarian way, and then efficiently translate and disseminate this new conceptualization of the evidence" (Dreher & Glasgow, 2011, p. 30).

■ Approach

This book is organized into three main parts, and scholarship is the foundation for all three. Part I describes the process of critical appraisal of research to support scholarship. Part II outlines the scholarship of administrative practice. Part III presents the scholarship of clinical practice.

Part I: Critical Appraisal of Research to Support Scholarship

Part I consists of six chapters that describe quantitative research, qualitative research, mixed methods research, data analysis, institutional review board procedure, and critical appraisal process of evidence-based research. Burns and Grove (2009) described the critical appraisal process of research as "a systematic, unbiased, careful examination of all aspects of a study to judge the merits, limitations, meaning, and significance" (p. 598).

Part II: Scholarship of Administrative Practice

Part II consists of six chapters that describe leadership; organizational systems; change; microsystems, macrosystems, and mesosystems; quality improvement: historical and future perspectives; and health policy. Chapters in Part II discuss quality improvement science and the process of integrating health policy into practice.

Part III: Scholarship of Clinical Practice

Part III consists of six chapters that describe philosophical and theoretical perspectives guiding inquiry, synthesis projects, translational research in the clinical setting, and dissemination of the evidence. The chapters discuss problem identification, evidence-based research, searching the literature, and incorporating evidence-based research into practice.

REFERENCES

American Association of Colleges of Nursing. (2006). *The essentials of doctoral education for advanced practice nursing.* Retrieved from http://www.aacn.nche.edu/DNP/pdf/Essentials.pdf

Bennett, M., & Gadlin, H. (2011, June). *Getting the most from research collaboratives: Applying the science of the team.* Keynote address presented at the Improvement Science Summit: Advancing Healthcare Improvement Research, San Antonio, TX.

Briere, R. (Ed.). (2001). *Crossing the quality chasm: A new health system for the 21st century.* Washington, DC: National Academies Press.

Burns, N., & Grove, S. K. (2009). *The practice of nursing research: Appraisal, synthesis, and generation of evidence* (6th ed.). St. Louis, MO: Saunders.

Dreher, M. H., & Glasgow, M. E. S. (2011). *Role development for doctoral advanced nursing practice.* New York, NY: Springer.

Edwards, N., Webber, J., Mill, J., Kahwa, E., & Roelofs, S. (2009). Building capacity for nurse-led research. *International Nursing Review, 56,* 88–94.

Elwell, J., & White, K. W. (2011). Integrative practitioner. In M. E. Zaccagnini & K. W. White (Eds.), *The doctor of nursing practice essentials: A new model for advanced practice nursing* (pp. 433–448). Burlington, MA: Jones & Bartlett Learning.

Freshman, B., Rubino, L., & Chassiakos, Y. R. (2010). *Collaboration across the disciplines in health care.* Sudbury, MA: Jones and Bartlett.

Goldman, S., & Kahnweiler, W. M. (2000). A collaborator profile for executives of nonprofit organizations. *Nonprofit Management and Leadership, 10,* 435–450.

Kreitzer, M. J., Kligler, B., & Meeker, W. C. (2009). *Health professions education and integrative health care.* Retrieved from http://www.iom.edu/~/media/Files/Activity%20Files/Quality/IntegrativeMed/Health%20Professions%20Education%20and%20Integrative%20HealthCare.pdf

Livesley, J., & Howarth, M. (2007). Integrating research evidence into clinical decisions. In J. V. Craig & R. L. Smyth (Eds.), *The evidence-based practice manual for nurses* (2nd ed., pp. 210–233). St. Louis, MO: Churchill Livingstone.

Polit, D. F., & Beck, C. T. (2012). *Nursing research: Generating and assessing evidence for nursing practice* (9th ed.). Philadelphia, PA: Lippincott Williams & Wilkins.

Porter-O'Grady, T., & Malloch, K. (2010). *Innovation leadership: Creating the landscape of health care.* Sudbury, MA: Jones & Bartlett.

Straus, D., & Layton, T. C. (2002). *How to make collaboration work: Powerful ways to build consensus, solve problems, and make decisions.* San Francisco, CA: Berrett-Koehler.

Suhonen, R., Saarikoski, M., & Leino-Kilpi, H. (2009). Cross-cultural nursing research. *International Journal of Nursing Studies, 46,* 593–602.

Tymkow, C. (2011). Clinical scholarship and evidence-based practice. In M. E. Zaccagnini & K. W. White (Eds.), *The doctor of nursing practice essentials: A new model for advanced practice nursing* (pp. 61–136). Sudbury, MA: Jones & Bartlett Learning.

Uhrenfeldt, L., Lakanmaa, R. L., Flinkman, M., Basto, M. L., & Attree, M. (2014). Collaboration: A SWOT analysis of the process of conducting a review of nursing workforce policies in five European countries. *Journal of Nursing Management, 22,* 485–498.

PART I

Critical Appraisal of Research to Support Scholarship

CHAPTER 1

Quantitative Research

■ Susan L. Neely-Barnes and Robin Lennon-Dearing ■

■ Objectives:

- Identify steps in the quantitative research process.
- Identify preexperimental, quasi-experimental, and experimental research studies when examining published research.
- Assess internal and external validity of various research designs.
- Recognize and understand the methodological issues in quantitative research designs.

■ Critical Appraisal

The goal of this chapter is to help readers understand the process of quantitative research so they can critically identify the usefulness of different studies for their own research or clinical practice. Appraising information critically and in a systematic way is important to practitioners' ability to base their clinical decisions on the research evidence. Healthcare providers must understand the basic process of quantitative research to distinguish the strengths and weaknesses of a study they may be evaluating.

■ Quantitative Research

Quantitative research involves a systematic process—the scientific method— to build knowledge. Quantitative research methods involve collecting numerical data to explain, predict, and/or control phenomena of interest. Data analysis is mainly statistical; it answers questions of what, and under what condition(s), specific independent variables predict or explain dependent variables through the use of numerical data suitable for statistical analysis (Solomon & Draine, 2010). Depending on the problem or issue under inquiry and after researchers have identified sufficient knowledge from a literature review, they begin with a research question or hypothesis (Keele, 2011). Whereas quantitative research questions look at the relationships among variables, quantitative hypotheses are predictions the researcher makes about the expected relationship among variables. The research design becomes the blueprint for the study—that is, how the study sample is selected and how the data are collected and analyzed (Keele, 2011). An overview of the basic steps in the quantitative research process is shown in **Box 1-1**.

When a problem of interest has been identified, the research process is applied to discover what is known about a topic and where knowledge gaps exist (Schmidt & Brown, 2012). The researcher then finds existing knowledge on a subject from a review of relevant literature. From what is learned in relation to the research problem from the literature review, a focused research question should follow (Yegidis & Weinbach, 2011). **Table 1-1** shows how the problem of interest has been narrowed to an answerable question and then to a hypothesis statement. A research hypothesis is stated as an answer to a research question (Yegidis & Weinbach, 2011).

The research hypothesis commonly states the type of relationship, as described in **Box 1-2**, between variables that it is presumed they have. Objective measurable data are then collected to confirm or refute a hypothesis (Schmidt & Brown, 2012).

In quantitative research studies, variables are numerical (Brown, 2014). Biophysical variables such as height, weight, blood pressure, and pulse may be measured directly. Conceptual variables have attributes or characteristics that differ in quantity or quality and describe people or things (Babbie, 2012), and they must be operationalized—that is, defined in terms that give precise indicators to be observed, and specify the level of those indicators (Rubin & Babbie, 2014). Tools used to measure conceptual variables are called instruments.

As shown in **Box 1-3**, the independent variable is what the researcher introduces and controls to measure its effect on the dependent variable (Yegidis & Weinbach, 2011). The dependent variable is the focus of the intervention and is what is measured. Confounding variables are factors that interfere with the relationship between the independent and dependent variable (Schmidt & Brown, 2012).

Box 1-1 Steps in Quantitative Research

1. Problem identification
2. Research question formulation
3. Literature review
4. Construction of hypothesis
5. Research design and planning
6. Data collection
7. Sorting and analysis of data
8. Specification of research findings
9. Interpretation of research findings
10. Dissemination of research findings
11. Use of findings by practitioner

Data from Yegidis, B. L., & Weinbach, R. W. (2009). *Research methods for social workers* (6th ed.). Boston, MA: Pearson.

Table 1-1   Study Example of a Research Question and a Research Hypothesis

Study	Research Question	Research Hypothesis
Schwindt, R. G., McNeils, A. M., & Sharp, D. (2014). Evaluation of a theory-based education program to motivate nursing students to intervene with their seriously mentally ill clients who use tobacco. *Archives of Psychiatric Nursing, 28,* 277–283.	What is the effect of a tobacco education program on the perceived competence and motivation of baccalaureate nursing students to intervene with severely mentally ill clients?	1. Students who complete an SDT-informed education program will perceive themselves as more competent to deliver tobacco dependence interventions. 2. Students who complete an SDT-informed education program will be more autonomously motivated to deliver tobacco dependence interventions.
Chapelain, P., Morineau, T., & Gautier, C. (2015). Effects of communication on the performance of nursing students during the simulation of an emergency situation. *Journal of Advanced Nursing, 71,* 2650–2659.	How is clinical performance affected by different forms of spontaneous team communications?	1. A message transmitted through an earpiece to nursing students would facilitate reflective thinking and consequently improve performance. 2. There would be some significant positive correlations between the communication in nurse teams and their performance.

SDT = Self-determination theory.

Box 1-2   Relationships Between Variables Expressed in Hypotheses Association

Certain value categories of X are found with certain value categories of Y.

Correlation   Higher values of X are found with higher values of Y and vice versa, or higher values of X are found with lower values of Y and vice versa.

Causation   Values or value categories of X cause values or value categories of Y.

Data from Yegidis, B. L. & Weinbach, R. W., 2011. *Research methods for social workers* (7th ed.). Reprinted by permission of Pearson Education, Inc., Upper Saddle River, NJ.

Research hypotheses suggest and test for relationships between variables. Relationships between variables can be positive, negative (inverse), or curvilinear. For example, in a study looking at the role of social networks and support as they

---

Box 1-3 Types of Variables

Independent Variable   This is manipulated by the researcher to influence the dependent variable; it also may be called the predictor variable.

Dependent Variable   This is the variable of primary interest to the researcher; it also may be called the outcome variable.

Confounding Variable   An extraneous third variable that influences the relationship between the independent and dependent variables.

Data from Yegidis, B. L. & Weinbach, R. W., 2011. *Research methods for social workers* (7th ed.). Reprinted by permission of Pearson Education, Inc., Upper Saddle River, NJ.

---

relate to symptoms of depression in women who have recently given birth, Surkan, Peterson, Hughes, and Gottlieb (2006) chose the Medical Outcomes Study Social Support Survey and a social network item as the independent variable and the Center for Epidemiologic Studies of Depression Scale as the dependent variable. Using the appropriate statistical analysis, the researchers found that both social networks and social support were independently and inversely correlated to symptoms of depression. Women who reported more social support from friends and family showed fewer depressive symptoms and reported lower scores on the measure for depression.

The strength and direction of a relationship, the *effect size*, between two variables can be statistically tested and reported using a correlation coefficient, such as Pearson's r. The direction of the relationship is positive (+1.0 is a perfect positive relationship) or negative (−1.0 is a perfect negative relationship). The closer the value gets to +1 or −1, the stronger the relationship; a value close or equal to 0 indicates no relationship (Brown, 2014). High correlation only implies a pattern in the relationship between variables; it does not equal causation (Brown, 2014).

■ Sampling

To answer the research question and test the research hypothesis, a researcher must define the population of interest. Studying an entire population of interest is usually prohibitive in terms of time, money, and resources, so a subset of a given population must be selected; this is called sampling (Yegidis & Weinbach, 2011). The method used for choosing a sample affects its representativeness of the population and thus the generalizability of results. There are two types of sampling: *probability* sampling and *nonprobability* sampling. Probability sampling means that all participants have the same chance of being chosen in the sample (Rubin & Babbie, 2014). Four probability sampling methods (see **Table 1-2**) are simple random sampling, stratified sampling, cluster sampling, and systematic sampling (Schmidt & Brown, 2012).

Table 1-2 Probability Sampling Methods

Method	Definition	Benefits and Limitations
Simple random sampling	Each subject has the same chance to be selected. Strategy used upholds randomization.	High probability that the sample will represent the population as long as sample size is sufficient.
Stratified random sampling	Strata must be mutually exclusive so a subject can be assigned to only one stratum. Random sampling used to select subject from each stratum.	High probability that the sample will represent the population if number of subjects in each stratum is sufficient.
Cluster sampling	Simple random sampling used first to select clusters and then select subjects within each cluster.	Greater potential for the sample to not represent the population depending on how the initial clusters are selected.
Systematic random sampling	Begin with random sampling and count the Nth subject on the list.	If bias occurs, this type of sampling is not as representative as the other three methods.

Data from (1) Haber, J. (2014). Sampling. In G. LoBiondo-Wood & J. Haber (Eds.), *Nursing research: Methods and critical appraisal of evidence-based practice* (pp. 230–234). Sudbury, MA: Jones and Bartlett; and (2) Wood, M., & Ross-Kerr, J. (2011). *Basic steps in planning nursing research: From question to proposal* (6th ed.). Sudbury, MA: Jones and Bartlett.

Nonprobability sampling (see **Table 1-3**) uses methods such as convenience sampling, quota sampling, purposive sampling, and snowball sampling (Schmidt & Brown, 2012). For some research studies, probability sampling is not possible or not feasible because of costs. In these situations, the researcher must rely on nonprobability methods. Research studies that use nonprobability methods can have scientific merit but will have limited generalizability to the larger population.

■ Data Collection

Quantitative data collection methods rely on structured data collection instruments that produce results that are easy to summarize, compare, and generalize. Four levels of measurement are used to quantify data, depending on what is being measured. Nominal measures differentiate between categories but do not place variables in any order or ranking. Ordinal measures rank categories in order but do not specify the distance between the categories. Interval measures use continuous data in which values are rank-ordered, and the distance between categories is equal. Ratio scales, the highest level of measurement, measure equal interval data and employ a fixed-point zero (Schmidt & Brown, 2012).

Table 1-3 Nonprobability Sampling Methods

Method	Definition	Benefits and Limitations
Convenience sampling	Inclusion criteria identified prior to selection of subjects. All subjects are invited to participate.	Because the sample is selected for ease of data collection, it may not be representative of the target population.
Quota sampling	Strata must be mutually exclusive so a subject can be assigned to only one stratum. Convenience sampling used to select subject from each stratum.	Because the sample within each stratum is selected using convenience sampling, it may not represent the population.
Purposive sampling	Researcher has sufficient knowledge of topic to select sample of experts. Researcher should identify criteria to include in selection of subjects.	Because the sample is selected by researcher, cannot generalize to population; generalizing the results is not an expected outcome.
Snowball sampling	Researcher selects initial subjects for study. Data saturation is reached.	Cannot generalize to population; generalizing the results is not an expected outcome.

Data from (1) Haber, J. (2014). Sampling. In G. LoBiondo-Wood & J. Haber (Eds.), *Nursing research: Methods and critical appraisal of evidence-based practice* (pp. 226–230). Sudbury, MA: Jones and Bartlett; and (2) Wood, M., & Ross-Kerr, J. (2011). *Basic steps in planning nursing research: From question to proposal* (6th ed.). Sudbury, MA: Jones and Bartlett.

Common data collection methods quantitative research include questionnaires, rating scales, and physiologic measures such as blood tests and vital signs (Keele, 2011). In this chapter, we provide a basic overview of issues of validity (see **Box 1-4**) and reliability (see **Box 1-5**) of measure. Readers are encouraged to consult other texts for in-depth reviews of measurement construction and measurement theory.

Reliability

Reliability measures the consistency and stability of responses over time in a standardized measurement instrument. Reliability does not ensure that measures are accurately measuring what researchers think they measure (Babbie, 2012). *Internal consistency reliability* is a measure of how closely items in a questionnaire measuring the same construct are related. Cronbach's alpha addresses overall average reliability, and items are considered to represent a similar construct when alpha is approximately 0.80.

■ Research Design

The value of evidence from a study depends on the design used. In quantitative research, a clearly defined step-by-step process is followed based on the research design chosen (Schmidt & Brown, 2012). The following pages review research designs (see **Table 1-4**) used as tools to answer research questions and test research hypotheses.

Box 1-4 Measurement Validity

Construct	It is *convergent* when results correspond to the results of methods measuring the same concept. It has *discriminant* validity when results do not highly correspond to other constructs as they do with measures of the same construct.
Content	Experts judge whether the measure covers the range of meanings within the concept.
Criterion-related or concurrent	Compares with an external measure of the same variable
Face Factorial	Appears to measure what the researcher intended. How many different constructs are measured and whether these are what the researcher intends to measure.

Data from Rubin, A., & Babbie, E. (2014). *Research methods for social work,* (8th ed.). Belmont, CA: Brooks/Cole Cengage.

Box 1-5 Reliability

Interrater reliability	The degree of agreement or consistency between raters.
Test-retest reliability	A measure that provides consistency in measurement over time.
Internal consistency reliability	This assesses the correlation of scores on each item with the of scores on the rest of the items. Cronbach's alpha should have a value of 0.80 or greater to be considered reliable.

Table 1-4 Research Types

Exploratory research	Preexperimental	Research is conducted to explore a topic about which little is known.
Descriptive research	Quasi-experimental	Descriptive research involves collecting data to test hypotheses or answer questions concerning the current status of the subjects of the study. Describes the variables. Lacks the element of random assignment.
Explanatory research	Experimental	Participants are assigned to groups based on some selected criterion often called an independent variable. At least one variable is manipulated so as to measure its effect on one or more dependent variables.

Data from Rubin, A., & Babbie, E. (2014). *Research methods for social work,* (8th ed.). Belmont, CA: Brooks/Cole Cengage.

■ Group Design

Group design is a commonly used technique in quantitative research and relatively well-known among students of research. When asked to design a research study, most students of quantitative methods will incorporate a group design. Group design is defined by Grinnell and Unrau (2011, p. 565) as "research design conducted with two or more groups of cases, or research participants, for the purpose of answering research questions or testing hypotheses." The method encompasses preexperimental, quasi-experimental, and experimental techniques. The most rigorous of group designs have an explanatory purpose to prove cause-effect relationships, whereas the least rigorous of these designs are used to generate or explore a theory.

There are many variations of group design. The more commonly used designs will be covered. Readers are encouraged to consult other texts for a more in-depth review.

Internal Validity

From the evidence-based practice perspective, rigorous group designs are more valued than less rigorous designs. This is because rigorous designs minimize threats to internal validity. Readers should remember that internal validity is concerned with the possibility that a change in the dependent variable (outcome) is the result of some cause other than the independent variable, that is, the target of the experiment. It is beyond the scope of this chapter to include an in-depth review of all threats to internal validity. Briefly, one should remember that respondents improve for many reasons other than the intervention or technique, that is, the target of the research experiment. It is possible that research subjects improve because they age (maturation), because they can better fill out the measure of the dependent variable (testing), or because they are exposed to an external event that caused the improvement (history). It is also possible that research subjects would have improved regardless of the experimental intervention (regression to the mean), or for other reasons not mentioned here.

Whereas internal validity refers to the confidence with which the study results can conclude that a treatment or intervention (independent variable) causes change in the dependent variable (see **Table 1-5**), external validity has to do with the generalizability of the research findings. Rubin and Babbie (2014) described external validity as "the extent to which we can generalize findings of a study to settings and populations beyond the study conditions" (p. 247). They also noted that "a study must be generalizable to some real-world settings." Characteristics of good quantitative research are presenting the research design and methods in enough detail that other researchers could replicate the study and obtain their own results (Durbin, 2004). Obtaining the same results through repeated experimentation by different researchers increases the value and worth of the findings (Durbin, 2004).

Table 1-5 Internal Validity

Threats to Internal Validity	*Maximizing Internal Validity*
Internal validity is the degree to which we can confidently conclude that the treatment caused the outcomes observed.	
History—Events occurring between repeated measurements.	Use a control group from the same population as the experimental group.
Maturation—Changes in participants that occur over time.	Use a control group and keep the study of short duration.
Testing—Change resulting from being measured; practice effect.	Use a research design that does not include a pretest or unobtrusive data collection.
Instrumentation—Changes in outcome because of equipment or human factors.	Use standardized instruments, administration, or data collection procedures.
Statistical regression—The natural tendency of very high or low scores to regress toward the mean during retest.	Avoid using extreme scores.
Mortality—Participants dropping out.	Use random assignment with large groups and follow-up with a portion of those who leave the study.
Selection of subjects—Choosing participants in such a way that groups are not equal before the experiment.	Use random selection and random assignment of subjects. If random selection and assignment are not possible, use certain other statistical techniques.

Preexperimental Design

The purpose of preexperimental designs is to explore new topics of research. Preexperimental designs rank low in the evidence-based practice hierarchy (Rubin & Babbie, 2014). Yet, the designs have an important role in testing new intervention approaches, evaluating programs, and generating theories. Examples of research questions that could be addressed using a preexperimental design include (a) Are patients leaving the hospital satisfied with discharge planning services? (b) Are patients in a health education program doing better than they were before they started?

▪ One-Shot Case Study

The one-shot case study is the most basic of group designs, so it is a good starting point. However, it is a weak design. Campbell and Stanley (1963) noted that these studies have a total absence of control and almost no scientific value. One-shot case studies are usually diagrammed as follows, with X standing for a stimulus such as an intervention, and O standing for an observation.

X   O

Despite the weakness of this study design, one-shot case studies are used quite frequently. In higher education, student evaluations of teaching are an example of this design. Many hospitals and social service agencies use this design to ask patients or participants about their knowledge or skills gained from a service. The problem with this design is that there are no points of comparison. We do not know the respondents' level of knowledge or skills prior to receiving the service, nor do we know how their current level of knowledge or skills compared with those of individuals who did not receive services. Many other options are available to provide a more rigorous design.

■ One-Group Pretest–Posttest

The one-group pretest–posttest design assesses the dependent variable before and after the stimulus or intervention is introduced. It is usually diagrammed as follows (Campbell & Stanley, 1963):

O_1 X O_2

This design has the advantage of establishing both time ordering and correlation. A researcher can use this design to demonstrate that the study group improved if scores are better at Observation 2 than they were at Observation 1. For reasons related to internal validity, this design cannot establish causality. For example, imagine that you are evaluating a diabetes education program for adolescents aged 12–15 years. You hypothesize that the program will improve healthy eating habits and reduce blood glucose levels. The program lasts for 1 year. You give a pretest at the beginning of the year and a posttest at the end of the year. You are able to establish that the adolescents' eating habits and blood glucose levels have improved. Did your program cause the change? There are several alternative explanations: (a) It could be that the adolescents' eating habits and management of their blood sugar improved because the adolescents matured and were 1 year older at the time of the posttest. (b) It could be that something extraneous occurred during that year that caused the change. For example, a popular show geared toward teens portrayed a young adult with diabetes. (c) It could be that the adolescents were referred when they were at their worst period of management, and they would have improved anyway. Without the presence of a control group, it is not possible to rule out these alternative explanations.

Quasi-Experimental Design

There are many situations in which it is not possible for researchers to use experimental designs. It may be unethical to deny treatment to a control group. Agency or hospital administration may not allow program participants to be randomly assigned.

In these situations, quasi-experimental designs can be used. Quasi-experimental designs usually involve assignment to two groups without randomization or the use of a comparison group in place of a control group. Although less rigorous than an experimental design, quasi-experimental designs are an improvement over preexperimental designs. Three common quasi-experimental approaches will be reviewed here. Readers interested in a more in-depth discussion of the approach should consult other texts (Cook & Campbell, 1979).

■ Nonequivalent Comparison Groups

Suppose that one high school in town has adopted a novel sex education curriculum. You as a researcher would like to evaluate this curriculum compared with the usual one, but the principal will not allow any students to be assigned to a control group. However, a high school across town has demographics similar to those of the one with the novel curriculum. The principal of this high school agrees to participate in your study and have students fill out the same pretest–posttest as the high school with the novel curriculum. In this example, you have a quasi-experimental design with nonequivalent comparison groups. You are not able to randomly assign the students to their conditions, but you hope that the two groups are similar enough to be comparable. This design is denoted:

$$O_1 \quad X \quad O_2$$
$$O_1 \qquad O_2$$

This use of the comparison group in this design addresses the concerns that students might have changed because of aging or an external event. Yet, some problems still remain in this design. The two groups were not randomly assigned. If their outcomes are different, we cannot rule out the possibility that demographic differences between the groups led to the change. Additionally, the comparison group is not a true control group. If the two groups have the same outcomes, we will be able to say that neither is superior, but we cannot answer the question of whether either approach is better than no education.

■ Time-Series Design

As mentioned, one concern in experimental research is that the intervention group may have changed regardless of the intervention. One of the ways of examining whether this is true is to administer multiple pretests before starting the intervention. By using multiple pretests, the researcher can detect whether there was a trend. In other words, was the group already engaged in a change process before the intervention started?

A more rigorous extension of the multiple pretest design is a time-series design. The time-series design allows the research to examine the question of whether there was a trend in the data both before and after the intervention. Opinions differ as to how many pretests and posttests are needed in a time-series design. In the example that follows, the dependent variable is measured four times before the intervention and four times after:

$$O_1 \quad O_2 \quad O_3 \quad O_4 \quad X \quad O_5 \quad O_6 \quad O_7 \quad O_8$$

To further increase the rigor, researchers can use a multiple time-series design. The multiple time-series design adds a nonequivalent comparison group. The non-equivalent comparison group gets the same number of observations of the dependent variable in the same time frame but does not receive the intervention. The multiple time-series design addresses the concern that an external event occurring simultaneous to the intervention could have influenced the dependent variable. It is usually denoted:

$$O_1 \quad O_2 \quad O_3 \quad O_4 \quad X \quad O_5 \quad O_6 \quad O_7 \quad O_8$$
$$O_1 \quad O_2 \quad O_3 \quad O_4 \quad \quad O_5 \quad O_6 \quad O_7 \quad O_8$$

■ Case-Control Studies

Many questions do not lend themselves to experimental designs. Suppose we want to understand what leads a person to become a perpetrator of child abuse, what contributes to becoming a high school dropout, or which health habits contribute to high blood pressure. Designing a controlled experiment to answer one of these questions may be difficult or even impossible. Though not as rigorous as an experimental design, a case control study is a good alternative. A case control study collects retrospective data from people who are and are not in the outcome condition and uses multivariate statistical analysis to compare the two groups and identify variables that may have contributed to the outcome condition. It is a more convenient and inexpensive way to collect outcome data than an experimental design. A downside of this design is that it relies on retrospective data. Some participants may have difficulty recalling events and circumstances of their early life, and many may not recall accurately.

Experimental Design

Experimental designs seek to answer explanatory research questions. In explanatory research, the investigator seeks to test hypotheses and explain how an independent variable influences a dependent variable. In an ideal experiment, it would be possible to say with certainty that an independent variable caused a dependent variable. It is unusual for a researcher in nursing or any medical or social science field to have sufficient control over the design of an experiment to produce the ideal (Grinnell, Unrau, & Williams, 2011). Yet, there are three criteria that can produce a high degree of certainty that an explanatory relationship exists, as follows (Rubin & Babbie, 2014):

- The independent variable (cause) should come before the dependent variable (effect) chronologically.
- The independent and dependent variables should be empirically related to each other.
- The relationship between the independent and dependent variables cannot be explained as the result of the influence of a third variable.

Two key techniques in experimental design separate it from preexperimental or quasi-experimental design. The first is the use of a *control group*. A control group is a set of research respondents who resemble the experimental group in every way except that they do not receive the target intervention of the research study (Rubin & Babbie, 2014). The second technique is *randomization*. Randomization is the assignment of respondents to either the experimental or control group at random. Techniques for randomization include flipping a coin, using a random numbers table, and assigning by an even or odd identification number (Rubin & Babbie, 2014). Without randomization, there is a chance that participants assigned to either an experimental or control group could be inherently different from each other. In other words, there is a risk for *selection bias*. The term *randomized controlled trial* used frequently in evidence-based practice refers to experimental group designs with both randomization and a control group. Three of the designs most commonly discussed in the research literature are reviewed here (see **Table 1-6**).

■ Pretest–Posttest Control Group Design

The first type of experimental design, sometimes known as the classic experimental design, is denoted as follows, with R signifying randomization to group:

$$R \quad O_1 \cdot X \quad O_2$$
$$R \quad O_1 \qquad O_2$$

The classic experimental design minimizes many threats to internal validity, including maturation, history, and selection bias. This design does not account for the problem of testing effects. It is possible that participants in both the experimental and control groups will improve simply because they are retested on the same measure and have improved in completing the measure. To address the problem of testing, a different design will be described next.

■ Solomon Four-Group Design

If researchers would like to know about pretest–posttest change but are concerned about the problem of testing effects, they can use the Solomon four-group design.

Table 1-6 Study Examples of Research Designs

Study	Research Design and Sampling	Instruments	Intervention	Findings
Wyatt, T. H., & Hauenstein, E. J. (2008). Pilot testing Okay With Asthma: An online asthma intervention for school-age children. *Journal of School Nursing, 24*(3), 145–150.	One-group pretest–posttest quasi-experimental design; convenience sample	The Asthma Information Quiz The Child Attitude Toward Illness Scale Given at baseline and 1 week and 2 weeks after the intervention	Okay With Asthma program	Significant improvements in asthma knowledge scores at the 1- and 2-week evaluations and significant improvements in attitude scores 2 weeks after the program
Park, J., Lee, N., Cho, Y., & Yang, Y. (2015). Modified constraint-induced movement therapy for clients with chronic stroke: Interrupted time series (ITS) design. *Journal of Physical Therapy Science, 27,* 963–966.	Time series design; assessments were performed five times in a 3-week period before and after intervention. No control group	Modified Barthel index (MBI) and the box and block test (BBT)	Modified constraint-induced movement therapy	Improved upper extremity functions and performance of daily living activities
Alexandropoulou, M. (2013). Evaluating a health educational first aid program for special education school personnel: A cluster randomized trial. *International Journal of Caring Sciences, 6,* 115–126.	Solomon-Four design; 5–7 schools randomized to each group with 32–54 participants per group	First aid questionnaire	Health educational first aid program for special education school personnel	Significant improvement in scores for the intervention groups

This is a highly regarded research design that involves dividing respondents into four groups: two are experimental, and two are control. One of the experimental groups and one of the control groups are pretested but not the other. It is denoted:

$$R \quad O_1 \quad X \quad O_2$$
$$R \quad O_1 \quad \quad O_2$$
$$R \quad \quad X \quad O_2$$
$$R \quad \quad \quad O_2$$

■ Alternative Treatment Design or Dismantling Study

Researchers often seek to compare alternative treatment approaches. For example, researchers may want to compare two drugs, two patient education programs, or two case management strategies. One method of comparing is to randomly assign participants to one of two groups: one receiving intervention A (X_A) and one receiving intervention B (X_B). Such a design could answer which of the two treatment alternatives is superior. However, what if the researcher is concerned that both treatments have no effect? To answer this question, a control group must be included in the study design. Then, the study would consist of three groups: one receiving intervention A, one receiving intervention B, and a final receiving no intervention. This would be denoted:

$$R \quad O_1 \quad X_A \quad O_2$$
$$R \quad O_1 \quad X_B \quad O_2$$
$$R \quad O_1 \qquad\quad O_2$$

A final design called a dismantling study can be used to explore which components of the intervention are needed to achieve the desired effect. In the first group, participants are randomly assigned to receive both intervention components A and B. In the second, participants receive only intervention A. In the third, participants receive only intervention B. The final group is a control group receiving no intervention. If either of the groups in the second or third rows shows as much improvement as the first group, the component in the second or third row would be all that is needed (Rubin & Babbie, 2014). This approach is denoted:

$$R \quad O_1 \quad X_{AB} \quad O_2$$
$$R \quad O_1 \quad X_A \quad O_2$$
$$R \quad O_1 \quad X_B \quad O_2$$
$$R \quad O_1 \qquad\quad O_2$$

An example of a dismantling study can be found in an article by Kroeze, Oenema, Dagnelie, and Brug (2008). This study examined a computed-tailored intervention aimed at reducing dietary fat intake among adults. The four conditions in the dismantling study were: (1) feedback on dietary fat intake, (2) feedback relative to one's peers, (3) the first two types of feedback plus practical suggestions on how to change fat intake, and (4) general information. Kroeze et al. found that the third condition, personal and peer feedback with practical suggestions, was effective in reducing fat intake among the high-risk populations. The first two conditions were effective only in changing intention to reduce fat intake.

■ Reactivity and Placebo Effects

All the experimental designs described earlier involve the use of a control group. The use of a control group introduces rigor in a study design to address many threats to internal validity. However, it also introduces problems of reactivity of study participants. It is possible that experimental group participants will improve simply because they are receiving additional attention that accompanies treatment. Another possibility is that control group participants will become frustrated with the study because they are not receiving treatment and drop out. On the other hand, control group participants may engage in compensatory rivalry, trying to find treatments elsewhere that mirror the one that the experimental group is receiving. All these possibilities threaten the validity of the study.

One option to address reactivity is to use a placebo. Use of a placebo has become standard practice in drug studies, but it also can be used in other types of intervention studies. Researchers who examine psychosocial or health education interventions may be concerned that the additional time and attention given to the experimental group over the control group will influence the outcome regardless of whether the intervention is effective. Thus, some researchers will introduce an alternative program for the control group that is not believed to have an impact on the dependent variables of interest. For example, Duru, Sarkisian, Leng, and Mangione (2010) completed a randomized controlled trial of a faith-based physical activity intervention for older African American women. Because the researchers were concerned about placebo effects, the control group received group lectures about topics important to seniors, such as financial planning. These group lectures were useful to the participants but were not expected to affect the outcome variables, such as body mass index and blood pressure.

■ Systematic Reviews and Meta-Analyses

From an evidence-based practice perspective, systematic reviews and meta-analyses hold the spot at the top of the hierarchy of research evidence. The purpose of systematic reviews and meta-analyses is to create an unbiased synthesis of the literature on a particular research question. The terms *systematic review* and *meta-analysis* are not synonymous, but the two techniques are highly compatible and can be used together to summarize a large body of research and generate new insights (Littell, Corcoran, & Pillai, 2008).

For example, Shah and Shah (2010) were interested in whether domestic violence during pregnancy has an adverse impact on the fetus. A literature review turned up a large number of studies. Some of the studies found that domestic violence increases risk, and others found no impact. How does one make sense of this variation in the literature? Shah and Shah used the systematic review process to search for literature and evaluate it. They used meta-analysis techniques to combine the results of multiple studies. Their conclusion was that domestic violence is associated with increased risk for low birth weight and preterm birth.

Systematic Review

A systematic review is a process of comprehensively locating and synthesizing the research on a particular question using organized, transparent, and replicable procedures (Littell, et al., 2008). The first step in the systematic review process is to develop a protocol. The first element of a protocol is a clearly formulated and answerable research question and a set of hypotheses. As part of the research question, there should be explicit inclusion and exclusion criteria to determine which studies are to be included in the review. These inclusion and exclusion criteria will specify problems or conditions, populations, interventions, settings, comparisons, outcomes, and study designs that are or are not to be included in the review. The protocol will specify the techniques to locate and screen studies. These techniques include search terms, databases and search engines to be used, and strategies to locate unpublished studies. When a systematic review is being prepared for inclusion in the Cochrane or Campbell Library, the protocol is submitted to and approved by peer review before the systematic review process begins. The final version of the approved protocol is posted online (Higgins & Green, 2011).

After the protocol has been formulated, the researchers locate and screen studies. Ideally, the researchers should keep a record of every abstract screened and the method by which it was retrieved. Database searches are usually the first step in a systematic review. Many systematic reviews will augment the database search with a hand search of 10–15 journals that frequently publish on the topic of review. Strong reviews will make every effort to locate unpublished studies. Methods for finding unpublished studies include reviewing proceedings of relevant conferences and searching the websites of government and nonprofit organizations that have an interest in the study topic. After the initial screening, two reviewers will read the study and determine whether it meets eligibility criteria for inclusion in the review. If the two reviewers disagree, a third usually breaks the tie.

After studies are located and screened, included studies are rated for study quality and data are extracted from the study. Data extraction involves recording the sample size and characteristics, the type of interventions used (if the focus of the research question is intervention), and the outcome variables and measures chosen. Study quality ratings are undertaken to assess whether there is any bias in the reporting of study outcomes. The *Cochrane Handbook* (Higgins & Green, 2011) recommends that reviewers assess the following types of bias: (a) selection bias—whether there were systematic differences in the composition of groups; (b) performance bias—whether there were systematic differences in care between the groups other than the intervention; (c) attrition bias—whether one group withdrew or dropped out at a higher rate than the other; (d) detection bias—whether there were systematic differences in outcome assessment because of unblinded assessment; and (e) reporting bias—whether there was a tendency to report only significant findings.

Meta-Analysis

Meta-analysis has been defined as "a set of statistical techniques for combining quantitative results from multiple studies to produce a summary of empirical knowledge on a given topic" (Littell et al., 2008, pp. 1–2). Meta-analysis is used after data have been extracted in the systematic review process. A meta-analysis produces an effect size, a measure of strength and direction of a relationship. Several different metrics can be used to estimate the effect size in a meta-analysis. When dependent variables are continuous, it is common to use standardized mean differences, also known as Cohen's *d*. When dependent variables are dichotomous, odds ratios or risk ratios are frequently the chosen metric.

Heterogeneity, or equivalence, across research studies can cross out the option of conducting a meta-analysis; however, even when statistical groupings are reasonable, this remains a problem. Proper testing for heterogeneity is necessary, except when it is evident at a glance "that effects are consistent in magnitude and direction" (Polit & Beck, 2012, p. 662). Creating a forest plot will achieve a visual assessment of heterogeneity. The effect sizes of the studies will be estimated with the graph and jointly with a 95% confidence interval around the estimates (Polit & Beck, 2012).

A researcher conducting a meta-analysis frequently needs to consider how bias in outcome reporting could have an impact on the effect size. Several methods can be undertaken to address bias. If the researcher is including studies that are randomized by group (e.g., family unit, school), the intraclass correlation coefficient may be needed to examine whether observations within clusters are independent. Reporting (publication) bias also may have an impact on the effect size. To address publication bias, researchers can use a funnel plot to examine the distribution of effect sizes across studies included in the review. If there is no bias, the funnel plot should be symmetrical. If bias is found, researchers can use the trim and fill method to impute the values of studies that are assumed missing because of publication bias and recalculate the effect size (Duval, 2005). Variation of rigor in study design and inclusion of small studies in the meta-analysis also may lead to bias. Again, researchers can use funnel plots to examine this bias. They also can calculate the effect size with and without the small or less rigorously designed studies (Littell et al., 2008).

■ Conclusion

Critical appraisal of research is a fundamental part of evidence-based practice. It begins with understanding the research process to carefully and systematically evaluate studies to judge their relevance for clinical practice. To determine significance of the research you are considering, examine the following areas:

- Does the study test a stated hypothesis?
- Who is being studied? How were participants selected?
- Is the research design appropriate for the research question/hypothesis?
- Is each feature of the research design clear and replicable?

- What measures were used, and how were the data collected?
- What are the results of the study, and are they statistically significant?

This chapter summarized the different types of quantitative research to support critical appraisal of studies to improve patient outcomes.

REFLECTIVE ACTIVITIES

1. How are variables operationalized?
2. Which variable—independent, dependent, or confounding—is the focus of the research study?
3. What key techniques separate experimental from nonexperimental research designs?
4. What research design would best compare two patient interventions (e.g., for lowering cholesterol)?
5. Why might a practitioner use a quasi-experimental research design in the practice setting?
6. How does a systematic review differ from a meta-analysis?

REFERENCES

Alexandropoulou, M. (2013). Evaluating a health educational first aid program for special education school personnel: A cluster randomized trial. *International Journal of Caring Sciences, 6*, 115–126.

Babbie, E. (2012). *The practice of social research* (13th ed.). Belmont, CA: Wadsworth.

Brown, S. J. (2014). *Evidence-based nursing: The research-practice connection* (3rd ed.). Burlington, MA: Jones & Bartlett Learning.

Campbell, D. T., & Stanley, J. C. (1963). *Experimental and quasi-experimental designs for research*. Chicago, IL: Rand McNally.

Chapelain, P., Morineau, T., & Gautier, C. (2015). Effects of communication on the performance of nursing students during the simulation of an emergency situation. *Journal of Advanced Nursing, 71*, 2650–2659.

Cook, T. D., & Campbell, D. T. (1979). *Quasi-experimentation: Design & analysis issues for field settings*. Chicago, IL: Rand McNally.

Durbin, C. G., Jr. (2004). How to come up with a good research question: Framing the hypothesis. *Respiratory Care, 49*(10), 1195–1198.

Duru, O. K., Sarkisian, C. A., Leng, M., & Mangione, C. M. (2010). Sisters in motion: A randomized controlled trial of a faith-based physical activity intervention. *Journal of the American Geriatrics Society, 58*, 1863–1869.

Duval, S. (2005). The trim and fill method. In H. R. Rothstein, A. J. Sutton, & M. Bornstein (Eds.), *Publication bias in meta-analysis: Prevention, assessment, and adjustments* (pp. 128–144). Chichester, England: Wiley.

Grinnell, R. M., Jr., & Unrau, Y. A. (2011). *Social work research and evaluation: Foundations of evidence-based practice* (9th ed.). New York, NY: Oxford University Press.

Grinnell, R. M., Jr., Unrau, Y. A., & Williams, M. (2011). Group-level designs. In R. M. Grinnell, Jr., & Y. A. Unrau (Eds.), *Social work research and evaluation: Foundations of evidence-based practice* (9th ed., pp. 258–283). New York, NY: Oxford University Press.

Higgins, J. P. T., & Green, S. (Eds.). (2011). *Cochrane handbook for systematic reviews of interventions* (Version 5.1.0). Chichester, England: Wiley. Retrieved from http://www.cochrane-handbook.org/

Keele, R. (2011). *Nursing research and evidence-based practice*. Sudbury, MA: Jones & Bartlett Learning.

Kroeze, W., Oenema, A., Dagnelie, P. C., & Brug, J. (2008). Examining the minimal required elements of a computer-tailored intervention aimed at dietary fat reduction: Results of a randomized controlled dismantling study. *Health Education Research, 23,* 880–891.

Littell, J. H., Corcoran, J., & Pillai, V. (2008). *Systematic reviews and meta-analysis.* New York, NY: Oxford University Press.

LoBiondo-Wood, G., & Haber, J. (2014). *Nursing research: Methods and critical appraisal for evidenced based practice,* (8th ed.). St. Louis, MO: Elsevier.

Park, J., Lee, N., Cho, Y., & Yang, Y. (2015). Modified constraint-induced movement therapy for clients with chronic stroke: Interrupted time series (ITS) design. *Journal of Physical Therapy Science, 27,* 963–966.

Polit, D. F., & Beck, C. T. (2012). *Nursing research: Generating and assessing evidence for nursing practice* (9th ed.). Philadelphia, PA: Lippincott Williams & Wilkins.

Rubin, A., & Babbie, E. (2014). *Research methods for social work* (8th ed.). Belmont, CA: Brooks/Cole Cengage.

Schmidt, N. A., & Brown, J. M. (2012). *Evidence-based practice for nurses: Appraisal and application of research* (2nd ed.). Burlington, MA: Jones & Bartlett Learning.

Schwindt, R. G., McNeils, A. M., & Sharp, D. (2014). Evaluation of a theory-based education program to motivate nursing students to intervene with their seriously mentally ill clients who use tobacco. *Archives of Psychiatric Nursing, 28,* 277–283.

Shah, P. S., & Shah, J. (2010). Maternal exposure to domestic violence and pregnancy and birth outcomes: A systematic review and meta-analysis. *Journal of Women's Health, 19,* 2017–2031.

Solomon, P., & Draine, J. (2010). An overview of quantitative methods. In B. Thyer (Ed.), *The handbook of social work research methods* (2nd ed., pp. 26–36). Thousand Oaks, CA: Sage.

Surkan, P., Peterson, K., Hughes, M., & Gottlieb, B. (2006). The role of social networks and support in postpartum women's depression: A multiethnic urban sample. *Maternal and Child Health Journal, 10*(4), 375–383.

Wood, M. J. & Ross-Kerr, J. C. (2011). *Basic steps in planning nursing research: From questions to proposal* (7th ed.). Boston, MA: Jones and Bartlett.

Wyatt, T. H., & Hauenstein, E. J. (2008). Pilot testing Okay With Asthma: An online asthma intervention for school-age children. *Journal of School Nursing, 24*(3), 145–150.

Yegidis, B. L., & Weinbach, R. W. (2009). *Research methods for social workers* (6th ed.). Boston, MA: Pearson.

Yegidis, B. L., & Weinbach, R. W. (2011). *Research methods for social workers* (7th ed.). Boston, MA: Pearson.

CHAPTER 2

Qualitative Research

■ HEATHER R. HALL ■

■ Objectives:

- Identify the process of qualitative research.
- Recognize the approaches used to collect data in qualitative research.
- Identify study methods (e.g., phenomenology, ethnography, historical research, grounded theory, and case study) when evaluating qualitative research.
- Describe trustworthiness in qualitative research.

■ The Process of Qualitative Research

The primary focus of this chapter is to explain the qualitative research process and its importance in the world of evidence-based practice (EBP). Entire books have been written to discuss qualitative research design. Therefore, it is beyond the scope of this chapter to examine qualitative research in depth. In this chapter, you will find details on, examples of, and references to additional materials to guide you through your study and the use of qualitative research.

Qualitative research brings together scientific and authentic life components to improve the understanding of a phenomenon (Barroso, 2010). A *phenomenon* is identified as the fundamental concept that the researcher is investigating. A phenomenon is the awareness that subjects are experiencing in the study and also involves emotional concepts such as pain, unhappiness, rage, irritation, and love (Creswell, 2007). Researchers from various disciplines may investigate the phenomenon from different viewpoints (Denzin & Lincoln, 2000; Strauss & Corbin, 1994).

Qualitative research has its philosophical foundation as realism, which makes it distinct from quantitative research (Marshall & Rossman, 2006; Munhall, 2007). Qualitative researchers question many of the practices concerning science and how knowledge is acquired. In qualitative research, an investigation procedure is applied to the examination used to investigate a social or human dilemma. The investigative procedure includes developing a complicated, holistic representation, evaluating information, describing opinions of participants, and performing the study in a natural location

(Creswell, 2007). Researchers apply an *emergent design* that consists of establishing an investigation on truths and perspectives expressed by participants. Neither the truths nor the perspectives were common knowledge of the researchers when they began their study (Lincoln & Guba, 1985).

Qualitative research varies by category, rationale, and value (Patton, 2002). Findings for qualitative research are discovered by using different data gathering processes: (1) open-ended interviews, (2) observations, and (3) written documents (Patton, 2002). Interviews generate quotations from individuals about their experiences, views, thoughts, and understandings. Information derived from observations includes comprehensive accounts of people's leisure interests, conduct, actions, and all the interpersonal and group dealings that constitute the structure of recognizable human practices and happenings. Evaluation of written documents consists of analyzing selected passages, quotes, or complete sections from executive, medical, or program registers; memos and letters; executive pamphlets and statements; personal journals; and open-ended replies to surveys and assessments (Patton, 2002).

A researcher's ability to communicate easily and effectively with participants determines the successfulness of qualitative research findings (Knox & Burkard, 2009). Researchers have the responsibility of developing trust with participants, showing value for participants' views, and remaining aware of the cooperation between the researcher and participants. Therefore, the researcher must have the capability to develop a relationship, be an active listener, and place emphasis on another individual's world of experience (Polkinghorne, 2005).

Qualitative research is an investigation process that examines the entire phenomenon, along with the views of the individuals involved rather than examining the association of cause and effect amid identified variables, as in quantitative research (Liehr & LoBiondo-Wood, 2006). Both qualitative and quantitative research methods are crucial to increasing and improving understanding of identified phenomena (Craig & Smyth, 2007; Munhall, 2007). Researchers may decide to combine qualitative research and quantitative research in one study to develop a mixed method research approach (Bryman, 2007). Regardless of the method chosen, for research findings to be valuable, concepts must be transferable from the research study to other circumstances, conditions, settings, or phenomena (Sandelowski, 2000).

Importance to Evidence-Based Practice

Administration of EBP necessitates the use of clinical treatments that are established on understandable, user-friendly current research (Porter-O'Grady, 2006). Until recent times, qualitative research was not believed to offer value to EBP and therefore caused problems for qualitative researchers.

If research findings from qualitative studies had no effect on EBP, organizations providing funds would be reluctant to support these studies and educational curricula or to place significance on qualitative research. Researchers who choose to conduct qualitative research should include ways to integrate findings into EBP (Burns & Grove, 2009; Sandelowski & Barroso, 2007).

Popay and Williams (1998) explained how findings of qualitative research provide insight into finding helpful EBP methods. They proposed that findings from qualitative research offer rationalization as to why a method is successful, clarify unanticipated outcomes, and create assumptions and theory. Qualitative research offers explanations for why people conduct their lives in a particular manner. Data emphasize consequences from various situations and surroundings in which the participants work or even receive health care (Popay & Williams, 1998).

■ Investigative Procedures

Researchers do not identify qualitative investigative design choices before beginning the study (Polit & Beck, 2012). Researchers must plan for diverse situations and conditions; when researchers understand the facts involved with schedules, locations, and communication, they can make informed decisions about the investigative design (Polit & Beck, 2012). An additional, distinct contrast in qualitative research is that differences may occur in the actual research settings and time frame choices. Polit and Beck asserted that giving researchers the flexibility of collecting data from various research settings allows data to be gathered in unpretentious, genuine settings that may help relax participants (e.g., home environment). Researchers have the choice of two different time frames when using qualitative research design: cross-sectional or longitudinal (Polit & Beck, 2012). Data are gathered from one place in *cross-sectional* design, whereas a qualitative *longitudinal* time frame (Auerswald et al., 2004) allows for data gathering for a longer period (Polit & Beck, 2012).

■ Sampling

Qualitative research designs are often criticized for the small number of participants or for their subjectivity. Disapproval of qualitative research is often based on misunderstandings of qualitative research aims and the methods used to generate distinctive, beneficial data for EBP by clinical professionals (Brown, 2012). Determining sample size in qualitative research does not follow one rule (Patton, 2002). Sample size depends on what the researcher desires to learn, the purpose of the study, useful data choices, trustworthiness of data, money available, and scheduled time constraints (Krueger & Casey, 2000; Patton, 2002).

Decisions concerning sampling are critical because a researcher cannot thoroughly study every applicable situation, incident, or person (Marshall & Rossman, 2006). There is no one rule related to sample size when using qualitative research design. A case study may include data from only one participant, especially when studying unfamiliar traditions, ethnicities, or customs (Patton, 2002). Safman and Sobal (2004) maintained that one to four participants are typically involved in health research, that focus group research averages 10 groups, and that observational research typically covers a time frame of 16 to 24 months.

Sample size for qualitative research is a point of discussion and disagreement for researchers. Burns and Grove (2009) offered additional information about sample size for qualitative research. The researcher must determine the number of participants by first establishing the quantity of data required for achieving an understanding of the subject or phenomenon. Patton (2002) emphasized that the strength of qualitative research depends on the capability of the researcher to gather, analyze, and disseminate data in a well-founded and trustworthy manner instead of placing the emphasis on the number of study participants. Sample size depends on reaching redundancy, *data saturation,* in data collection (Boeije, 2007; Lincoln & Guba, 1985). Four significant criteria are important in determining sample size that results in data saturation: (a) scope of research project, (b) type of subject to be studied, (c) usefulness of data gathered, and (d) research design (Marshall & Rossman, 2006; Munhall, 2007; Patton, 2002).

Multiple approaches used to select samples for qualitative research include convenience sampling, snowball sampling, purposive sampling, and theoretical sampling (Polit & Beck, 2012). *Convenience sampling* refers to individuals volunteering their time to participate in the study. *Snowball sampling* involves participants referring other individuals to enroll in the study. *Purposive sampling* involves the researcher's intentional choice of individuals or groups of people who will help the study (Polit & Beck, 2012). *Theoretical sampling* is essential to the grounded theory approach in qualitative research (Patton, 2002). This strategy does not include selecting groups prior to conducting the research; however, groups are chosen as needed based on theoretical significance for the purpose of allowing categories to emerge from the data (Polit & Beck, 2012). The sample selection is based on the probability of representing a theoretical construct (Patton, 2002). Tappen (2011) concluded that qualitative research participants consist of a biased sample but also stated that the bias is both purposeful and helpful to the research study. Morse (2006) differentiated between what Tappen (2011) called purposeful bias and a bias that could occur inadvertently. Bias that can occur accidentally consists of (a) placing too much confidence in a small number of participants, (b) concentrating on impressive incidents instead of the daily lives of participants, and (c) presenting too much of the researcher's involvement in researched actions (Morse, 2006). Documentation of actions and recordings should indicate the researcher's involvement in the actions studied if the researcher is required to take part in any activities (Tappen, 2011).

■ Collection of Data in Qualitative Research

The researcher's ability to collect important data influences the data's value in qualitative research. Arranging data in an organized manner initiates the data analysis procedure (Creswell, 2007). Burns and Grove (2009) suggested conducting a pilot study to determine the best data collection method. The researcher executes four primary tasks during the data collection process: (a) choose participants, (b) collect data, (c) preserve research management as presented in research design, and (d) resolve predicaments that jeopardize research findings (Burns & Grove, 2009). Regardless of the data collection method used, the researcher's ability to communicate with participants is paramount in determining qualitative research validity and trustworthiness (Marshall & Rossman, 2006).

Regardless of training or schooling, some people should not attempt to conduct qualitative research. Marshall and Rossman (2006) asserted that without the ability to connect, communicate, and share with participants, the researcher will not be successful in completing a qualitative design study that yields accurate findings. Therefore, if talking with people does not rate at the top of the researcher's effective qualities, the researcher should not use a qualitative research design.

When the researcher makes the choice to use a qualitative research design, the data collection process begins. Neither the interview process nor the observational process should be attempted until the researcher has studied each procedure carefully and prepared to implement the method properly. Each participant provides data to the research through an *interview*, a process in which the participant furnishes the researcher with details, figures, and other essential data (Bernard, 2006). Interviews are most often performed between researcher and participants, either face to face, by telephone (Bernard, 2006), or by computer (Mann & Stewart, 2002). The interview process is not to be taken lightly. The researcher should prepare carefully for the interview and study interview methods before creating the interview plan (Briggs, 1986; Converse & Presser, 1986; Dillon, 1990; Fowler, 1990; McLaughlin, 1990).

Observation is one data collecting process used in qualitative research (Patton, 2002). The observation method demands preparation and instruction before the researcher begins to use the process. Instruction for becoming a competent observer consists of (a) being attentive to what is being said and what is being seen, (b) writing skills that include specific narratives, (c) learning to write detailed field notes, (d) attaining the ability to distinguish important information from irrelevant information, (e) employing meticulous techniques to authenticate and corroborate observations, and (f) conveying the researcher's views while expressing self-understanding of strengths and weaknesses of such views (Patton, 2002).

Tappen (2011) maintained that the researcher needs to learn and use organizational methods while collecting data that will serve to not only control the order of data collected but also assist in the data analysis process. Some suggestions given by Tappen for organization of data include (a) making notations on records that include date, time, location, and informant; (b) the researcher's views concerning informants' actions; (c) the researcher's opinions concerning the interview or observation; (d) direct quotes from informants; and (e) the researcher's understanding and analysis of initial interpretations. The researcher is cautioned to record interviews by using exact language used by the informant. Use precise quotes; do not make grammatical corrections. Make notes about phrases that are accentuated or an informant's reluctance to speak (Tappen, 2011).

Some researchers prefer to use computer software created for use with qualitative research. Gibbs (2007) advised that not all researchers are comfortable using the software programs. According to Gibbs, some researchers reported that using the software caused them to feel less connected to the recorded information and to the study participants. Researchers must realize that software programs aid only in evaluating data; software will not reason, ponder, imagine, or assume (Gibbs, 2007).

Focus group interviews are commonly used to study issues related to human health. A focus group interview consists of a group of at least five people gathered to discuss a specific phenomenon. The session includes a moderator, who leads the discussion using questions related to specific topics. These planned sessions use the dynamics of the group to access the rich material with limited costs. The questioning route (also known as the interview guide) used by the researcher is significant to a focus group being effective (Stewart, Shamdasani, & Rook, 2007). Neely-Barnes, Graff, Roberts, Hall, and Hankins (2010) conducted a descriptive, qualitative study using eight focus groups with 45 parents of children diagnosed with autism, cerebral palsy (CP), Down syndrome, and sickle cell disease. Two focus group interviews were conducted for each diagnosis. This study explored the perceptions of parents related to their communication with siblings of children diagnosed with the four disorders, which have an identified or suspected genetic basis (Neely-Barnes et al., 2010).

Qualitative research can be conducted as a pilot study. Hall and Graff (2010) conducted a pilot study using focus group interviews with parents of children with autism. This study provided parents with the opportunity to describe their parenting concerns related to autism and identified techniques that parents can use to assist with parental challenges.

■ Data Analysis and Interpretation of Findings

Coding

Coding in qualitative research occurs in three phases, which are labeled descriptive, interpretive, and explanatory (Burns & Grove, 2009). *Descriptive codes* explain how the researcher intends to control and deal with all recorded data. Descriptive coding is the easiest process of organization and categorization, and researchers often choose this coding method in the early phases of analyzing data. When using descriptive coding, the researcher aims to keep the language similar to the original terminology used by study informants in the interview phase (Burns & Grove, 2009).

As the data collection process progresses and the researcher acquires more understanding into the procedure, he or she advances past cataloging recorded accounts.

The researcher begins to use *interpretive coding* to connect significance and consequence to informants' explanations (Burns & Grove, 2009).

Explanatory coding is the type of code developed late in the process of collecting data. This late stage of coding occurs when the researcher begins to sort out significances that are natural to the phenomena studied. Explanatory codes allow the researcher to make associations between data and the theory that is materializing (Burns & Grove, 2009).

Analysis of Focus Groups Data

Analysis of data gathered from focus groups is complicated because the researcher is required to perform analysis and make associations of individual participants' responses and the entire focus group's responses (Morgan, 1995). It is paramount to the trustworthiness of the study that the researcher conscientiously focus on not only the topics discussed by focus groups but also the agreement or disagreement on the topics among focus group participants. Likewise, opinions that differ from those of the majority of the focus group should not be ignored, but analyzed. In addition, participants often give communications nonverbally; these actions are important and should be included in the analysis (Morgan, 1995).

When the researcher reaches the analysis stage of the process, he or she begins to find answers to the research question or questions that caused the original interest (Burns & Grove, 2009). Experience should not be underestimated. If possible, the researcher should find someone familiar with the method of qualitative research being conducted. A researcher has the greatest opportunity to learn, investigate, and analyze the qualitative research method of choice by teaming with an experienced researcher (Morse, 1997; Sandelowski, 1997).

■ Methods of Qualitative Research

This chapter focuses on five commonly used qualitative research methods: phenomenology, ethnography, historical research, grounded theory, and case study (see **Table 2-1**). The reader will discover that the methods have likenesses, but they also have variations that make them distinctly different. Data for each method require the written word instead of numbers. Data analysis must be performed on the *text,* with the data collected as written words from interviews or observations. Regardless of the multiple similarities, each qualitative method was theoretically developed for a unique purpose as a means to study a phenomenon (Cohen, 2006).

■ Phenomenological Research

Phenomenological research is the method of discovering and structuring the meaning of human incidents through interviews with people actually involved in the real-life experience (Creswell, 2007; Polit & Beck, 2012). The researcher's objective is to become truly aware of and comprehend the significance and consequences of the

Table 2-1 Qualitative Research Methods

	Data Collection	Data Source	Data Analysis
Phenomenology	Unstructured interviews; new questions emerge as the data evolve	Individuals	Inductive analysis; data collection and analysis occur simultaneously
Ethnography	Documents, interviews, observation	Individuals within a culture	Ongoing throughout the data collection process
Historical	Firsthand account interviews, pictures, newspapers	Individuals or in documentation	Criticism and themes in the data
Grounded theory	Interviews, observation	Individuals	Systemic coding (open, axial, and selective)
Case study	Questionnaires, interviews, observation, participant journals	Individuals or groups	Patterns and themes in the data

Data from Boswell, C., & Cannon, S. (2011). *Introduction to nursing research: Incorporating evidence-based practice* (2nd ed.) Sudbury, MA: Jones & Bartlett Learning.

phenomena as they are described by the participant. The researcher is expected to *bracket* (put aside) personal biases when involved in the phenomenological research process (Creswell, 2007; Polit & Beck, 2012).

Researchers using phenomenology look for individuals who have lived or who are living the phenomenon to be studied (Creswell, 2007). The researcher collects either written or oral data from participants, and the number of interviews depends on the researcher's chosen analysis method. The researcher may present questions in writing and request written responses or schedule an interview during which the conversation is tape-recorded. *Data saturation,* hearing the same themes over again with no new categories, normally determines the number of interviews used by the researcher and indicates that the research should conclude (Liehr & LoBiondo-Wood, 2006).

Example of Phenomenological Research

Hill, Higgins, Dempster, and McCarthy (2009) used interpretive phenomenological analysis to analyze the transcripts collected during a study focused on the understanding of fathers of children with acute lymphoblastic leukemia related to their family role during their child's diagnosis and treatment. The following themes surfaced: (a) adjustment to diagnosis, (b) experiencing the nature of maternal protection, (c) making every effort to have normalcy, (d) and providing and accepting support (Hill et al., 2009).

Phenomenological Data Collection

Data collection for a phenomenological study involves extended interviews with participants. Typically, participants are asked to convey their experiences with the phenomenon being studied while the researcher collects and stores the information communicated by each participant (Tilley, 2011). Burns and Grove (2009) insisted that the researcher can use more than one method or a combination of methods to collect data when using the phenomenological research process by engaging both behaviors and intuiting. *Intuiting* involves the researcher concentrating all attentiveness and enthusiasm on strengthening understanding of the phenomenon of concern (Burns & Grove, 2009).

One method for collecting phenomenological data includes interviewing participants. The researcher must be patient and supportive in permitting the participants to use as much time as needed for them to present comprehensive explanations of their experiences. Instead of verbally communicating experiences, participants could be allowed to supply the researcher with a written account of their encounters with the phenomenon (Burns & Grove, 2009).

The researcher plays an important role in another method for collecting data for phenomenology research, including the researcher in the phenomenon. The researcher participates in the experience as an observer concerning all behaviors, the setting, and the researcher's reactions to what is occurring. The researcher takes notes, tape-records, or videotapes (Burns & Grove, 2009).

Phenomenological Data Analysis

Multiple data analysis techniques exist when using phenomenological research methods. Even though there are differences in the techniques, a pattern moves from the description stated by the participant and is then synthesized by the researcher with all descriptions from participants. Analysis of phenomenological research findings requires the researcher to present the reader with data that begin with the research question. Then the researcher leads the reader through the research process, which includes examples of participants' responses and the researcher's explanation. Last, the researcher provides the reader with an account that expands and integrates the participants' experiences with the phenomenon of concern. Phenomenological research findings are presented to the reader in an explanatory narrative that both justifies the use of the qualitative research and explains the phenomenon studied through the experiences of participants (Liehr & LoBiondo-Wood, 2006).

■ Ethnographic Research

Ethnography is the study of either a whole cultural or social group or a person or persons within the group (Wolcott, 1995). Ethnographic research originated when researchers began seeking information about cultures that differed from their own (Wolf, 2007). An ethnographer enters an unfamiliar cultural or social group and accepts the challenge of presenting accurate data from a group member's interpretation (Agar, 1986). To completely immerse themselves into a different culture, some ethnographers choose to move into the new world, study the speech and speak the dialect of the new culture, and involve themselves in every part of the culture. Researchers provide narratives that describe from their point of view every detail of the lives of the people studied, including their social networking, principles, and other actions (Wolf, 2007).

Chambers (2003) maintained that ethnography concentrates on scientific reports and explanations of cultural or social groups and organizations. The ethnographic study is established largely on the researcher's field experiences collected by examination of the participating sample through surveillance over an extended period. *Fieldwork* is a closely controlled method of questioning that allows an ethnographer to personally gather data over a broad period. Well-organized fieldwork blends skills and knowledge of the proficient ethnographer for a narrative to be constructed that gives the reader an awareness of the different culture studied (Wolcott, 1995). During the fieldwork, the ethnographer watches, listens, asks questions, and documents actions and conversations of participants for the purpose of creating the culture through words for readers (Creswell, 2007; Tedlock, 2000; Thomas, 1993).

Before the researcher is allowed to enter the new society, he or she must earn the respect of a chief member of the group, the *gatekeeper*. Until the gatekeeper believes that the researcher is honorable and trustworthy, the group will not participate (Creswell, 2007). Once the researcher gains entrance into the group and is accepted, reliable research documentation can be collected. The researcher is now ready to move forward with prepared research inquiry concerning the life, roles, and behaviors of the cultural or social group (Liehr & LoBiondo-Wood, 2006).

Example of Ethnographic Research

Neufeld, Harrison, Hughes, and Stewart (2007) conducted an ethnographic research study to identify interactions that were nonsupportive among 59 women who were caregivers in diverse circumstances. Participants included mothers of premature infants, mothers of children diagnosed with asthma or diabetes, and caregivers for an adult member of the family with cancer or dementia. The participants who provided care in all circumstances stated that they experienced the following interactions considered nonsupportive: (a) unconstructive support, (b) unproductive support, or (c) deficient anticipated support. The participants' interaction evaluation was based on individual expectations and their perspectives of the circumstances (Neufeld et al., 2007).

Ethnographic Data Collection

Ethnographic research begins with choosing a civilization, subculture, or racial group to study and the setting in which the group will be studied (Tappen, 2011). Ethnography requires the researcher to observe the participants or become engrossed in the situation, interview the participants, and explain the culture of the participants (Crabtree & Miller, 1992). Ethnography research requires the inclusion of a group of people living in the culture and experiencing the phenomenon involved in the research (Liehr & LoBiondo-Wood, 2006). Research participants include either informants who provide researchers with common knowledge among the cultural group or *key informants* who impart significant knowledge concerning the phenomenon under investigation (Creswell, 2007).

Ethnographers gather data in the field—fieldwork—by literally going to the locations where the culture is actually being lived by the people. The researcher transcribes fieldwork into *field notes*. Gathering fieldwork and transcribing data into field notes often require an extended time frame. As long as the research is in progress, the ethnographer remains in contact with the study group by joining in the members' interests, leisure time activities, cultural events, and required specific locations. The researcher strives to become part of the group to better understand the culture (Sanjek, 1990).

Information gathered from interviewing participants is recorded by the researcher while the interview is in process or directly after. The researcher may choose to record data by either writing or recording. If the researcher senses that a participant is hesitant to answer if notes or recordings of any kind are in process, the researcher should record notes after the interview. The participant's permission must be acquired before any interview taping can proceed (Burns & Grove, 2009).

Transcription of interviews must be word-for-word precise because the transcriptions serve as data for establishing significance. Significant statements are categorized into clusters that denote themes that are shared in all participants' narratives. Themes develop a thorough explanation of the phenomenon, and the participants should be permitted to go through all data for accurateness (Riemen, 1998). Management of data includes producing and arranging data files, studying tests, and forming of preliminary coding (Creswell, 2007).

Ethnographic Data Analysis

Data analysis for ethnographic research is similar to data analysis for the grounded theory research method in that data are gathered and evaluated concurrently. In addition, data analysis starts with choosing main categories or domains and then listing less significant categories or domains under the main headings (Liehr & LoBiondo-Wood, 2006). The ethnographer clarifies and interprets data while continuing to search for meanings. When analysis is complete and findings can be explained, the ethnographer organizes a report and/or lecture to present findings. Data are to be stored in transcribed forms (Creswell, 2007). Ethnographic research produces a vast amount of data (e.g., observations, interviews, photographs).

■ Historical Research

Historical research is a systematic attempt to study past life experiences by gathering, assembling, classifying, and evaluating data. One important objective of the researcher is to bring forth historical data to look for ways to direct present and future experiences. Findings allow the reader to understand what occurred in the past and modify life practices in an attempt to prevent unwanted past experiences from reoccurring (Liehr & LoBiondo-Wood, 2006).

The researcher may choose to use a biography format as historical research; however, before documenting events in a person's life, the researcher must receive permission to do so (Creswell, 1998). After the researcher gathers historical data about the biographer's life, data interpretation begins. The researcher develops a theory about the person's life experiences and past and present influences in his or her life. The researcher then develops an abstract that emphasizes the person's life practices and the significance and consequences of these practices as stated in the documentation. Last, findings in documentation that focused on actions, theories, and practices discussed in the research should be presented (Creswell, 1998).

Example of Historical Research

Wood (2009) used historical research methods to study the function of surgical nurses in preventing sepsis in wounds. In addition, an aim of this study was to identify how this role was represented in nursing literature during the period preceding the use of antibiotics, 1895 to 1935. During this time, trained nurses working in the surgical clinical setting were seen as supporters of surgeons' efforts to prevent wound sepsis; however, nurses were blamed when a patient was diagnosed with wound sepsis. More use of sterilized dressing supplies, decreased dependence on needless antiseptics, and fewer rigorous processes preparing the supplies for surgery were the greatest changes important to awareness and practice. The literature associated the nurse with the surgeon, instead of the patient. The relationship between the nurse and surgeon should not be interpreted as being "subservient." Surgeons were seeking support and a meticulous approach from nurses. This research provides evidence for nurses related to not only the lasting characteristics of clinically based understanding and practice but also how others may not be quick to change (Wood, 2009).

Historical Research Data Collection

Data that provide the sample for historical research could consist of written documents, videotapes, interviews with participants who provide firsthand accounts, pictures, and other relics pertinent to the historical research. The historical researcher must be specific about the historical incident of concern to use only artifacts that provide crucial data for the studied incident. Data sources are considered to be primary or secondary. *Primary sources* include eyewitnesses to the historical event. Primary sources are expected to supply researchers with more trustworthy information than a secondary source (Christy, 1975). *Secondary sources* supply data that have been conveyed to them about the phenomenon. The further an informant is from being an eyewitness to an event, the more untrustworthy the information becomes (Liehr & LoBiondo-Wood, 2006).

Historical Research Data Analysis

The evidence retrieved using historical research methods is evaluated using two forms of criticism: *external* and *internal* (Polit & Beck, 2012). The data's authenticity is evaluated using external criticism. Evaluating the value of the evidence of historical data is internal criticism. The purpose of the internal criticism is to judge the content.

Truth of the data is the foundational issue (Polit & Beck, 2012). Being familiar with the specific historical period is crucial for assessing reliability (Liehr & LoBiondo-Wood, 2006). Data collection and analysis are simultaneous processes in historical research (Polit & Beck, 2012).

■ Grounded Theory Research

Grounded theory was developed for the purpose of studying communication and relations in social groups (Glaser & Strauss, 1967). Grounded theory is considered the most popular and often used qualitative research method across many disciplines and branches of learning (Bryant & Charmaz, 2008). Parker (2006) defined *theory* as a notion or idea that gives details or describes happenings, sheds light on opinions, explains associations, and predicts effects or conclusions. Corbin (2009) maintained that grounded theory is differentiated from other qualitative research methods in that the objective is the development of theory grounded in facts. Qualitative research is particularly effective as a resource for grounded theory. Grounded theory is produced from fieldwork data collected through the researcher's observations and interviews in natural settings instead of in a laboratory (Patton, 2002). Research questions for grounded theory concentrate on fundamental social practices that generally concern the influencing of human behavior (Liehr & LoBiondo-Wood, 2006).

The foundation for grounded theory is the use of communication with participants to learn about how they identify and relate to a particular phenomenon in their lives and how their ideas and principles are associated with their actions (Burns & Grove, 2009). The grounded theory method is particularly advantageous when the accepted knowledge comes from a speculative viewpoint and fails to adequately give an explanation of what is happening (Wuest, 2007). In grounded theory research, the researcher produces a theoretical plan about a phenomenon. The theoretical plan describes details concerning selected proceedings, communications, or procedures (Burns & Grove, 2009).

Grounded theory research is achieved through the compilation of interview records, numerous field visits to collect theoretical samples, continual evaluation of data, and the creation of a context-specific hypothesis (Strauss & Corbin, 1990). Although the researcher reviews some literature for the study, the researcher does not prepare a thorough literature study. The researcher allows the theory to surface from collected data so that it serves as an indicator of related principles fundamental to social practices researched. The theory that materializes is created from the collected information (Liehr & LoBiondo-Wood, 2006).

Interaction is the focal point of observation in the qualitative research grounded theory method (Burns & Grove, 2009). Individuals produce realism as a result of assigning significance to circumstances and conditions, which develops into the foundation for achievement. When people participate together in social living, groups assign meanings and exchange these meanings with their latest associates by socializing with them. Interaction may guide the way to innovative and novel values, and the outcome could be a person or persons with a new identity of self (Burns & Grove, 2009).

Example of Grounded Theory Research

Davis et al. (2010) conducted a study using grounded theory. The aims of this study were to (a) investigate the quality of life (QOL) of mothers and fathers of children (aged 3 to 18 years) diagnosed with CP and (b) determine if caring for children with CP changes from child years to teenage years. The participants of this study were 24 mothers and 13 fathers of children with CP, with different levels of severity. A wide range of QOL resulted among parents. The following are affected while caring for children diagnosed with CP: (a) physical health, (b) social contentment, (c) autonomy and independence, (d) family strength, and (e) monetary solidity (Davis et al., 2010).

Grounded Theory Methodology Data Collection

Grounded theory research data collection is referred to as fieldwork (Burns & Grove, 2009). Participants are chosen for the study because of their capacity to play a part in the development of the theory. Participant grouping, which may begin as homogeneous, will become more heterogeneous as the theory grows (Tappen, 2011).

The researcher may typically use observation of participants as the data collection method. Concentration during observation should be directed at group interactions targeted toward the researched phenomenon. Researchers may choose to interview participants to allow them to express viewpoints (Burns & Grove, 2009).

Coding Grounded Theory

The researcher begins data analysis by using collected data for open coding. *Open coding* requires the researcher to use data collected from informants and observations and create about six categories that will develop into major themes in the research study (Strauss & Corbin, 1990). Any category not directly related to the phenomenon of concern is not included in the coding process (Wuest, 2007). The fundamental actions required for developing categories consist of continual evaluation of data, codes, and categories (Kelle, 2008).

After the categories are selected, the researcher recognizes and names the principal phenomenon and initiates the investigation into the association among categories using *axial coding* (Creswell, 2007). The researcher searches for situations that affect the principal phenomenon, the conditions that influence methodologies, and the significance of accepting the methodologies. Then the researcher establishes a *coding paradigm,* a hypothetical standard that allows the associations of the axial coding to be viewed and studied (Creswell, 2007). The last step involves *selective coding*: the researcher acquires the model to develop hypotheses in which the categories are interrelated (Creswell, 2007).

Grounded Theory Analysis

Open coding calls for the researcher to scrutinize data meticulously and evaluate likenesses and differences (Strauss & Corbin, 1990). During the entire grounded theory process, the *constant comparative method*, in which data are constantly compared, is used. As codes or categories become apparent during the process, the researcher finds that they may enlarge or they may be minimized and become a component of another category. As the theorist continues through this process, a theory is developed. Therefore, in grounded theory research, the processes of data collection, coding, analyzing, and theory development have a mutual connection (Strauss & Corbin, 1990).

To interpret findings of grounded theory research, the researcher furnishes details of the process and reasoning of the method and describes the theory developed. Researchers are encouraged to use diagrams and charts as well as detailed narrative to report their findings and show how the data are associated (Liehr & LoBiondo-Wood, 2006). At the completion of the study, the researcher is required to put all data in safe keeping, including all notes, transcripts, and computer data (Creswell, 2007).

■ Case Study Research

Case study research involves the investigator examining both irregularities and harmonies of a particular circumstance or phenomenon. A case study can consist of quantitative and/or qualitative data, but it is identified by the center of attention being placed on one personal situation (Stake, 2000). An investigator generally prefers to examine an organization or routine practice, such as an activity, episode, curriculum, or several people. Before an investigator can secure contact with the study sample, he or she must obtain the trust of those involved (Creswell, 2007).

Case study research can consist of one case study, multiple case studies, or a series of case studies (Tappen, 2011). Each case study requires the researcher to examine the situation or phenomena, document data that are either relevant to the inquiry or explicatory of the circumstances or phenomena, and record a narrative explanation of each case (Tappen, 2011). An *intrinsic case study* provides an improved perception of the case. An *instrumental case study* allows the researcher to look more closely at a topic or subject of concern or to question a generality (Stake, 2000).

Example of Case Study Research

Krausz and Meszaros (2005) conducted a single case study to identify and comprehend how a mother's life is affected by having a child with autism, to analyze

(continues)

themes that have formed her life, to identify adaptation stages of parents of children with autism, and to develop meanings that others may benefit from based on the experiences of the participants. This study was written in narrative form and documented the heartbreaking process of acceptance related to the child's developmental condition. In-depth interviews were conducted during the data collection process. Eleven themes emerged consistently from the data; falling apart was the one new theme, and two strategies related to coping were apparent (Krausz & Meszaros, 2005).

Case Study Data Collection

Case study data are collected through the use of interviews, observations, reexamination of documentation, and other techniques used to allow the researcher to understand the phenomenon. The researcher is required to do whatever needs to be done to collect the necessary data (Liehr & LoBiondo-Wood, 2006).

Case Study Data Analysis

Liehr and LoBiondo-Wood (2006) maintained that the case study account depends on proper analysis of data and an appropriate explanation of research findings. When the researcher has completed the process of examining recorded data, connecting relationships among data collected from all resources, and beginning to develop significance of data, the case study story begins. The researcher is responsible for considering all data pertinent to the phenomenon studied and presenting findings that accurately reflect research results (Liehr & LoBiondo-Wood, 2006).

The case study research findings typically do not include research activities; therefore, interpretation of findings by the reader may be difficult (Liehr & LoBiondo-Wood, 2006). According to Stake (2000), findings for case study research are included in other segments of the study: (a) sequential progress of the research, (b) the researcher's account of the case study, (c) the explanation of case components, and (d) the emphasis of the case study attributes.

■ Trustworthiness in Qualitative Research

A necessary component in both qualitative and quantitative research is quality (Tappen, 2011). However, the precise definition of quality that is considered to be high has created a discussion among researchers. Scholars have debated the issue of whether rigor and validity should be used to identify quality in qualitative research (Polit & Beck, 2012). Rigor has been defined as the strength of the research design and the appropriateness of the method to answer the questions (Morse, 2003). Some scholars consider different criteria to classify rigor in the qualitative research process; therefore, they argue for the need to use other terms

(Tappen, 2011). However, rigor has been used to express the attributes related to the qualitative research process (Barroso, 2010; Davies & Dodd, 2002). Morse, Barrett, Mayan, Olson, and Spiers (2002) stated that "without rigor, research is worthless, becomes fiction, and loses its utility" (p. 2).

Framework: Lincoln And Guba

Lincoln and Guba (1985) developed a framework of criteria to identify quality in qualitative research. Trustworthiness is used as the central concept in the framework to appraise the rigor of the qualitative study and is a priority to scholars evaluating the research. The following four criteria for trustworthiness are equivalent to the criteria of reliability and validity in quantitative research design: credibility, dependability, confirmability, and transferability (Lincoln & Guba, 1985). Guba and Lincoln (1994) developed a fifth criterion, authenticity, following comments from others; it is a developing concept.

Credibility is a principal goal in qualitative research (Lincoln & Guba, 1985). Polit and Beck (2012) described credibility as the assurance in data truth and the analysis of the data. Credibility includes conducting the study in a manner that increases the confidence in the results and following a method to exhibit credibility in the dissemination of the findings (Lincoln & Guba, 1985).

Dependability is the strength or reliability of data through time and circumstances. Credibility cannot be achieved if dependability is absent (Lincoln & Guba, 1985).

Confirmability is the comparison between at least two researchers regarding the accuracy, significance, or meaning of the data (Lincoln & Guba, 1985). Confirmability is related to the data representing the information the participants described. In addition, data interpretations should not be created by the researcher. Data findings must describe the participants' words and the setting of the study, not the researcher's perceptions (Polit & Beck, 2012).

Transferability is related to the findings being applicable in other locations or groups of people. The researcher should offer adequate data to evaluate the applicability in other settings (Lincoln & Guba, 1985).

Authenticity is the researcher reasonably providing certainty (Guba & Lincoln, 1994). In a report, the authenticity is suggested when the tone of participants' lives is portrayed as their lives are truly lived. When the reader has increased sensitivity to the data descriptions of the topic being addressed, authenticity has been achieved (Polit & Beck, 2012).

■ Strategies to Increase Quality

Multiple strategies are used to increase the quality of qualitative research (Polit & Beck, 2012). The strategies to be discussed are (a) prolonged engagement, (b) persistent observation, (c) triangulation, (d) member checking, and (e) peer debriefing.

Lincoln and Guba (1985) described prolonged engagement as a vital component in determining the credibility of a study. Prolonged engagement includes the researcher spending quality time during the data collection process to increase his or her knowledge of the participants and guarantee data saturation. Researchers need to participate in persistent observation to enhance quality. Persistent observation includes the researchers paying attention to the specific details of a discussion among participants significant to the study (Lincoln & Guba, 1985). Triangulation uses multiple references to establish truth and data, and conclusions can be cross-checked (Denzin, 1978; Polit & Beck, 2012; Tappen, 2011). In the data analysis phase, different viewpoints are provided regarding the same phenomenon; this enhances credibility by strengthening the conclusions (Patton, 2002). An essential method to establish the credibility of data in qualitative research is member checking (Lincoln & Guba, 1985). Member checking involves the researchers offering participants feedback related to the analysis of data and recording their responses. Participants should confirm the researchers' analysis of data provided during the data collection process (Lincoln & Guba, 1985; Polit & Beck, 2012). Peer debriefing includes meetings between the researchers and their peers to evaluate the characteristics of the study. During these meetings, the researchers are open to questions of other researchers who are not invested in the study and who have experience in a specific research process or with the research topic (Polit & Beck, 2012).

■ Meta-Synthesis

Qualitative meta-synthesis was recognized in the 1970s as a vital advancement in research (Sandelowski & Barroso, 2007). A meta-synthesis is a form of a systematic review relevant to qualitative research (Polit & Beck, 2012). Erwin, Brotherson, and Summers (2011) stated that meta-synthesis is a planned method to synthesize and understand data across studies using qualitative research methods. The process involves distinct phases that allow the researcher to identify a research question. The researcher will "search for, select, appraise, summarize, and combine evidence to address the research question" (Erwin et al., 2011, p. 191). The findings of qualitative studies conducted on a specific topic are systematically reviewed and integrated. A meta-synthesis provides researchers an opportunity to put together findings from qualitative research important to the practice setting (Barroso, 2010; Polit & Beck, 2012).

For example, Bertero and Chamberlain (2007) conducted a meta-synthesis using 30 qualitative research reports related to the diagnosis of breast cancer and the treatments affecting the self. Self aspects were identified as affected by the breast cancer diagnosis and the necessary treatment: (a) knowledge of individual mortality, (b) existing with an unsure confidence, (c) confirmation of attachment, and (d) giving a new definition to self. Women who are diagnosed with breast cancer become accustomed to their life as a patient (Bertero & Chamberlain, 2007).

■ Disseminating Research Findings

Tappen (2011) advised researchers not to believe their research is finished when they have completed the analysis process. According to Tappen, the research process is unfinished until the researcher reveals findings not only to funders of the research but also to colleagues, other interested groups, and the general public. If the research is funded, the researcher must communicate with the funder before reporting findings. Often, the funders may request that findings be reported in a particular way (Tappen, 2011).

Tappen (2011) further cautioned the researcher concerning reporting findings to groups or the general public who may be interested in findings. Scientific terminology must be changed in a manner that the general public can understand and glean information from it. The researcher must relate findings in the current study with findings previously reported; relating findings either confirms or refutes previous findings. Results must be duplicated for readers to believe that the findings confirm that the research should be used in EBP (Tappen, 2011).

Researchers should write notes about their views, feelings, and opinions concerning situations that occur during the progression of the research procedure because the same conditions may not arise again (Lempert, 2008; Stern, 2008). A new investigator may find that one of the hardest aspects of the research process centers is the need for simultaneous data collection, evaluation, and theory development (Wiener, 2008). However, unless the researcher remembers to write notes and code data from the beginning of the process, he or she will become inundated with data. Too many times, researchers have failed to complete the research process of publishing findings because they were weighted down with too many notes and tapes that had remained untouched for too long (Wiener, 2008).

■ Conclusion

Qualitative research procedures are specifically designed to gain perceptions into particular, personal knowledge and an understanding of social practices. Qualitative research also provides insight into complicated, personal truths that cannot be separated, influenced, and inspected the way physical certainties can. The awareness of human practices, encounters, and social relationships that is generated by qualitative research techniques cannot be attained using procedures that condense human attributes to statistics and the circumstances of human existence to being labeled as variables (Brown, 2012).

REFLECTIVE ACTIVITIES

1. Describe qualitative research as an investigation of human experiences in naturalistic settings, pursuing meanings that inform theory, practice, instrument development, and further research.

2. How does data saturation determine sample size compared to power analyses associated with quantitative studies. In fact, qualitative researchers also identify the need for larger samples without offering explanations as to the rationale for needing a greater number of participants (Cohen, Kahn, & Steeves, 2002).
3. Describe qualitative research methods to include five basic elements: identifying the phenomenon, structuring the study, gathering the data, analyzing the data, and describing the findings.
4. How can qualitative research data be managed through the use of computers? How will the researcher interpret those data?
5. Using Lincoln and Guba's (1985) framework of criteria related to quality (i.e., credibility, dependability, confirmability, transferability, and authenticity) choose a qualitative study to appraise the trustworthiness of the qualitative inquiry.

REFERENCES

Agar, M. H. (1986). *Speaking of ethnography.* Beverly Hills, CA: Sage.

Auerswald, C. L., Greene, K., Minnis, A., Doherty, L., Ellen, J., & Padian, N. (2004). Qualitative assessment of venues for purposive sampling of hard-to-reach youth: An illustration in a Latino community. *Sexually Transmitted Diseases, 31*(2), 133–138.

Barroso, J. (2010). Qualitative approaches to research. In G. LoBiondo-Wood & J. Haber (Eds.), *Nursing research: Methods and critical appraisal for evidence-based practice* (7th ed., pp. 100–125). St. Louis, MO: Mosby.

Bernard, H. R. (2006). *Research methods in anthropology: Qualitative and quantitative approaches* (4th ed.). Lanham, MD: AltaMira Press.

Bertero, C., & Chamberlain, W. M. (2007). Breast cancer diagnosis and its treatment affecting the self: A meta-synthesis. *Cancer Nursing, 30*(3), 194–202.

Boeije, H. (2007). A purposeful approach to the constant comparative method in the analysis of qualitative interviews. In S. Sarantakos (Ed.), *Data analysis* (pp. 265–285). Los Angeles, CA: Sage.

Boswell, C., & Cannon, S. (2011). *Introduction to nursing research: Incorporating evidence-based practice* (2nd ed.). Sudbury, MA: Jones & Bartlett Learning.

Briggs, C. L. (1986). *Learning how to ask: A sociolinguistic appraisal of the role of the interview in social science research.* Cambridge, England: Cambridge University Press.

Brown, S. J. (2012). *Evidence-based nursing: The research-practice connection* (2nd ed.). Burlington, MA: Jones & Bartlett Learning.

Bryant, A., & Charmaz, K. (2008). Grounded theory research: Methods and practices. In A. Bryant & K. Charmaz (Eds.), *The SAGE handbook of grounded theory* (pp. 31–57). Thousand Oaks, CA: Sage.

Bryman, A. (2007). Barriers to integrating quantitative and qualitative research. *Journal of Mixed Methods Research, 1*(8), 8–22. Doi:10.1177/2345678906290531

Burns, N., & Grove, S. K. (2009). *The practice of nursing research: Appraisal, synthesis, and generation of evidence* (6th ed.). St. Louis, MO: Mosby.

Chambers, E. (2003). Applied ethnography. In N. K. Denzin & Y. S. Lincoln (Eds.), *Collecting and interpreting qualitative materials* (pp. 389–418). Thousand Oaks, CA: Sage.

Christy, T. E. (1975). A methodology of historical research. *Nursing Research, 24*(3), 189–192.

Cohen, M. Z. (2006). Introduction to qualitative research. In G. LoBiondo Wood & J. Haber (Eds.), *Nursing research: Methods and critical appraisal for evidence-based practice* (6th ed., pp. 131–147). St. Louis, MO: Mosby.

Cohen, M., Kahn, D., & Steeves, R. (2002). Making use of qualitative research. *Western Journal of Nursing Research, 24*(4), 454–471.

Converse, J. M., & Presser, S. (1986). *Survey questions: Handcrafting the standardized questionnaire.* Newbury Park, CA: Sage.

Corbin, J. (2009). Taking an analytic journey. In J. M. Morse, P. M. Stern, J. Corbin, B. Bowers, K. Charmaz, & A. E. Clarke. *Developing grounded theory: The second generation* (pp. 35–53). Walnut Creek, CA: Left Coast Press.

Crabtree, B. F., & Miller, W. L. (1992). *Doing qualitative research.* Newbury Park, CA: Sage.

Craig, J. V., & Smyth, R. L. (2007). *The evidence-based practice manual for nurses* (2nd ed.). Philadelphia, PA: Churchill Livingstone.

Creswell, J. W. (1998). *Qualitative inquiry and research design: Choosing among five traditions.* Thousand Oaks, CA: Sage.

Creswell, J. W. (2007). *Qualitative inquiry and research design: Choosing among five traditions* (2nd ed.). Thousand Oaks, CA: Sage.

Davies, D., & Dodd, J. (2002). Pearls, pith, and provocation: Qualitative research and the question of rigor. *Qualitative Health Research, 12*(2), 279–289.

Davis, E., Shelly, A., Waters, E., Boyd, R., Cook, K., & Davern, M. (2010). The impact of caring for a child with cerebral palsy: Quality of life for mothers and fathers. *Child: Care, Health and Development, 36*(1), 63–73. Doi:10.1111/j.1365-2214.2009.00989.x

Denzin, N. K. (1978). *Sociological methods.* New York, NY: McGraw-Hill.

Denzin, N. K., & Lincoln, Y. S. (2000). *Handbook of qualitative research* (2nd ed.). Thousand Oaks, CA: Sage.

Dillon, J. T. (1990). *The practice of questioning.* New York, NY: Routledge.

Erwin, E. J., Brotherson, M. J., & Summers, J. A. (2011). Understanding qualitative metasynthesis. *Journal of Early Intervention, 33*(3), 186–200.

Fowler, F. J. (1990). *Standardized survey interviewing: Minimizing interviewer-related error.* Newbury Park, CA: Sage.

Gibbs, G. R. (2007). *Analyzing qualitative data.* London, England: Sage.

Glaser, B., & Strauss, A. (1967). *The discovery of grounded theory: Strategies for qualitative research.* Piscataway, NJ: Aldine Transaction.

Guba, E., & Lincoln, Y. (1994). Competing paradigms in qualitative research. In N. Denzin & Y. Lincoln (Eds.), *Handbook of qualitative research* (pp. 105–117). Thousand Oaks, CA: Sage.

Hall, H. R., & Graff, J. C. (2010). Parenting challenges in families of children with autism: A pilot study. *Issues in Comprehensive Pediatric Nursing, 33*(4), 187–204. Doi:10.3109/01460862.2010.528644

Hill, K., Higgins, A., Dempster, M., & McCarthy, A. (2009). Fathers' views and understanding of their roles in families with a child with acute lymphoblastic leukaemia: An interpretive phenomenological analysis. *Journal of Health Psychology, 14*(8), 1267–1280. Doi:10.1177/1359105309342291

Kelle, U. (2008). The development of categories: Different approaches in grounded theory. In A. Bryant & K. Charmaz (Eds.), *The SAGE handbook of grounded theory* (pp. 191–213). Los Angeles, CA: Sage.

Knox, S., & Burkard, A. (2009). Qualitative research interviews. *Psychotherapy Research, 19*(4–5), 566–575. Doi:10.1080/10503300802702105

Krausz, M., & Meszaros, J. (2005). The retrospective experiences of a mother of child with autism. *International Journal of Special Education, 20*(2), 36–46.

Krueger, R. A., & Casey, M. A. (2000). *Focus groups: A practical guide for applied research* (3rd ed.). Thousand Oaks, CA: Sage.

Lempert, L. B. (2008). Asking questions of the data: Memo writing in the grounded theory tradition. In A. Bryant & K. Charmaz (Eds.), *The SAGE handbook of grounded theory* (pp. 245–264). Thousand Oaks, CA: Sage.

Liehr, P. R., & LoBiondo-Wood, G. (2006). Qualitative approaches to research. In G. LoBiondo-Wood & J. Haber (Eds.), *Nursing research: Methods and critical appraisal for evidence-based practice* (6th ed., pp. 148–175). St. Louis, MO: Mosby.

Lincoln, Y. S., & Guba, E. G. (1985). *Naturalistic inquiry.* Newbury Park, CA: Sage.

Mann, C., & Stewart, F. (2002). *Internet communication and qualitative research: A handbook for researching online.* Thousand Oaks, CA: Sage.

Marshall, C., & Rossman, G. B. (2006). *Designing qualitative research* (4th ed.). Thousand Oaks, CA: Sage.

McLaughlin, P. (1990). *How to interview: The art of asking questions* (2nd ed.). North Vancouver, British Columbia, Canada: International Self-Counsel Press.

Morgan, D. L. (1995). Why things (sometimes) go wrong in focus groups. *Qualitative Health Research, 5*(4), 516–523.

Morse, J. M. (1997). Learning to drive from a manual? *Qualitative Health Research, 7*(2), 181–183.

Morse, J. M. (2003). A review committee's guide for evaluating qualitative proposals. *Qualitative Health Research, 13,* 833–851. Doi:10.1177/1049732303013006005

Morse, J. M. (2006). It is time to revise the Cochrane criteria. *Qualitative Health Research, 16*(3), 315–317.

Morse, J. M., Barrett, M., Mayan, M., Olson, K., & Spiers, J. (2002). Verification strategies for establishing reliability and validity in qualitative research. *International Journal of Qualitative Methods, 1*(2), Article 2. Retrieved from http://www.ualberta.ca/~iiqm/backissues/1_2Final/pdf/morseetal.pdf

Munhall, P. L. (2007). *Nursing research: A qualitative perspective* (4th ed.). Sudbury, MA: Jones and Bartlett.

Neely-Barnes, S. L., Graff, J. C., Roberts, R. J., Hall, H. R., & Hankins, J. S. (2010). "It's our job": Qualitative study of family responses to ableism. *Intellectual and Developmental Disabilities, 48*(4), 245–258. Doi:10.1352/1934-9556-48.4.245

Neufeld, A., Harrison, M. J., Hughes, K., & Stewart, M. (2007). Non-supportive interactions in the experience of women caregivers. *Health and Social Care in the Community, 15*(6), 530–541.

Parker, M. E. (2006). *Nursing theories and nursing practice* (2nd ed.). Philadelphia, PA: F. A. Davis.

Patton, M. Q. (2002). The nature of qualitative inquiry. In M. Q. Patton (Ed.), *Qualitative research & evaluation methods* (3rd ed., pp. 3–29). Thousand Oaks, CA: Sage.

Polit, D. F., & Beck, C. T. (2012). *Nursing research: Generating and assessing evidence for nursing practice* (9th ed.). Philadelphia, PA: Lippincott Williams & Wilkins.

Polkinghorne, D. E. (2005). Language and meaning: Data collection in qualitative research. *Journal of Counseling Psychology, 52*(2), 137–145. Doi:10.1037/0022-0167.52.2.137

Popay, J., & Williams, G. (1998). Qualitative research and evidence-based healthcare. *Journal of the Royal Society of Medicine, 91*(Suppl. 35), 32–37.

Porter-O'Grady, T. (2006). A new age for practice: Creating the framework for evidence. In K. Malloch & T. Porter-O'Grady (Eds.), *Introduction to evidence-based practice in nursing and health care* (pp. 1–29). Sudbury, MA: Jones and Bartlett.

Riemen, D. J. (1998). A phenomenology: The essential structure of a caring interaction—Doing phenomenology. In J. W. Creswell (Ed.), *Qualitative inquiry and research design: Choosing among five traditions* (pp. 271–295). Thousand Oaks, CA: Sage.

Safman, R. M., & Sobal, J. (2004). Qualitative sample extensiveness in health education research. *Health Education & Behavior, 31,* 9–21.

Sandelowski, M. (1997). "To be of use": Enhancing the utility of qualitative research. *Nursing Outlook, 45*(3), 125–132.

Sandelowski, M. (2000). Combining qualitative and quantitative sampling, data collection, and analysis techniques in mixed-method studies. *Research in Nursing & Health, 23*(3), 246–255. Doi:10.1002/1098-240X(200006)

Sandelowski, M., & Barroso, J. (2007). *Handbook for synthesizing qualitative research.* New York, NY: Springer.

Sanjek, R. (1990). *Fieldnotes: The makings of anthropology.* Ithaca, NY: Cornell University Press.

Stake, R. E. (2000). Case studies. In N. K. Denzin & Y. S. Lincoln (Eds.), *Handbook of qualitative research* (2nd ed., pp. 435–454). Thousand Oaks, CA: Sage.

Stern, P. N. (2008). On solid ground: Essential properties for growing grounded theory. In A. Bryant & K. Charmaz (Eds.), *The SAGE handbook of grounded theory* (pp. 114–126). Thousand Oaks, CA: Sage.

Stewart, D. W., Shamdasani, P. N., & Rook, D. W. (2007). *Focus groups: Theory and practice* (2nd ed.). Applied Social Research Methods Series Volume 20. Thousand Oaks, CA: Sage.

Strauss, A., & Corbin, J. (1990). *Basics of qualitative research: Grounded theory procedures and techniques.* Newbury Park, CA: Sage.

Strauss, A., & Corbin, J. (1994). Grounded theory methodology: An overview. In N. Denzin & Y. Lincoln (Eds.), *Handbook of qualitative research* (pp. 273–285). Thousand Oaks, CA: Sage.

Tappen, R. M. (2011). *Advanced nursing research: From theory to practice.* Sudbury, MA: Jones & Bartlett Learning.

Tedlock, B. (2000). Ethnography and ethnographic representation. In N. K. Denzin & Y. S. Lincoln (Eds.), *Handbook of qualitative research* (2nd ed., pp. 455–486). Thousand Oaks, CA: Sage.

Thomas, J. (1993). *Doing critical ethnography.* Newbury Park, CA: Sage.

Tilley, D. S. (2011). Qualitative research methods. In C. Boswell & S. Cannon (Eds.), *Introduction to nursing research: Incorporating evidence-based practice* (2nd ed., pp. 193–216). Sudbury, MA: Jones & Bartlett Learning.

Wiener, C. (2008). Making teams work in conducting grounded theory. In A. Bryant & K. Charmaz (Eds.), *The SAGE handbook of grounded theory* (pp. 294–310). Thousand Oaks, CA: Sage.

Wolcott, H. F. (1995). *The art of fieldwork.* Walnut Creek, CA: AltaMira Press.

Wolf, Z. R. (2007). Ethnography: The method. In P. L. Munhall (Ed.), *Nursing research: A qualitative perspective* (4th ed., pp. 293–330). Sudbury, MA: Jones and Bartlett.

Wood, P. J. (2009). Supporting or sabotaging the surgeon's efforts: Portrayals of the surgical nurse's role in preventing wound sepsis, 1895–1935. *Journal of Clinical Nursing, 18*(19), 2739–2746. Doi:10.1111/j.1365-2702.2009.02895.x

Wuest, J. (2007). Grounded theory: The method. In P. L. Munhall (Ed.), *Nursing research: A qualitative perspective* (4th ed., pp. 239–271). Sudbury, MA: Jones and Bartlett.

CHAPTER 3

Mixed Methods Research

■ J CAROLYN GRAFF ■

■ Objectives:

- Discuss the emergence, purpose, and characteristics of mixed methods research.
- Describe the designs and decisions related to selecting a design in mixed methods research.
- Discuss issues related to research questions, sampling, measurement, and analysis in mixed methods research.
- Consider opportunities for conducting mixed methods research.

■ Introduction

Mixed methods has emerged in the social and behavioral sciences during the past two decades, joining qualitative and quantitative methods of scholarly inquiry as the "third research community" (Teddlie & Tashakkori, 2009, p. 4). Quantitative researchers typically focus on numeric data and analyses; qualitative researchers typically focus on narrative data and analyses; and mixed methods researchers focus on numeric and narrative data and analyses. The paradigm or worldview that researchers work in is most often consistent with their beliefs about the nature of reality, their philosophical views, and the scientific field or scholarly community they are part of. In other words, researchers tend to work from perspectives that allow them to explore and examine the problems and issues that are consistent with their own beliefs and views and that are most important to their scholarly community (Teddlie & Tashakkori, 2009).

Quantitative researchers most often work from the positivist paradigm or the postpositivist paradigm. Research conducted from positivism is expected to be objective, free of values, hypothesis driven, and measurable. Positivists use deductive reasoning and seek to find causes that precede, or occur at the same time as, effects. The postpositivist paradigm has replaced positivism (Schwandt, 1997) or follows positivism as "the (current) predominant philosophy for (quantitative) research in the human sciences" (Teddlie & Tashakkori, 2009, p. 69). Research consistent with postpositivism is influenced by researchers' values and their chosen theory or conceptual framework. According to the postpositivist paradigm, facts cannot necessarily prove a theory and determine a cause. Reality is socially constructed, and internal and external validity are both important.

Qualitative researchers work mostly from the constructivist (or interpretivist) paradigm, which supports the notion that there are many realities that are constructed as the researcher engages with participants. Realities are constructed by participants and researchers who seek to understand participants' points of view. Observations of reality are influenced by researchers' values. Multiple realities exist, and our understanding of these realities is constructed individually and socially. Constructivists believe that determining a connection between cause and effect is impossible; therefore, description of reality is important. Qualitative researchers engage in inductive reasoning as they work from units of data toward a theory, or as they work from the specific or particular to the general. Statements about reality are limited to the time and context of the study, so generalizability is limited to transferability of results from one context to another (Teddlie & Tashakkori, 2009).

Philosophical differences between positivist/postpositivist and constructivist paradigms contributed to tension, or "paradigm wars" (Tashakkori & Teddlie, 1998, p. 3), between qualitative and quantitative researchers. "Qualitative researchers stress the socially constructed nature of reality, the intimate relationship between the researcher and what is studied, and . . . emphasize the value-laden nature of inquiry . . . [Qualitative researchers note that] quantitative studies emphasize the measurement and analysis of causal relationships between variables, not processes . . . within a value-free framework" (Denzin & Lincoln, 2008, p. 14).

As social science grew and evolved during the 1960s and 1970s, scholars began debating issues around quantitative methods. For example, Cook and Campbell (1979) and Cronbach (1982) discussed the importance of the research setting. Their debate focused on a controlled setting that was important to positivists and a natural setting that was important to constructivists (Tashakkori & Teddlie, 1998).

By the 1990s, support for mixed methods increased as the contribution of both quantitative and qualitative methods to address complex research problems became more evident and the number of mixed methods studies increased. Researchers began pointing to the similarities between the qualitative and quantitative approaches and calling for recognition that the divide between qualitative "purists" and quantitative "purists" was exaggerated (Tashakkori & Teddlie, 1998).

Howe (1988) proposed that the paradigm pragmatism replace the debate around an incompatibility between qualitative and quantitative methods. Similar points that compatibility and partnership could exist between these two methods were made by others (Brewer & Hunter, 1989; Reichardt & Rallis, 1994). Many social and behavioral scientists have beliefs that are distinct and separate from positivism, postpositivism, or constructivism. Pragmatism allows researchers to "study what interests and is of value to (them), study it in the different ways that (they) deem appropriate, and use the results in ways that can bring about positive consequences within (their) value system" (Tashakkori & Teddlie, 1998, p. 30).

Working from the pragmatist paradigm, mixed methods researchers accept the idea that qualitative and quantitative methods are indeed compatible (Howe, 1988). These researchers are not required to choose between qualitative or quantitative methods. Instead, they determine how both qualitative and quantitative methods will answer their research questions. Inductive and deductive reasoning are used, and hypotheses may be proposed. Mixed methods researchers work with participants from an objective or subjective point of view, depending on whether they are engaged in the qualitative or quantitative aspect of the study. Values play an important role in determining what mixed methods researchers study, how the study is designed, and how data are analyzed (Tashakkori & Teddlie, 1998).

Pragmatists view reality from two perspectives. One reality is consistent with the positivists' and postpositivists' views of reality. That is, there is a reality outside the human that can be observed, measured, and understood to some extent. Pragmatists' second perspective of reality is that there is no one truth, but there are several explanations of reality. Researchers who are pragmatists choose the best explanation that makes sense within their value system. Cause and effect relationships exist but are changing and difficult to identify. Internal validity and credibility are important to pragmatists. Regarding generalization of findings, pragmatists place importance on external validity and transferability of findings, along with the idea that hypotheses are tied to time and context (Teddlie & Tashakkori, 2009).

■ Purpose and Characteristics of Mixed Methods Research

Greene, Caracelli, and Graham (1989) identified the purposes of mixed methods research as triangulation, complementarity, development, initiation, and expansion based on their reviews of mixed methods studies. Triangulation of qualitative and quantitative methods (Jick, 1979; Patton, 1980) is considered an antecedent to mixed methods as it is known today (Creswell, 2011). Triangulation involves the use of qualitative and quantitative methods in an effort to reach convergence of findings. Complementarity refers to the use of qualitative and quantitative methods to examine the overlapping and different facets of a phenomenon in order to obtain a more meaningful understanding of the phenomenon. Development involves using one method after the other so that the first method guides the second in terms of decisions made about sampling, measurement, and implementation. Initiation occurs in mixed methods when paradoxes are discovered; consistencies and discrepancies in qualitative and quantitative findings are compared and analyzed for new perspectives and insights that can yield new questions. Expansion occurs as qualitative and quantitative components are included in a study to increase its scope and breadth.

Greene et al. (1989) also identified characteristics of mixed methods designs that can be useful to researchers as they determine which mixed methods design will be used. These characteristics include methods, phenomena, paradigms, status, implementation independence, implementation timing, and study (see **Table 3-1**). Greene et al.

Table 3-1 Characteristics of Mixed Methods Designs

Characteristic	*Explanation/Rationale*
Methods—How similar or different qualitative and quantitative methods are to each other in form, assumptions, strengths, and limitations.	A structured interview and survey with closed-ended questions are similar, whereas an unstructured interview and standardized patient satisfaction survey are different.
Phenomena—Whether or not the qualitative and quantitative methods will explore or examine the same or different phenomena.	A standardized patient satisfaction survey measures. the degree to which patients are satisfied with healthcare services, and the unstructured interview is used to understand how the healthcare setting contributes to satisfaction or lack of satisfaction.
Paradigms—The extent to which the qualitative and quantitative methods are carried out in the same or different paradigms.	Although quantitative and qualitative approaches represent differing paradigms, research often includes multiple methods from both qualitative and quantitative approaches. The range may extend from quantitative and qualitative methods representing one paradigm to all qualitative methods representing one paradigm and all quantitative methods representing another paradigm.
Status—The extent to which the qualitative and quantitative methods are equally important to the purpose of the study.	Qualitative methods may be more important than quantitative methods, or vice versa.
Implementation independence—The extent to which qualitative and quantitative methods are conceptualized, designed, and implemented through interaction or independently.	This is represented by a continuum that ranges from complete interaction of qualitative and quantitative methods to complete independence.
Implementation timing—The extent to which the qualitative and quantitative methods are conducted simultaneously or sequentially.	In addition to either simultaneous or sequential timing, a qualitative method may be used at the beginning of a study, followed by a quantitative method, with simultaneous use of the qualitative or quantitative method at the end.
Study—Categorical—One study or more than one study.	The research includes one or more than one study.

Data from Greene, J. C., Caracelli, V. J., & Graham, W. F. (1989). Toward a conceptual framework for mixed-method evaluation designs. *Educational Evaluation and Policy Analysis, 11*, 255–274.

contributed to an increased understanding of mixed methods research as they focused on purpose, paradigm issues, data analysis strategies, and usefulness.

Creswell and Plano Clark (2011) identified core characteristics of mixed methods research. The researcher:

- Collects and analyzes persuasively and rigorously both qualitative and quantitative data (based on research questions)

- Mixes (or integrates or links) the two forms of data concurrently by combining them (or merging them), by having one build on the other sequentially, or by embedding one within the other
- Gives priority to one or to both forms of data (in terms of what the research emphasizes)
- Uses these procedures in a single study or in multiple phases of a program of study
- Frames these procedures within philosophical worldviews and theoretical lenses
- Combines the procedures into specific research designs that direct the plan for conducting the study. (p. 5)

Mixed methods research offers a practical approach to addressing research problems and questions and the potential for increased applicability because these problems and questions are examined in different ways. After considering the purposes of mixed methods and the characteristics that can be useful in determining which design to use, specific types of designs will be discussed, and selected studies exemplifying these designs will be presented.

■ Mixed Methods Designs

Key principles to follow when designing a study include (a) deciding on the type of design; (b) identifying the design approach to use; (c) matching the design to the study's problem, purpose, and questions; and (d) being clear about the reason for using mixed methods (Creswell & Plano Clark, 2011, p. 54). Deciding on the type of design means that the researcher makes a decision about using qualitative and quantitative methods before the research is started (fixed mixed methods design) or adds a second method after the study has begun (emergent mixed methods design). Creswell and Plano Clark's (2011) design approaches are typology based and dynamic, and they include classifications that come from different disciplines or fields and use different terminology to describe similar designs. Their dynamic approach to mixed methods design focuses on a process that considers and interrelates components of research design instead of selecting a design from existing classifications. Following this approach, researchers consider how the components of the design need to be considered throughout the research. The dynamic approach is most easily used by experienced researchers. Researchers using a mixed methods design for their study should know both qualitative and quantitative research and methods associated with both. Rigorous procedures should be following for both components of the mixed methods design (Creswell, 2015).

Matching the design to the research problem, purpose, and questions is a crucial aspect of mixed methods research design. Recalling that the pragmatist paradigm serves as the philosophical base for mixed methods, researchers choose the design that best addresses the research problem and research questions. Researchers should thoughtfully generate the research problem and research questions and use sound reasoning when selecting a design.

Mixed Methods Designs Terminology

The mixed methods research notation system was developed by Morse (1991) and is still used in mixed methods research. The Morse notation system (**Box 3-1**) indicates whether the project has a qualitative (QUAL) or quantitative (QUAN) orientation, which aspect of the research design is dominant (QUAL or QUAN) and which is less dominant (qual or quan), and whether the projects are carried out simultaneously (QUAL + quan) or sequentially (QUAN → qual).

Different terminology is used by some researchers who have built on the Morse system. Teddlie and Tashakkori (2009) consider the term *parallel mixed designs* to be

---

Box 3-1   Terminology for Mixed Methods Research Designs

Notations

QUAL indicates a qualitatively oriented project
QUAN indicates a quantitatively oriented project
+ indicates projects that are conducted simultaneously
→ indicates projects that are conducted sequentially
Uppercase (QUAL or QUAN) indicates a dominant project
Lowercase (qual or quan) indicates a less dominant project

Simultaneous designs

QUAL + qual indicates a qualitatively oriented, qualitative simultaneous design
QUAN + quan indicates a quantitatively oriented, quantitative simultaneous design
QUAL + quan indicates a qualitatively oriented, qualitative and quantitative simultaneous design
QUAN + qual indicates a quantitatively oriented, quantitative and qualitative simultaneous design

Sequential designs

QUAL → qual indicates a qualitatively oriented project followed by a second qualitative project
QUAN → quan indicates a quantitatively oriented project followed by a second quantitative project
QUAL → quan indicates a qualitatively oriented project followed by a quantitative project
QUAN → qual indicates a quantitatively oriented project followed by a qualitative project

Data from Morse, J. M. (1991). Approaches to qualitative-quantitative methodological triangulation. *Nursing Research, 40*(1), 120–123.

Morse, J. M. (2003). Principles of mixed methods and multimethod research design. In A. Tashakkori & C. Teddlie (Eds.), *Handbook of mixed methods in social and behavioral research* (pp. 189–208). Thousand Oaks, CA: Sage..

more inclusive than *simultaneous designs*. They noted that the term *parallel mixed methods design* allows for QUAL and QUAN data to be collected at the same time or at slightly different times. For practical reasons, researchers may be unable to collect data at the same time or simultaneously. Creswell and Plano Clark (2011) have expanded the Morse notation system to include an embedded method in a larger design and implementation of methods in a recursive process.

Decision On Mixed Methods Design

Researchers must decide (a) if the study will involve one method (QUAL or QUAN) or mixed methods (QUAL and QUAN), (b) if the study includes one phase or multiple phases, (c) how the mixing of QUAL and QUAN methods will occur, and (d) if the mixing of methods occurs across all stages of the study. A phase refers to the process of carrying out the study, that is, formulating the research question (conceptualization), collecting and analyzing data (experiential stage), and interpreting results (inferential stage; Tashakkori & Teddlie, 2003).

Studies with a one-method design use one method and one phase (i.e., a QUAN design or a QUAL design with one phase) or one method and two phases (i.e., a parallel one-method study or a sequential one-method study). Using the Morse notation system, a parallel one-method study is depicted as QUAN + QUAN or as QUAL + QUAL. A sequential one-method study is depicted as QUAN → QUAN or as QUAL → QUAL.

A mixed methods design is seen in studies with two methods and one phase (i.e., one phase conversion design) or two methods and multiple phases (i.e., parallel mixed design, sequential mixed designs, conversion mixed design, and multilevel mixed design). The one-phase conversion design refers to a study that involves a single phase, that is, the conceptualization, experiential, and inferential stages are carried out as one study. Conversion of data occurs when data originally collected as QUAN data are converted to narrative data for qualitative analysis (qualitized). Conversion of data can also occur when data originally collected as QUAL data are converted to numeric data for statistical analysis (quantitized).

Parallel mixed designs involve two phases: one phase involves QUAL, and the other phase involves QUAN, or vice versa. The QUAL and QUAN phases occur simultaneously or with a slight time lapse between each phase. The two parallel phases are somewhat independent of each other. One phase includes QUAL questions, data collection, and data analysis, and one phase includes QUAN questions, data collection, and data analysis. The QUAL and QUAN phases are planned and carried out to answer similar aspects of a main research question. Researchers draw conclusions or make inferences based on the data from each phase, and they integrate their conclusions from the QUAL and QUAN phases to make a meta-inference (Teddlie & Tashakkori, 2009, p. 152). In the parallel mixed design, researchers may ask research questions to confirm existing thinking and to explore and generate new ideas. The QUAN phase may confirm existing ideas, and the QUAL phase may explore new ideas; both the QUAL and the QUAN phases can be exploratory. As previously noted, a slight lapse in time between each phase may be the result of practical issues such as the research team's inability to collect QUAL and QUAN data at the same time, or the research question may necessitate a time interval between each phase. Using the Morse notation system, the parallel mixed design study with an equal orientation for both phases would be depicted as QUAL + QUAN. The parallel mixed methods design in which the qualitative phase dominates would be depicted as QUAL + quan; the design in which the quantitative phase is dominant would be depicted as QUAN + qual.

Sequential mixed designs are used in studies in which one phase occurs after the other phase (i.e., QUAL → QUAN or QUAN → QUAL). The findings from the first phase lead to the development of the second phase. The researcher draws final conclusions based on the data from both phases. Research questions and data collection and analysis for the second phase evolve from the first phase. The second phase of the study is carried out to further explain or confirm the findings from the first phase (Tashakkori & Teddlie, 2003). The iterative sequential mixed methods design is a more complicated sequential mixed design in which there are more than two phases (e.g., QUAN → QUAL → QUAN; Teddlie & Tashakkori, 2009).

A conversion mixed design is used in studies in which the collected data are qualitized or transformed from QUAN to QUAL, or when the collected data are quantitized or transformed from QUAL to QUAN. Therefore, the collected data are analyzed both qualitatively and quantitatively. Related aspects of the same research questions are answered using both the qualitative data and the quantitative data.

The multilevel mixed design may be parallel or sequential. QUAN data are collected from one level, and QUAL data are collected from a different level. The data are analyzed by level, and the results for the QUAN level and the QUAL level are used to formulate the conclusions. These conclusions are then integrated to create meta-inferences. For example, QUAL data on patient safety may be collected at the patient level or from individual patients, and QUAN data on patient safety may be collected at the unit level or from hospital units. The QUAL data and the QUAN data are analyzed separately. Inferences are made about patients from the patient-level data, and inferences are made about the hospital units from the hospital unit-level data. These inferences are integrated to generate conclusions that represent both the patient- and the hospital-unit levels of data.

■ Mixing Qualitative and Quantitative Phases

Mixing a study's QUAL and QUAN phases refers to the integration of the qualitative and quantitative phases. Morse and Niehaus (2009) described the point at which the quantitative and qualitative phases are mixed as the point of interface. Mixing can occur at the point of a study's design, data collection, data analysis, results, and interpretation (Creswell, 2015). Integrating the QUAL and QUAN methods can occur at one or all methodological and analytical stages, with the "most dynamic and innovative"

(Teddlie & Tashakkori, 2009, p. 146) designs being mixed across stages. These two mixed methods researchers indicated that the parallel designs (QUAN + qual or QUAL + quan) are the most popular designs. They referred to these parallel designs as quasi-mixed, whereas Morse (1991, 2003) referred to these designs as dominant or less dominant.

Once researchers have settled on conducting a mixed methods study, they must choose the best design for their study. Building on the work of Creswell (2003) and Morgan (1998), Teddlie and Tashakkori (2009) developed a seven-step process for selecting the appropriate design in mixed methods research (**Table 3-2**). Researchers

Table 3-2   Process for Selecting an Appropriate Mixed Methods Design

Step	*Explanation*
1. Determine if the research questions require one method or a mixed method design.	Research questions that can be answered by either QUAL or QUAN data can be addressed by a one-method design. Research questions that require both QUAL and QUAN to answer the questions require a mixed methods design.
2. Be aware that a number of typologies of mixed methods research designs exist and know how to access information about them.	Accessing the original presentations of mixed methods designs can provide detailed information about the design and its characteristics.
3. Select the best available mixed methods research design, realizing that a design may eventually need to be generated for the study.	It is important to look for the most appropriate or one best available research design instead of the "perfect fit" for a study. Designs may need to be combined or created for a study.
4. Be aware of the criteria emphasized by each of the mixed methods design typologies and of the implications for a study.	For example, criteria for the typology proposed by Creswell (2003) are implementation, priority, stage of integration, and theoretical perspective.
5. List the general criteria before selecting the specific criteria that are most important to the study.	General criteria for mixed methods typologies include number of methods (QUAL and/or QUAN), number of phases, implementation process, stage of integrating methods, priority of QUAL or QUAN, functions of the research study, and theoretical perspective.
6. Apply the selected criteria to potential designs to select the best research design for the study.	Determining the research design that is most consistent with the desired qualities on the selected criteria will likely result in the best design for the study.
7. Because there may be no one best design for a given study, a new mixed methods design may need to be developed at the beginning or during the evolution of the study.	Mixed methods studies may change as the research progresses and yields more phases than were originally planned or includes phases that change in importance.

Data from Teddlie, C., & Tashakkori, A. (2009). *Foundations of mixed methods research: Integrating quantitative and qualitative approaches in the social and behavioral sciences.* Los Angeles, CA: Sage., pp. 163–164.

can use this process as a guide to identifying the best research design for their study or generating a new design that will address the research questions.

■ Research Questions, Sampling, Data Collection, and Analysis

After identifying the design that will be used for mixed methods, researchers select appropriate sampling, data collection, and analysis strategies to answer the research questions. Recognizing that research questions guide the mixed methods design and methods, the following section focuses on generating research questions in mixed methods research.

Research Questions

Mixed methods research questions, like research questions in QUAN or QUAL research, are generated to address a phenomenon that needs to be understood or better understood. A review of the literature is carried out when researchers have identified the focus of their research and before the initiation of or during the research process. In mixed methods, the research questions require narrative and numeric information. Two or more questions are generated; at least one question elicits narrative data (QUAL), and at least one question elicits numeric data (QUAN). Along with the QUAN research question, a research hypothesis may be generated to reveal predictions about the phenomenon before the study begins. For a study using the parallel mixed design, research questions will be generated before the study begins; for a study using a sequential mixed design, additional research questions may emerge as the study progresses. Research questions for mixed methods designs should include an overarching or mixed methods question that addresses both the QUAL and QUAN questions, or separate QUAL and QUAN questions are generated along with a mixed methods question that reflects integration of the QUAL and QUAN questions. Careful thinking about the mixed methods design used in the study will assist with developing the mixed methods question (Creswell, 2015). At least one research question should justify the need for using both QUAL and QUAN methods (Teddlie & Tashakkori, 2009).

Sampling

Mixed methods sampling requires an understanding and acknowledgment of the sampling strategies that occur in QUAN and QUAL research. Probability sampling techniques are used most often in QUAN research to obtain a sample that most accurately represents the entire population. Purposive sampling techniques are used mainly in QUAL research to select participants or other units of study who can provide or yield data that will address the research questions. Although convenience sampling is sometimes used in QUAL and QUAN research, it includes samples that are the most available to the researcher; these may not be representative of the population being studied and may yield biased data. Because techniques for mixed methods include choosing participants for a study using both probability and purposive sampling, a comparison of purposive and probability sampling techniques is presented in **Table 3-3**.

Mixed methods sampling includes characteristics of both purposive and probability sampling. Combining sampling techniques for QUAL and QUAN methods requires thoughtful attention and creativity. When generating samples for the QUAN

Table 3-3 Comparison Between Purposive and Probability Sampling Techniques

Dimension of Contrast	Purposive Sampling	Probability Sampling
Other names	Purposeful sampling Nonrandom sampling QUAL sampling	Scientific sampling Random sampling QUAN sampling
Overall purpose of sampling	To generate a sample that will address research questions	To generate a sample that will address research questions
Issue of generalizability	Seeks a form of generalizability (transferability)	Seeks a form of generalizability (external validity)
Number of techniques	At least 15 specific techniques (nominally, groups under three general types)	Three basic techniques with modifications
Rationale for selecting cases/units	To address specific purposes related to the research questions; selection of cases deemed most informative in regard to research questions	Selection of cases that are collectively representative of the population
Sample size	Typically small (usually 30 or fewer cases)	Large enough to establish representativeness (usually at least 50 units)
Depth/breadth of information per case/unit	Focuses on depth of information generated by the cases	Focuses on breadth of information generated by the sampling units
Time of sample selection	Before the study begins, during the study, or both	Before the study begins
Selection method	Uses expert judgment	Often applies mathematical formulas
Sampling frame	Informal sampling frame somewhat larger than sample	Formal sampling frame typically much larger than sample
Form of data generated	Focuses on narrative data, though numeric data can also be generated	Focuses on numeric data, though narrative data can also be generated

Reproduced from Teddlie, C. B., & Tashakkori, A. (2008). In Foundations of mixed methods research: Integrating quantitative and qualitative approaches in the social and behavioral sciences (p. 179). Sage Publishers, Inc.

phase of mixed methods studies, researchers typically seek to obtain samples that are representative of the population. When generating samples for the QUAL phase, researchers typically seek to establish samples that will provide information at multiple levels of meaning, or a "thick description" (Geertz, 1973). Using mixed methods, the researcher aims to generate a sample that is representative and that also provides meaningful information. In mixed methods research, decisions about sampling are usually made before the study begins; however, sequential mixed designs may result in the need to make sampling decisions during the study.

In the absence of an established classification or typology for mixed methods sampling strategies, Teddlie and Tashakkori (2009) discussed strategies for sampling and mixed methods designs from the perspectives of probability and purposive sampling. Their provisional typology of mixed methods sampling strategies includes (a) basic, (b) sequential, (c) parallel, (d) multilevel, and (e) multiple mixed methods sampling strategies. The first three strategies will be discussed.

A basic mixed methods sampling technique is stratified purposive sampling. This involves identifying subgroups in a population and then selecting cases (participants) from each subgroup in a purposive manner. Researchers can then identify characteristics for the subgroups and compare and contrast across the subgroups. Purposive random sampling involves selecting a random sample of a small number of units (participants) from a larger population (Kemper, Stringfield, & Teddlie, 2003). Random selection of this sample reflects probability sampling, and the smaller number of participants selected reflects purposive sampling.

Using sequential mixed methods sampling, researchers select units of analysis (e.g., participants) by using probability and purposive sampling strategies, one after another. That is, probability sampling for the QUAN phase is followed by purposive sampling for the QUAL phase (QUAN → QUAL), or vice versa (QUAL → QUAN). This sampling method is used often, with the QUAN → QUAL procedure being the most frequent (Teddlie & Tashakkori, 2009).

Parallel mixed methods sampling refers to use of probability and purposive sampling strategies concurrently or with a slight time lapse between each phase. A probability sampling is used to produce data for the QUAN phase, and purposive sampling produces data for the QUAL phase. These two sampling procedures are used to generate separate sets of data. Parallel mixed methods sampling can also occur when the participants are selected using both probability and purposive sampling (Teddlie & Tashakkori, 2009). Researchers use the sample derived from probability and purposive sampling to test a hypothesis for the QUAN phase and to answer a research question in the QUAL phase. Using the Morse notation system, parallel mixed methods sampling is represented as QUAN + QUAL or QUAL + QUAN.

Data Collection

Mixed methods researchers use strategies that are the same as those used by researchers engaged only in QUAN research and by those engaged only in QUAL research.

That is, mixed methods researchers use strategies such as observation, unobtrusive measures, focus groups, interviews, questionnaires, and tests (Johnson & Turner, 2003). They need to have an understanding of both QUAN and QUAL data collection strategies.

When used in mixed methods research, the strategies mentioned obviously require a blending or combining to yield the data that researchers are trying to obtain. For example, data collected through observation can include a procedure that has open-ended prompts to elicit free response, and close-ended items that require a preestablished response. For unobtrusive measures such as documents and artifacts, both nonnumeric and numeric data will be sought. Focus group scripts may include both open-ended questions to elicit narrative data and other questions that elicit numeric data. Interviews may include open-ended interview questions to yield narrative data and closed-ended questions with preestablished responses. Questionnaires may include items that require responding to preestablished or predetermined categories and open-ended items that require narrative responses. Standardized tests or tests developed by a researcher that include closed-ended items may be used along with open-ended essay items (Teddlie & Tashakkori, 2009).

Researchers conducting mixed methods studies seek permission from institutions (i.e., institutional review boards), organizations, key individuals within organizations, and participants who will provide their own data or representatives who can provide data about participants. When qualitative research requires researchers to spend an amount of time with participants to collect data, researchers may need to gain formal and/or informal permission from a gatekeeper. Creswell and Plano Clark (2011) described the gatekeeper as "an individual in the organization supportive of the proposed research who will, essentially, 'open up' the organization" (p. 175).

The quality of data collected by researchers conducting mixed methods studies is determined to an extent by the standards of quality established for the QUAL and QUAN phases. Valid and credible QUAL and QUAN data will contribute to high-quality data in the mixed methods study. Differences in what represents quality in QUAL and QUAN data can present challenges to mixed methods researchers. Data quality in QUAN research is based on validity and reliability, whereas data quality in QUAL research is based on credibility and dependability. Teddlie and Tashakkori (2009) noted that QUAN researchers "evaluate (or often fail to evaluate) their data quality in terms of data/measurement validity (whether the data represent the constructs they were assumed to capture) and data/measurement reliability (whether the data consistently and accurately represent the constructs under examination)" (p. 209). Qualitative researchers discuss validity of data in terms of its trustworthiness and credibility.

Trustworthiness refers to findings that are "worth paying attention to" (Lincoln & Guba, 1985, p. 290) and is divided into credibility, dependability, transferability, and confirmability. With credibility, researchers evaluate whether the findings are credible interpretations of the participants' data; credibility is similar to internal validity in QUAN research. Dependability is related to reliability and evaluates the quality of the integration of data collection, data analysis, and formulation of a conclusion or theory. Transferability is considered a form of external validity and refers to the degree to which findings can apply or transfer to situations outside the study that generate the findings. Confirmability is a measure of the extent to which study findings are supported by the data (Lincoln & Guba, 1985; Rolfe, 2006).

There is not consistent agreement on quality in qualitative research in the discipline of nursing; therefore, the two basic questions posed by Teddlie and Tashakkori (2009) offer guidance to mixed methods researchers regarding the QUAL phase of their study. The first question focuses on measurement validity/credibility and reads, "Am I truly measuring/recording/capturing what I intend to, rather than something else?" (p. 209). The second question focuses on measurement reliability/dependability and reads, "Assuming that I am measuring/capturing what I intend to, is my measurement/recording consistent and accurate (i.e., yields little error)?" (p. 209). Teddlie and Tashakkori noted that researchers' difficulties answering these two questions are often the basis of controversy around research findings.

Measurement validity and credibility is often an issue in health research because the attributes being measured cannot be observed, but must be measured indirectly. Instruments chosen to measure an attribute should obtain data from participants that provide essential information about that attribute. Face validity of a measurement instrument (i.e., the extent to which an instrument looks as if it is measuring the attribute it is supposed to measure) does not replace construct validity (i.e., the extent to which an instrument measures the attribute or construct). Researchers can ask others who are considered experts to help determine if an instrument is measuring the attribute(s) it is supposed to measure. Additional information on methods for determining validity of data collection measures used during the QUAN and QUAL phases of research is available (Morse, Barrett, Mayan, Olson, & Spiers, 2002; Shadish, Cook, & Campbell, 2002; Teddlie & Tashakkori, 2009).

Determining measurement validity in the QUAN phase of a mixed methods study can be accomplished by evaluating content, convergent, concurrent, predictive, and discriminant validity. Determining reliability in the QUAN phase of a mixed methods study can be accomplished by using techniques such as test-retest reliability, split half reliability, parallel forms reliability, and interrater reliability.

As mentioned earlier, validity in the QUAL phase of a mixed methods study can be determined using trustworthiness criteria established by Lincoln and Guba (1985). Teddlie and Tashakkori (2009) identified six strategies that can be used to determine the trustworthiness of QUAL data: (a) prolonged engagement (spending enough time with participants to establish trust, learn about the participants, and check for misinformation), (b) persistent observation (helping the researcher to use his or her observations to address his or her research questions), (c) triangulation techniques (using multiple sources, methods, and investigators to best represent the reality or realities of the participants), (d) member checks (asking participants to verify the researchers' interpretations and representations of their reality—events, phenomena), (e) thick descriptions (analyzing multiple levels of meaning of reality—events, phenomena), and (f) reflexive journal (generating a diary in which researchers record information about themselves, their use of self as an instrument, and the research method).

Data Analysis

Mixed methods data analysis requires knowledge of strategies used to analyze QUAL and QUAN data. QUAL data analysis involves an inductive process in which researchers work to address research questions. These questions may involve generating new ideas and theories; explaining phenomena; exploring associations between attitudes, behaviors, and experiences; developing typologies and classifications; and developing conceptual definitions (Green & Thorogood, 2014). QUAL data analysis is iterative in that there is a movement between data collection and data analysis so that analysis may be occurring shortly after data collection begins. QUAL data analysis is eclectic (Teddlie & Tashakkori, 2009), as noted in the statement, "There are many ways of analyzing qualitative data" (Coffey & Atkinson, 1996, p. 3). Although Miles, Huberman, and Saldana (2014) described a focused method of data analysis (i.e., data reduction, data display, and conclusion drawing/verification) in their text, *Qualitative Data Analysis: A Methods Sourcebook,* they advised researchers "to look behind any apparent formalism and seek out what is *useful* in your own work" (p. 7).

Thematic content analysis is likely the most commonly used data analysis approach reported in QUAL health research (Green & Thorogood, 2014). Using this approach, the content of data is analyzed to generate and categorize recurring themes. Data are coded and categorized until themes are identified or emerge. Grounded theory involves a cyclical process in which data are collected and analyzed, and a coding scheme is developed; additional data collection and analysis may be needed until saturation is reached and there are no new constructs emerging. There is movement back and forth between the emerging theory and data or constant comparison (Glaser & Strauss, 1967; Strauss, 1987). Narrative analysis is conducted "to see how respondents in interviews impose order on the flow of experience to make sense of events and actions in their lives" (Riessman, 1993, p. 2). Narrative, or the practice of storytelling (Green & Thorogood, 2014), is analyzed in terms of "how it is put together, the linguistic and cultural resources it draws on, and how it persuades the listener of authenticity" (Riessman, 1993, p. 2).

The number of computer software programs available to assist with QUAL data analysis has increased, and the quality and efficiency of this software have improved to provide sophisticated methods of managing and organizing data. Mixed methods researchers should be aware of advantages and disadvantages of software programs and their usefulness for a given research study. Researchers should select software that supports rigorous QUAL data analysis. Computer Assisted Qualitative Data Analysis or CAQDAS refers to a range of software programs that help with management and analysis of qualitative data. The CAQDAS

Networking Project at the University of Surrey maintains a website that provides support, training, and information about software programs designed to assist with qualitative data analysis.

QUAN data are analyzed using various statistical techniques. Descriptive statistics summarize data to allow researchers to better understand the data trends. Inferential techniques are typically used to test hypotheses and further examine the descriptive statistics results. Univariate statistical analysis examines the association between one variable that is the focus of the analysis or dependent variable, and one or more variables that are independent variables and possible predictors of the dependent variable. Multivariate statistical analysis examines the association between at least two sets of variables, multiple dependent variables and multiple independent variables. Last, QUAN data can be analyzed using parametric or nonparametric statistics. Parametric statistics require that data meet rigorous assumptions to include variable measurement on an interval or ratio scale. Nonparametric statistical analyses are used with nominal and ordinal scale data and do not involve the rigorous assumptions needed with parametric statistical analyses.

Mixed methods data analyses involve QUAN and QUAL data analyses that are "combined, connected, or integrated in research studies" (Teddlie & Tashakkori, 2009, p. 263). There are numerous classifications of data analysis strategies (Caracelli & Greene, 1993; Creswell, 2015; Creswell & Plano Clark, 2007; Creswell & Plano Clark, 2011; Greene, 2007; Hesse-Biber, 2010; Onwuegbuzie & Teddlie, 2003; Rao & Woolcock, 2003; Teddlie & Tashakkori, 2009). The following discussion on mixed methods data analysis will follow the typology of mixed methods designs proposed by Teddlie and Tashakkori. Four components of their typology (i.e., parallel, sequential, conversion, and multilevel mixed data analysis) will be discussed here.

Parallel mixed data analysis involves QUAN analysis of data using statistical techniques appropriate for the variables, and QUAL analysis of data using qualitative analysis approaches appropriate for the data and the research question. The two analyses are conducted independent of each other and provide information about the phenomenon through connecting, combining, or integrating the findings from the QUAN analysis and from the QUAL analysis.

Sequential mixed data analysis is conducted when the QUAL and QUAN phases of a study are in chronological order. For example, QUAL → QUAN analysis indicates that the QUAN analysis emerges from the QUAL analysis, and QUAN → QUAL analysis indicates that the QUAL analysis emerges from the QUAN analysis. An iterative sequential mixed analysis occurs when a sequential design has more than two phases. Examples are QUAN → QUAL → QUAN or QUAL → QUAN → QUAL → QUAN. An interesting note is that sequential mixed data analysis can result in the development of data categories or classifications. Teddlie and Tashakkori (2009) discussed the strategy proposed by Caracelli and Green (1993), in which one set of data yields a set of categories that is used when analyzing the second set of data.

Conversion mixed data analysis occurs when data are converted from one form (numeric or narrative) to the other form (narrative or numeric). As mentioned earlier, converting QUAL data into numeric data is referred to as quantitizing, and converting QUAN data into narrative or another type of QUAL data is referred to as qualitizing. Most often, QUAL data are quantitized or are converted into narrative categories that are assigned numbers. Teddlie and Tashakkori (2009) described the simplest qualitizing technique as one that involves identifying groups of values within the distribution of values on numeric data. These groups of numeric data are examined for meaning, and narrative categories are created based on the meaning of the groups.

Multilevel mixed data analysis involves the use of QUAL and QUAN data analysis at different levels within a study. For example, QUAL analysis may be used at one level (e.g., health provider), and QUAN analysis is used at the other level (e.g., hospital). When more than two levels are included in a study, QUAL analysis is always conducted for one of the levels, and QUAN analysis is always used for one of the remaining levels. For example, QUAN analysis is conducted at the patient level, QUAL analysis is conducted at the health provider level, and QUAN analysis is conducted at the clinic level.

▪ Conclusion

Mixed methods research has gained increasing acceptance as complex healthcare issues demand that healthcare providers have "conceptually sound, holistic knowledge" (Carroll & Rothe, 2010, p. 3479) to guide practice, policy, and research. As reflected in the quotation at the beginning of this chapter, new ideas that are needed badly enough will be accepted. Similarly, mixed methods research is an idea that has been badly needed and is being accepted. The number of research articles using a mixed methods design and the number of journals devoted to mixed methods research has been steadily increasing. Similarly books on action research (Ivankova, 2015), nursing (Andrew & Halcomb, 2009), program design and evaluation (Nastasi & Hitchcock, 2016), and social work (Watkins & Gioia, 2015) are advancing mixed methods research. Plano Clark and Ivankova (2016) have published a guide to the field of mixed methods research that includes a proposed conceptual framework for the field. International recognition of mixed methods research is growing as mixed methods conferences are being hosted annually in the United Kingdom and membership in the Mixed Methods International Research Association, an international community of mixed methods researchers, is growing.

Emerging from paradigms with differing philosophical perspectives, mixed methods research addresses critical healthcare problems using both qualitative and quantitative research methods. The research-based evidence resulting from studies using mixed methods will guide healthcare providers to improve healthcare quality and patient outcomes. Mixed methods research examples are presented in **Table 3-4**. The references at the end of this chapter serve as a beginning point for students and scholars to gain additional, in-depth information on mixed methods research.

Table 3-4 Mixed Methods Research Studies

Study Citation	Design
Brazier, A., Cooke, K., & Moravan, V. (2008). Using mixed methods for evaluating an integrative approach to cancer care: A case study. *Integrative Cancer Therapies, 7*(1), 5–17.	Sequential
Carr, E. C. (2009). Understanding inadequate pain management in the clinical setting: The value of the sequential explanatory mixed method study. *Journal of Clinical Nursing, 18*(1), 124–131.	Sequential
Giesbrecht, E. M., Ripat, J. D., Quanbury, A. O., & Cooper, J. E. (2009). Participation in community-based activities of daily living: Comparison of a pushrim-activated, power-assisted wheelchair and a power wheelchair. *Disability & Rehabilitation Assistive Technology, 4*(3), 198–207.	Parallel
Hodgkin, S. (2008). Telling it all: A story of women's social capital using a mixed methods approach. *Journal of Mixed Methods Research, 2*(3), 296–316.	Sequential
Jones, J., Nijman, H., Ross, J., Ashman, N., Callaghan, P. (2014). Aggression on haemodialysis units: A mixed method study. *Journal of Renal Care, 40*(3), 180–193.	Sequential
Jack, S. M., Sheehan, D., Gonzalez, A., MacMillan, H. L., Catherine, N., & Waddell, C. (2015). British Columbia Health Connections Project process evaluation: a mixed methods protocol to describe the implementation and delivery of the Nurse-Family Partnership in Canada. *BMC Nursing, 14*(47). Doi:10.1186/s12912-015-0097-3	Parallel
McTaggart-Cowan, H. M., O'Cathain, A., Tsuchiya, A., & Brazier, J. E. (2012). Using mixed methods research to explore the effect of an adaptation exercise on general population valuations of health states. *Quality of Life Research, 21*(3), 465–473.	Sequential
McCann, E., & Sharek, D. (2014). Survey of lesbian, gay, bisexual, and transgender people's experiences of mental health services in Ireland. *International Journal of Mental Health Nursing, 23*, 118–127.	Sequential
Mortenson, W. B., Miller, W. C., & Miller-Pogar, J. (2007). Measuring wheelchair intervention outcomes: Development of the wheelchair outcome measure. *Disability & Rehabilitation Assistive Technology, 2*(5), 275–285.	Conversion
Myers, K. K., & Oetzel, J. G. (2003). Exploring the dimensions of organizational assimilation: Creating and validating a measure. *Communication Quarterly, 51*(4), 438–457.	Sequential
Pomeroy, S. E. M., & Cant, R. P. (2010). General practitioners' decision to refer patients to dietitians: Insight into the clinical reasoning process. *Australian Journal of Primary Health, 16*(2), 147–153.	Sequential
Raine, K. D., Plotnikoff, R., Nykiforuk, C., Deegan, H., Hemphill, E., Storey, K., . . . Ohinmaa, A. (2010). Reflections on community-based population health intervention and evaluation for obesity and chronic disease prevention: The Healthy Alberta Communities project. *International Journal of Public Health, 55*(6), 679–686.	Multi-layered
Van Staa, A. (2011). Unraveling triadic communication in hospital consultations with adolescents with chronic conditions: The added value of mixed methods research. *Patient Education & Counseling, 82*(3), 455–464.	Sequential
Wiecha, J. L., Nelson, T. F., Roth, B. A., Glashagel, J., & Vaughan, L. (2010). Disseminating health promotion practices in after-school programs through YMCA learning collaborative. *American Journal of Health Promotion, 24*(3), 190–198.	Sequential
Wittink, M. N., Barg, F. K., & Gallo, J. J. (2006). Unwritten rules of talking to doctors about depression: Integrating qualitative and quantitative methods. *Annals of Family Medicine, 4*(4), 302–309.	Parallel

REFLECTIVE ACTIVITIES

1. Describe paradigms supporting quantitative, qualitative, and mixed methods research.
2. Identify processes involved in implementing mixed methods research using a parallel, sequential, conversion, or multilevel design.
3. How would the use of mixed methods research address a clinical practice problem and policy issue?

REFERENCES

Andrew, S., & Halcomb, E. J. (Eds.). (2009). *Mixed methods research for nursing and the health sciences.* West Sussex, UK: Wiley-Blackwell.

Brewer, J., & Hunter, A. (1989). *Multimethod research: A synthesis of styles.* Newbury Park, CA: Sage.

Caracelli, V. J., & Greene, J. C. (1993). Data analysis strategies for mixed-method evaluation designs. *Educational Evaluation and Policy Analysis, 15,* 195–207.

Carroll, L. J., & Rothe, J. P. (2010). Levels of reconstruction as complementarity in mixed methods research: A social theory-based conceptual framework for integrating qualitative and quantitative research. *International Journal of Environmental Research and Public Health, 7,* 3478–3488.

Coffey, A., & Atkinson, P. (1996). *Making sense of qualitative data: Complementary research strategies.* Thousand Oaks, CA: Sage.

Cook, T. D., & Campbell, D. T. (1979). *Quasi-experimentation: Design and analysis issues for field settings.* Boston, MA: Houghton Mifflin.

Creswell, J. W. (2003). *Research design: Qualitative, quantitative, and mixed methods approaches.* Thousand Oaks, CA: Sage.

Creswell, J. W. (2011). Controversies in mixed methods research. In N. K. Denzin & Y. S. Lincoln (Eds.), *The SAGE handbook of qualitative research* (4th ed., pp. 269–284). Thousand Oaks, CA: Sage.

Creswell, J. W. (2015). *A concise introduction to mixed methods research.* Los Angeles, CA: Sage.

Creswell, J. W., & Plano Clark, V. L. (2007). *Designing and conducting mixed methods research.* Thousand Oaks, CA: Sage.

Creswell, J. W., & Plano Clark, V. L. (2011). *Designing and conducting mixed methods research* (2nd ed.). Los Angeles, CA: Sage.

Cronbach, L. J. (1982). *Designing evaluations of educational and social programs.* San Francisco, CA: Jossey-Bass.

Denzin, N. K., & Lincoln, Y. S. (2008). The discipline and practice of qualitative research. In N. K. Denzin & Y. S. Lincoln (eds.), *The landscape of qualitative research* (pp. 1–43). Los Angeles, CA: Sage.

Geertz, C. (1973). *The interpretation of cultures: Selected essays.* New York, NY: Basic Books.

Glaser, B., & Strauss, A. (1967). *The discovery of grounded theory: Strategies for qualitative research.* Chicago, IL: Aldine Press.

Green, J., & Thorogood, N. (2014). *Qualitative methods for health research* (3rd ed.). Los Angeles, CA: Sage.

Greene, J. C. (2007). *Mixing methods in social inquiry.* San Francisco, CA: Jossey-Bass.

Greene, J. C., Caracelli, V. J., & Graham, W. F. (1989). Toward a conceptual framework for mixed-method evaluation designs. *Educational Evaluation and Policy Analysis, 11,* 255–274.

Hesse-Biber, S. N. (2010). *Mixed methods research: Merging theory with practice.* New York, NY: Guilford Press.

Howe, K. R. (1988). Against the quantitative-qualitative incompatibility thesis or dogmas die hard. *Educational Researcher, 17*(8), 10–16.

Ivankova, N. V. (2015). *Mixed methods applications in action research: From methods to community action.* Los Angeles, CA: Sage.

Jick, T. D. (1979). Mixing qualitative and quantitative methods: Triangulation in action. *Administrative Science Quarterly, 24,* 602–611.

Johnson, R. B., & Turner, L. (2003). Data collection strategies in mixed methods research. In A. Tashakkori & C. Teddlie (Eds.), *Handbook of mixed methods in social and behavioral research* (pp. 297–320). Thousand Oaks, CA: Sage.

Kemper, E., Stringfield, S., & Teddlie, C. (2003). Mixed methods sampling strategies in social science research. In A. Tashakkori & C. Teddlie (Eds.), *Handbook of mixed methods in social and behavioral research* (pp. 273–296). Thousand Oaks, CA: Sage.

Lincoln, Y. S., & Guba, E. G. (1985). *Naturalistic inquiry.* Beverly Hills, CA: Sage.

Miles, M. B., Huberman, A. M., & Saldana, J. (2014). *Qualitative data analysis: A methods sourcebook* (3rd ed.). Los Angeles, CA: Sage.

Morgan, D. L. (1998). Practical strategies for combining qualitative and quantitative methods: Applications to health research. *Qualitative Health Research, 8*(3), 362–376.

Morse, J. M. (1991). Approaches to qualitative-quantitative methodological triangulation. *Nursing Research, 40*(1), 120–123.

Morse, J. M. (2003). Principles of mixed methods and multimethod research design. In A. Tashakkori & C. Teddlie (Eds.), *Handbook of mixed methods in social and behavioral research* (pp. 189–208). Thousand Oaks, CA: Sage.

Morse, J. M., Barrett, M., Mayan, M., Olson, K., & Spiers, J. (2002). Verification strategies for establishing reliability and validity in qualitative research. *International Journal of Qualitative Methods, 1*(2), 1–19.

Morse, J. M., & Niehaus, L. (2009). *Mixed methods design: Principles and procedures.* Walnut Creek, CA: Left Coast Press.

Nastasi, B. K., & Hitchcock, J. H. (2016). *Mixed methods research and culture-specific interventions: Program design and evaluation.* Los Angeles, CA: Sage.

Onwuegbuzie, A., & Teddlie, C. (2003). A framework for analyzing data in mixed methods research. In A. Tashakkori & C. Teddlie (Eds.), *Handbook of mixed methods in social and behavioral research* (pp. 351–384). Thousand Oaks, CA: Sage.

Patton, M. Q. (1980). *Qualitative evaluation and research methods.* Newbury Park, CA: Sage.

Plano Clark, V. L., & Ivankova, N. V. (2016). *Mixed methods research: A guide to the field.* Los Angeles, CA: Sage.

Rao, V., & Woolcock, M. (2003). Integrating qualitative and quantitative approaches in program evaluation. In F. J. Bourguignon & L. Pereira de Silva (Eds.), *Evaluating the poverty and distribution impact of economic policies* (pp. 165–190). New York, NY: The World Bank.

Reichardt, C. S., & Rallis, S. F. (1994). Qualitative and quantitative inquiries are not incompatible: A call for a new partnership. In C. S. Reichardt & S. F. Rallis (Eds.), *The qualitative-quantitative debate: New perspectives* (pp. 85–92). San Francisco, CA: Jossey-Bass.

Riessman, C. K. (1993). *Narrative analysis.* Newbury Park, CA: Sage.

Rolfe, G. (2006). Validity, trustworthiness and rigour: Quality and the idea of qualitative research. *Journal of Advanced Nursing, 53*(3), 304–410.

Schwandt, T. (1997). *Qualitative inquiry: A dictionary of terms.* Thousand Oaks, CA: Sage.

Shadish, W., Cook, T. D., & Campbell, D. T. (2002). *Experimental and quasi-experimental designs for general causal inference.* Boston, MA: Houghton Mifflin.

Strauss, A. (1987). *Qualitative analysis for social scientists.* Cambridge, England: Cambridge University Press.

Tashakkori, A., & Teddlie, C. (1998). *Mixed methodology: Combining qualitative and quantitative approaches.* Thousand Oaks, CA: Sage.

Tashakkori, A., & Teddlie, C. (Eds.). (2003). *Handbook of mixed methods in social and behavioral research.* Thousand Oaks, CA: Sage.

Teddlie, C., & Tashakkori, A. (2009). *Foundations of mixed methods research: Integrating quantitative and qualitative approaches in the social and behavioral sciences.* Los Angeles, CA: Sage.

Watkins, D. C., & Gioia, D. (2015). *Mixed methods research.* New York, NY: Oxford University Press.

CHAPTER 4

Data Analysis

■ Madhuri S. Mulekar, Kenda Jezek, and Sharon M. Fruh ■

■ Objectives:

- Discuss the merits of data analysis methods.
- Describe different data collection techniques and compare their limitations.
- Summarize statistical analysis techniques for both qualitative and quantitative data.

■ Importance of Data Analysis

Data analysis is part of the process of searching for answers to the questions that generated the research project. The nurse researcher makes clinical observations, ponders those observations, reviews current literature, identifies related clinical guidelines, and evaluates nursing practice in view of current research. Research questions arise within the context of clinical practice, and research aims to answer those questions.

Clinical practice based on research findings is considered to be evidence-based. For example, Sully, Baltzan, Wolkove, and Demers (2012) recognized that there was no pulmonary rehabilitation (PR) assessment model that linked an individual patient's responses to a PR program. Yet, differences among individuals determine which program components are relevant to each patient's needs. Realizing that there was little understanding of the relationship between individual patient needs and PR outcomes, Sully et al. collected data from focus groups, medical records, and the literature review. Analysis of those data resulted in a patient rehabilitation needs assessment model that links consequences of chronic obstructive pulmonary disease (COPD) with a patient's needs, knowledge, motivation, expectations, and goals.

Thus, asking the right question(s) is the first step of the research process. The question(s) drive the study purpose, the data collection methodology, and type of data analysis. This chapter provides an overview of quantitative and qualitative data analysis.

Data analysis is critical for providing structure and meaning to collected information. Analysis consists of methods for dealing with information, such as data collected through direct observations, surveys, interviews, and other measurements. The goal of data analysis is to extract as much information as possible and summarize it for decision-making. Different analysis methods provide select information; hence, often multiple analysis methods are necessary to extract information from data. Consulting with a statistician and an experienced researcher during the planning phase of research is strongly recommended because the selection of appropriate methods for data collection and analysis depends on the type of data desired and the research questions to be answered—that is, hypotheses of interest. A statistician can help with the design of the study so that collected data will lead to answers to questions of interest. Researchers plan the entire research process, including identifying data analysis methods, prior to beginning any research project.

Within the qualitative paradigm, the researcher is an essential instrument of data collection and data analysis (Bailey, 1996; Jacelon & O'Dell, 2005; Lincoln & Guba, 1985; Sharts-Hopko, 2002). For example, in focus group discussions, the researcher and the participants, both questing for truth and meaning, are partners in the research process; this relationship is critical to obtaining and interpreting dependable data. By telling their stories, participants invite the researcher to share in their experiences. The researcher must be credible, trustworthy, nonjudgmental, and open to the participants' narratives. Just as a nurse calibrates instruments that assess physical data, so must the researcher calibrate his or her own assumptions about investigations, a process known as *bracketing*. Each researcher brings *a priori* knowledge, values, beliefs, and biases to the research process. Therefore, a researcher needs to bracket or set aside personal assumptions throughout the research process—particularly during data collection and analysis, thereby recognizing that others' experiences or cultures may vary from his or her own. However, paradoxically, it is the researcher's personal experiences and beliefs that enable him or her to thoughtfully analyze the data and interpret the findings.

General Principles

Some general principles are applicable to research projects. They are related to the following actions: (a) theorizing, (b) data collection, (c) data management, (d) active waiting, (e) data analysis, and (f) writing research findings. Each of these principles is discussed in this chapter, with examples. Emphasis is on collecting and analyzing data.

■ Theorizing

Theorizing creates a link between data analysis and theory, thus providing structure and applicability for findings and connecting them with the greater body of knowledge (Morse & Field, 1985, p. 128). Theories comprise concepts and statements of relationship among the concepts. Theories vary in stages of development, and these stages reflect various purposes of theory: to describe, explain, predict, or control. Some research studies generate theory that describes or explains phenomena; others test theories for the purpose of predicting or controlling phenomena.

Research that generates theory is used when little is known about a phenomenon. For example, Riemen (1986) interviewed patients about their experiences of caring and noncaring interactions with nurses. Then, based on analysis of patient interviews (*qualitative data*), he defined a caring nurse-client interaction.

▪ Data Collection

After the researcher theorizes about the unknown characteristics of the population of interest, he or she collects data to determine if data support the theory. Data may contribute to the process of developing new knowledge in many different ways— for example, by estimating unknown population characteristics, by generating a new theory or supporting an existing theory, or by estimating unknown relations that can be used for predictions.

Population Versus Sample

Data are collected from either a population or a sample. A *population* is the entire set of units under consideration for which conclusions are to be made based on the study—that is, "the entire aggregation of cases that meet specified criteria" (Polit & Beck, 2006, p. 259). A *sample* is part of the population studied. The population to which we intend to apply the results of the study is known as the *target population,* and the population from which data are collected is known as the *sampled population.* It is desirable to have the target population the same as the sampled population, but in some cases, they might differ. The sampled population is also referred to as the *accessible population*—that is, "the population that is feasible for the researcher to access" (Gillis & Jackson, 2002, p. 497).

The research purpose identifies the population. For example, Dirksen and Epstein (2008) conducted an exploratory study "to describe the efficacy of cognitive behavioral therapy for insomnia on fatigue, mood and quality of life in breast cancer survivors" (p. 666). Therefore, the *target population* is breast cancer survivors. Because it is impossible to study all breast cancer survivors, the researchers decided to select a *sample.* They recruited subjects via newspaper notices, breast cancer support groups, and physician referral from a subset of the population: "breast cancer survivors recruited in the southwestern United States of America (USA)" and who were "women, 18 years of age or older, with a diagnosis of stages I, II or III breast cancer who were at least 3 months post-completion of primary cancer treatment and without current evidence of disease" (p. 666). Therefore, the *accessible* or *sampled population* consists of those members of the target population who learned of the researchers' recruitment efforts via newspapers, support groups, or physicians and met the specified criteria. Ultimately, a *sample* of 72 breast cancer survivors participated in that study.

Population characteristics are known as *parameters.* Calculations derived from the data are known as *statistics.* Often parameter values are unknown, and statistic values are used to estimate or make inference about parameter values. For example, Fruh et al. (2012) conducted a study to estimate the perceptions and practices of nurse practitioners (NPs) in the United States regarding the benefits of family meals. In this study, the population of interest is all NPs in the United States. But NPs who attended a statewide continuing education conference in the Midwest constituted the sampled population, and 142 participants who completed the survey constituted a sample. The researchers were interested in estimating "the percent of NPs that spend less than 40% of their time educating families on the benefits of family meals," that is, the parameter. Of course the parameter value is unknown, but 76% of NPs (a statistic) in a sample of 142 reported spending less than 40% of their time educating families on the benefits of family meals. In practice, we use this statistic to estimate the unknown parameter value and thus conclude that 76% of NPs in the United States spend less than 40% of their time educating families on the benefits of family meals.

Data obtained from a sample are generalizable to the target population only if the sample is representative of the population. Random sampling is the technique for ensuring that every unit within a population or target population has an equal chance for inclusion. Randomization ensures that subjects with different biopsychosocial characteristics in the population will be represented in the sample. Any sampling scheme that depends on subjective judgment instead of random selection is likely to suffer from a *judgment bias*. For example, a doctor may decide not to include a subject in a weight-loss study because he or she knows the eating habits of this subject and suspects that the person is less likely to lose weight—an unwanted result. If the target population differs from the sampled population, the results will suffer *exclusion bias* because of systematic exclusion of part of the population from the sample. For example, in the previously cited study by Dirksen and Epstein (2008), if there are systematic differences among those breast cancer survivors who read newspaper notices, attend breast cancer support groups, and see a physician who refers them versus those who do not, the excluded group will have no representation in the sample, and the results will be biased. Note that those who pay attention to such notices are also likely to follow the physician-recommended lifestyle and thereby are likely to have a better quality life than those who do not.

In evidence-based practice, the nurse must understand the implications of selection of sampling methods when evaluating findings. If samples used are those of volunteers or of convenience, the findings from such samples may be applicable only to the actual samples. It is important to note that in such studies, confounding factors over which the researcher has no control may lead to biased results.

Methods for Obtaining Data

The key to decision-making regarding the accuracy of data is that measurement tools must be valid and reliable. A valid tool measures what it is supposed to measure with a reasonable degree of accuracy. A reliable tool obtains consistent results with repeated measures (stability), reflects the same variable (internal consistency), and yields the same results among different observers or different forms of the instrument (equivalence) (Gillis & Jackson, 2002). Suppose a researcher interested in estimating participants' clinical knowledge administers a survey instrument that requests information about a person's educational level (high school, bachelor's, master's, doctorate, and so on). Will these data on participants' education level provide a reasonably accurate measure of participants' clinical knowledge?

There are different methods of data collection, and the types of conclusions that can be made from the data change depending on the method used for data collection. For example, cause-effect conclusions can be drawn from experiments but not from observational studies.

Census and Survey Sampling

Collection of data from all units in the population is referred to as *census*. The U.S. Census Bureau conducts a census of all U.S. citizens every 10 years. An example of a census is contacting all nurses in a hospital for their opinion about a hospital policy and applying the conclusions only to that hospital. However, it is not possible to use census as a data collection technique for every study. For example, if the American Nurses Association is interested in assessing opinions of nurses about 8-hour versus 12-hour workdays, a census would require contacting every nurse in the country. The task of contacting all nurses (probably in thousands) in the country and analyzing the data would be excessively time-consuming and costly. However, collecting data from a randomly selected sample of nurses across the country would be both time- and cost-effective, and findings would be generalizable to the population. Although named so, the U.S. Census Bureau does not collect all data through census; the Bureau uses many different types of sample surveys for data collection.

With survey sampling, data are collected from a sample to obtain information about a population. For example, to check a patient's glucose level, one does not need to draw all blood (i.e., census) from the patient and test it. A drop (i.e., a sample) is drawn and tested. It is assumed that the blood sample is similar to the rest of the blood in the body—that is, the nontested population. Samples can be surveyed via paper-and-pencil surveys, online (web-based) surveys, email surveys, telephone surveys, personal surveys, chart surveys, medical tests, and so on.

Focus Groups and Individual Interviews

Individual interviews and focus groups are particularly useful during the initial stages of research, when little is known about the phenomenon of inquiry. Individual interviews are typically more efficient at data gathering, whereas focus groups are typically more cost-effective. They are not substitutes for one another because they yield different information about the target population. Individual interviews can result in rich or thick data that are essential to credible research findings and judgments about the "transferability" of findings to other individuals or contexts, whereas the focus group can provide data through group dynamics.

The interviewer must keep the interviewee focused yet be open to new information about the individual's experiences. The interviewee must have the opportunity to thoroughly relate his or her experience. Interviewers often use semistructured interviews combined with open-ended questions or comments. Depending on the research purpose and timeline, some researchers schedule more than one interview with each participant, often in an effort to verify or amplify information.

Researchers may choose to conduct focus groups—that is, interview several persons at one time. The biggest drawback of focus groups is that some individuals may not express their personal opinion when in the presence of others or may conform to the popular opinion, thereby biasing the study results. When conducting focus groups, a researcher needs to pay special attention to the group dynamics to ensure everyone's participation and keep the group on task.

To obtain reliable data, Lincoln and Guba (1985, p. 327) recommended that the researcher keep a daily self-reflexive journal to include (a) the daily schedule and logistics of the study; (b) a personal diary that provides the opportunity for catharsis, reflection on what is happening in terms of one's own values and interests, and speculation about growing insights; and (c) a methodological log in which methodological decisions and accompanying rationales are recorded.

Experiments and Observational Studies

An *experiment* is a planned activity designed to compare different environments or interventions known as *treatments* in which subjects are assigned to different environments or interventions randomly; responses to interventions are then observed and compared. An experimental study is considered the gold standard for the study of cause-effect relationships. At minimum, an experimental study involves two groups: two treatment groups, or a treatment group and a control group. Random assignment ensures that biopsychosocial characteristics are distributed evenly across groups and therefore assumes some control for biological, psychological, and social variation among the groups (or environments). The treatments or interventions are applied only to the treatment groups. Except for interventions, the control group is subject to all the factors that affect the treatment group. Thereafter, the researcher determines if outcomes for the treatment group vary from those of the control group. Differences between the groups are considered to be related to the intervention, because all other factors are controlled by randomization.

For example, Qi, Resnick, Smeltzer, and Bausell (2011) conducted a randomized controlled trial to study the effectiveness of a self-efficacy program to prevent osteoporosis among Chinese immigrants. The sample comprised 110 Chinese immigrants whom the researchers randomly assigned to either the treatment group (which received the self-efficacy program) or the control group (which received none).

A study that lacks any one of the essentials for true experimental design is called a *quasi-experimental study*. For example, at the University of South Alabama (USA) Medical Center, in order to compare the effectiveness of Transforming Care at the

Bedside (TCAB) strategies with the traditional methods, one hospital floor was assigned to TCAB and the other to the traditional methods, thereby creating two different environments or treatments (Dearmon et al., 2013). The outcomes from both floors were recorded over a predetermined period and compared at the end of the study period. This research design has a treatment (TCAB) and both a treatment group and a control group. However, random assignment of patients to groups is missing.

An *observational study* is a data collection activity in which the researcher plays the role of an observer. The researcher has no control over the assignment of treatments to subjects and merely observes the effect of treatments without influencing environments. Data collection in observational studies includes such activities as reading charts or other documents, including newspapers, magazines, websites, and books. Findings from observational studies cannot be generalized to the target population because observational studies often use volunteers or a convenience sample, such as nurses on duty, rather than a random sample selected from all nurses.

Qualitative and Quantitative Data

Data are qualitative or quantitative. *Qualitative data* (also known as categorical data) are expressed in words and phrases that are distilled into themes and descriptions that describe or explain the phenomena of inquiry. Although qualitative data are not presented numerically, a researcher may assign numerical values to demographic data relevant to a qualitative research study. For example, a researcher might use numbers to code participants' gender, marital status, social class, sexual orientation, and so on, to facilitate analysis of the sample's characteristics. Although assigned a number, these characteristics still represent categorical data. *Quantitative data* are represented numerically.

Both types of data—qualitative and quantitative—are equally valuable. Each may contribute to building a body of nursing knowledge. Both types of data may be collected within a singular study. For example, to evaluate the differences in weight control behaviors between overweight adolescents who lost weight and those who did not, Boutelle, Liney, Neumark-Sztainer, and Story (2009) measured weight (in kilograms) and body mass index (BMI) for each subject in their study. To obtain sex- and age-adjusted BMI, they recorded the gender and age (in years) of each subject. Subjects responded "yes/no" to 32 questions about weight control strategies. Therefore, the variables—age, weight, and BMI—resulted in quantitative data, whereas gender (male/female) and subjects' "yes/no" responses to weight control strategies or behaviors resulted in categorical data.

A research study does not have to be solely based on quantitative or qualitative data. In fact, most studies involve the use of methods based on both quantitative and qualitative data, as described by the earlier example of a study by Boutelle et al. (2009). Choice of data type depends on the question to be answered and the design of the study. Use of both types of data collection methods often provides greater depth and breadth to the research findings.

Quantitative data can be discrete or continuous. *Discrete* data take only countable values such as the number of patients examined or the number of tablets dispensed in which gaps exist between possible values. *Continuous* data take all possible values in some range, such as weight, height, and blood pressure of patients. The measuring device usually puts limits on the continuous data observed—for example, the weight of a patient recorded to the nearest kilogram or the height recorded to the nearest inch.

Qualitative data can be classified as nominal or ordinal. *Nominal* data are categorical data for which order of the categories is arbitrary, such as gender of subject, which can be described to as 1 = male and 2 = female, or 1 = female and 2 = male. *Ordinal* data are categorical data for which a logical ordering exists—for example, month, which can be described as 1 = January, 2 = February, . . . and 12 = December. Any other ordering of months would be illogical.

Quantitative data can be classified as interval or ratio data. *Interval* data are numerical data measured on a scale in which equal intervals at different points on the scale are equal, and the zero point in an interval scale is arbitrary. For example, temperature measured on a Fahrenheit scale indicates that the difference in temperatures at 10° and 12° is the same as the difference in temperatures at 75° and 77°. A *ratio* scale is similar to an interval scale except that the ratio scale has a true zero point—for example, height and weight of a person, which have true zero points.

Research studies are designed to collect univariate, bivariate, or multivariate data. The data resulting from a study is *univariate* if only one measurement per experimental unit is taken, such as BMI measurement for each woman in the study or heart rate recorded for each admitted patient. Occasionally more than one measurement is taken for each experimental unit. Two measurements per unit result in *bivariate* data, and more than two measurements per unit result in *multivariate* data. To arrive at valid conclusions, the analysis techniques selected need to be appropriate for the type of data collected.

Data Collection From Human Subjects

Many healthcare providers are involved in research projects that require collection of a great mix of quantitative and qualitative data from human subjects, and such projects need special attention. Strict federal rules aim to ensure the safety and protection of all human subjects involved in research studies, particularly vulnerable populations such as children, the elderly, and prisoners; these rules apply to the type of data that can be collected, the data collection and management methods used, and the dissemination of information resulting from the project.

■ Data Management

A system for data management is essential to the process of analyzing data. Research generates a great deal of data that may overwhelm a researcher who has given no forethought to managing the data. Thoughtfulness in regard to data management will pay big dividends as data analysis proceeds.

Organizational skills are fundamental to data management. A researcher should select a data management system that matches his or her style or habits and is accessible by the selected analysis system. When working with qualitative data, some researchers use color highlighters to code portions of texts, significant statements, or themes, whereas others use a system of index cards sorted into various theme categories. Alternatively, some researchers put important texts and ideas in computer files using programs such as Microsoft Excel and Access. Maintaining a copy or backup file is important to avoid accidental loss of data.

No matter which data management system is selected, the researcher should have a method of maintaining all records, including transcriptions and theme categories. If any data or records are coded, the researcher should leave a trail so they can be traced back to the original supporting data or records. Records should also be organized systematically so that another researcher could easily audit them to verify the findings.

■ Active Waiting

The concept *active waiting* is described as "striking a balance throughout a research project between moving forward and advancing the research process and, on the other hand, allowing adequate time for the full development of each aspect of the research" (Hunt, 2010, p. 69). Rushing through the research process may result in inadequate data collection, premature closure of data analysis, and specious findings or interpretations. In contrast, lingering without active engagement stifles progression of the research process and may result in the researchers becoming bogged down or abandoning the study altogether. To avoid such digressions, researchers are advised to maintain a strong orientation to the fundamental question and avoid settling for superficialities and falsities (Van Manen, 1990, p. 33).

■ Data Analysis

Data analysis, which is planned prior to data collection, is directed toward answering the original research question and achieving the study purpose. Many different data analysis techniques have been developed that are specific to the type of data collected. Here we discuss only a few.

Summarizing Quantitative Data

Collected data are seldom in a format useful for estimation or inference and need to be summarized. Three commonly used summary methods are tabular, graphical, and numerical.

Tabular Methods

The *frequency distribution* is one type of tabular summary method that typically gives a list or grouping of possible values for data and the corresponding frequencies of occurrence. Sometimes researchers also add proportions, percentages, and

Table 4-1 Distribution of Ethnicity of Subjects in the Study

Ethnicity	Frequency (n = 130)	Percentage
White	77	59.2%
African American	17	13.1%
Mixed	19	14.6%
Other	17	13.1%

Boutelle et al. (2009)

Table 4-2 Distribution of Number of Live Births per Participant

Number of Live Births	Frequency	Percentage	Cumulative Percentage
0	78	11.50%	11.50%
1	302	44.54%	56.04%
2	173	25.52%	81.56%
3	82	12.09%	93.65%
4	29	3.98%	97.63%
5	9	1.33%	98.96%
6	5	0.74%	99.70%
7	2	0.29%	99.99%

(Vincent et al., 2009)

cumulative percentages to tables as needed. For example, **Table 4-1** shows the frequency distribution of ethnicity of subjects in the study by Boutelle et al. (2009). **Table 4-2** shows the frequency distribution of number of live births by subjects participating in one study conducted by the obstetric and gynecologic department at the USA (Vincent et al., 2009). It shows that 173 (or 25.52%) participants reported exactly two live births and 81.56% reported at most two live births.

Graphical Methods

Charts or pictorial representation of data or data summary are useful for the communication of results. However, graphical methods are subjective and should be used with caution. There are many types of charts, and advancing technology has made it easier to present complicated data in a user-friendly manner. Bar charts (**Figure 4-1**), pie charts (**Figure 4-2**), and line charts (**Figure 4-3**) are useful for summarizing categorical data. On the other hand, histograms (**Figure 4-4**), line charts, boxplots (**Figure 4-5**), timeplots (**Figure 4-6**), and scatterplots (**Figure 4-7**) are useful to summarize numerical data.

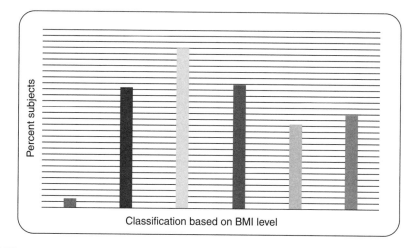

■ Figure 4-1 A Bar Chart of Subject Classification Based on BMI Level

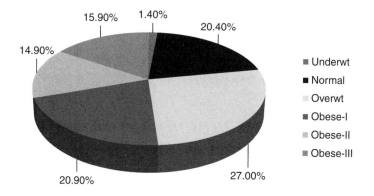

■ Figure 4-2 A Pie Chart of Subject Classification Based on BMI Level

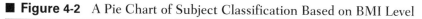

The bar chart (see Figure 4-1) classifying subjects based on their BMI level shows that the majority of subjects of the study (Vincent et al., 2009) are either overweight or obese. Barely 20% of subjects are in the normal weight category, and a negligible amount are underweight. The same data displayed using a pie chart (see Figure 4-2) clearly indicate the size of each BMI group in the sample by the size of the pie wedge. The same sample stratified by the ethnicity of the subject in the line chart (see Figure 4-3) indicates differences in BMI classification by ethnicity. The African American group of participants reported the highest percentage of obese women, and the Other ethnic group reported the highest percentage of normal-weight women. In regard to obesity, Caucasians closely followed African Americans, and in the normal-weight category, they were close to those in the Other category.

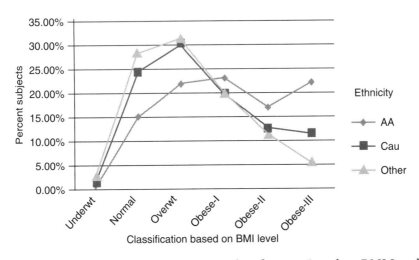

▪ Figure 4-3   A Line Chart of Subject Classification Based on BMI Level by Ethnicity

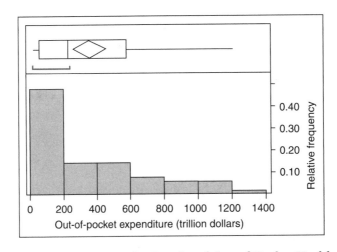

▪ Figure 4-4   A Histogram and a Boxplot of Out-of-Pocket Healthcare Expenditure

The histogram (see Figure 4-4) for healthcare expenditures summarized by Statistical Abstracts of the United States (U.S. Census Bureau, 2010) shows the distribution of out-of-pocket healthcare expenditures for individuals over 47 years of age. It is right-skewed, indicating many years with lower out-of-pocket expenditures and fewer years with high expenditures. The timeplot (see Figure 4-5) shows that insurance and out-of-pocket healthcare expenditures have increased exponentially over time.

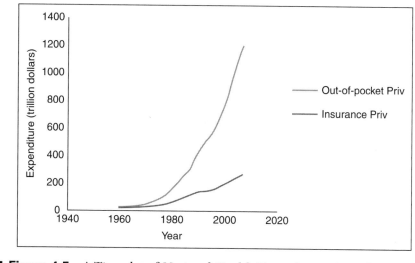

■ **Figure 4-5** A Timeplot of National Health Expenditure, Out-of-Pocket and Insurance (1960–2007)

However, compared with insurance expenditures, the out-of-pocket expenditures have increased at a much faster rate during the study's time period. The scatterplot (see Figure 4-6) shows that as insurance expenditure on health care increased, so did the out-of-pocket expenditure. The histogram and the boxplot of BMI levels of subjects (Vincent et al., 2009) show the right-skewed nature of distribution, with quite a few outliers identified by squares on the higher end of the box plot (see Figure 4-7). This means that several subjects are extremely obese compared to the rest of the subjects in the study.

Different charts provide different information about data. The histogram (see Figure 4-4) shows the shape of the distribution but fails to indicate trend over time. On the other hand, the time plot (see Figure 4-5) shows the trend in expenditure over 48 years but fails to describe the shape of the distribution. Similarly, the boxplot identifies outliers but fails to identify the unimodal nature of the distribution. A boxplot would have failed to identify gaps in data or multiple peaks were they present, but a histogram would have identified them successfully.

Numerical Methods

Although graphical summaries are attractive for publications and presentations, they are also less precise and subjective. The numerical summaries provide a number or a group of numbers representing data and are less likely to be affected by the researcher's opinions and abilities. Proportions and percentages are the most commonly used numerical summary measures for categorical data. For example, as Table 4-1 shows, 14.6% of subjects in the study were of mixed ethnic origins. Many different

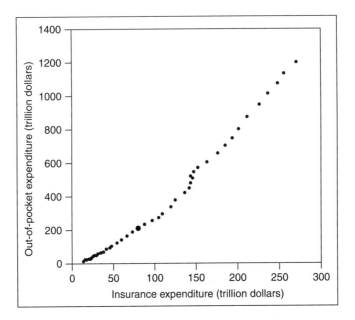

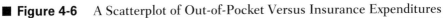

▪ **Figure 4-6** A Scatterplot of Out-of-Pocket Versus Insurance Expenditures

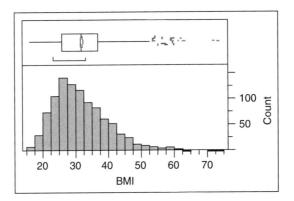

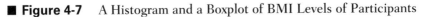

▪ **Figure 4-7** A Histogram and a Boxplot of BMI Levels of Participants

numerical summary measures exist to describe numerical data. The three major types are measures of central tendency, measures of variation, and measures of position.

Measures of Central Tendency

The mean and median are commonly used measures of central tendency. The *mean* indicates the balancing point, and the *median* is the middle value. For symmetrically distributed data, both mean and median are usually similar, but for asymmetric data with outliers, median provides a better representative for data than the mean.

Measures of Variation

The range, standard deviation (SD), and interquartile range (IQR) are commonly used measures of variation. The *range* is the distance between the largest and the smallest measurements; *standard deviation* is the average distance between measurements and the mean; and *IQR* is the range of the middle 50% data. The range depends only on two extreme measurements, whereas the SD takes into account all measurements. The square of SD, known as *variance,* is also used commonly in research. Note that SD is measured in the same units as the data, but variance is measured in the squared units of data.

Measures of Position

Quartiles and percentiles are the most commonly used measures of position. *Quartiles* divide the data set into four equal parts, whereas *percentiles* divide the data set into 100 equal parts. The second quartile and the 50th percentile are also known as the median, and the difference between the first and third quartiles gives the IQR.

For example, a study conducted at the USA (Vincent et al., 2009) enrolled 1000 women, and, among many different measurements, their BMI was also recorded. The lowest BMI level recorded for this group of women was 15.66, and the highest was 73.32 (**Table 4-3**) resulting in a range of 73.32 to 15.66 = 57.66. The mean BMI level, 31.78, is higher than the median, 30.27, because of the influence of outliers on the higher end (see Figure 4-7). The 90th percentile of BMI is equal to 43.2, which means that at least 90% of the subjects in the study had a BMI level of 43.2 or lower. The same study resulted in a first quartile of BMI equal to 25.8—that is, at least 25% of the subjects had a BMI level of at most 25.8. It means that approximately 75% of the subjects in the study were overweight or obese. The third quartile is 36.64—that is, at least 75% of the subjects had BMI levels at or below 36.64. The IQR for BMI is

Table 4-3 Summary Statistics for BMI Measurements

	BMI		*BMI*
Maximum	73.32	Mean	31.78
90%	43.22	Std dev	8.52
75% (3rd quartile)	36.64	Std err mean	0.27
50% (Median)	30.27	Upper 95% of mean	32.31
25% (1st quartile)	25.75	Lower 95% of mean	31.26
10%	22.15	N	1,000
Minimum	15.66		

(Vincent et al., 2009)

calculated as 36.64 to 25.75 = 10.89, and it shows that the BMI levels of the middle 50% of women are within a short range. Note that the IQR value is much smaller than the range because IQR does not depend on outliers on the higher end, whereas the range does. Note that in the boxplot (see Figure 4-7), the box is drawn from the first quartile to the third quartile. Thus, the box length gives the IQR, and the dividing line in the box is the median.

Normal Distribution

Normal distribution is a commonly used distribution by researchers, not because it occurs more commonly in practice, but because the analysis techniques based on the assumption of normality are easy to apply. Also, for many analysis techniques, the assumption of normality is a robust assumption—that is, it does not need to be strictly satisfied. Some variation from normality does not affect the validity of the results of such procedures.

Normal distribution is a continuous, symmetric, bell-shaped distribution. Technically, it covers the range of the entire number line ($-\infty$, ∞), but almost all of the distribution (99.7%) falls within three SDs of the mean, that is, in the range (mean − 3 SD, mean + 3 SD). Because of the symmetry of normally distributed data, the mean and the median are very close. **Figure 4-8** is a histogram of body temperatures (F) recorded for 130 subjects and shows a distribution that is fairly symmetric and bell-shaped without any outliers (Shoemaker, 1996). Also, the mean is almost the same as the median (**Table 4-4**). It is reasonable to assume that the body temperatures are approximately normally distributed, with a mean of 98.25 and SD of 0.73. Therefore, analysis techniques based on the assumption of normality can be used. On the other hand, the distribution of out-of-pocket healthcare expenditure (see Figure 4-4) clearly shows that the assumption of normality of expenditures will not be valid, and the decision-making tools based on the assumption of normality should be avoided.

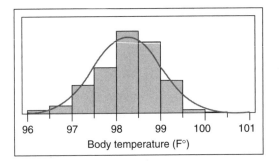

■ **Figure 4-8**   Distribution of Body Temperatures (in Fahrenheit)

Table 4-4   Summary Statistics for Body Temperatures (in Fahrenheit)

	Body Temperature
Maximum	100.80
Minimum	96.30
Median	98.30
Mean	98.25
Std Dev	0.73
N	130

Estimation and Inferential Statistics

The two most commonly used data analysis techniques are estimation and inference. *Estimation* is obtaining an educated guess of the unknown population characteristic—that is, parameter. *Inference* is making a decision about the unknown population characteristic. The *parametric techniques* involve estimating or making inference about the parameters, whereas the nonparametric techniques are useful to make inference about the population in general. The *nonparametric techniques* involve making inference about parameters without assuming any specific characteristics or distribution for the population.

Confidence Intervals for Population Mean and Proportion

The unknown parameters are estimated using confidence intervals, which provide a range of values as a possible guess for unknown parameters with a specific amount of confidence attached to it. For example, in the BMI study, data are available from 1000 subjects; however, the mean BMI level of the population of women seen at the USA clinics (a parameter) is unknown (Vincent et al., 2009). It can be estimated from the BMI data using a confidence interval. From Table 4-3, we know that a 95% confidence interval for mean BMI is (31.26, 32.21)—that is, we are 95% confident that the mean BMI of the population of women attending the USA clinic is between 31.26 and 32.31. In other words, this interval gives a range of plausible values for the unknown mean BMI with a 95% confidence. Note that there is still a 5% chance that our estimate is wrong.

The mean is not the only parameter estimated in practice. Another commonly estimated parameter of interest is the proportion of the population with certain characteristics. For example, in the study by Vincent et al. (2009), we may be interested in estimating the proportion of women with no live births in the population served by the USA clinics. The data indicate that 78 of 680 participants had no live births (see Table 4-2), which leads to a 95% confidence interval for the proportion of women with no live births (0.15, 0.21). It means that we are 95% confident that the proportion of women served by the USA clinics with no live births is between 0.15 and 0.21—that is, any value in this range is a plausible population proportion.

Testing Hypothesis About Mean or Proportion

Sometimes researchers are interested in making an inference about the population using information collected from the sample. Inference procedures use deductive reasoning. The researcher starts with a specific statement about the population characteristic—that is, the research hypothesis that differs from the status quo statement about the population characteristic. The hypothesis is typically developed within a conceptual framework or theory. Then the researcher designs a study to determine if data support the hypothesis and, using the outcome of study (i.e., data), makes a judgment as to whether the findings support the hypothesis. The likelihood of observing sampled value or the more extreme value is calculated, assuming that the status quo is true. This probability is known as a *p-value*. It indicates if the findings are true representations of reality or just chance occurrence. For decision-making, a researcher often chooses a *level of significance* of 0.05, meaning that the researcher is willing to take a 5% chance of making a wrong decision (i.e., sets the probability of accepting the wrong statement about the population based on data). A finding with a p-value < 0.05 is considered an indication that the sampled data are significantly different from the hypothesized statement about status quo, thus statistically significant. The smaller p-value is considered significant because it gives the likelihood of occurrence of extreme outcomes when the status quo situation is true. However, one must also consider practical significance in decision-making, which might lead to a different decision compared with the statistical significance.

For example, Vincent et al. (2009) were interested in knowing if the majority of the population of women seen by USA clinics are obese. A research hypothesis can be developed in terms of the proportion of women who are obese and tested using collected data. Research hypothesis: The proportion of obese women is more than 0.5 (i.e., more than 50% women in the target population are obese).

The data show that 512 of 1000 women (51.2%) who participated in the study were obese. Is this percentage significantly higher than 50% to consider it a majority, or it is just a sampling variation so that another sample of 1000 women could possibly result in lower than 50% obese women? An approximate z-test for proportion resulted in p-value $= 0.2239$; this means that if 50% of women in the population are obese, the likelihood of getting at least 51.2% obese women in a sample of 1000 is 0.2239. The likelihood of approximately 22% does not indicate such a rare event. So, at a 5% level of significance ($\alpha = 0.05$), we can conclude that the current sample does not provide sufficient evidence to conclude that the majority of the population is obese. The data fail to support our research hypothesis at a 5% level of significance.

Comparing Two Population Means

The earlier example described making inference about a characteristic of one population. Sometimes, researchers are interested in comparing characteristics of two or more populations. For example, Shoemaker (1996) recorded body temperatures and heart rates of a group of men and women. The questions that we might be interested

Table 4-5   Comparison of Measurements for Male and Female Subjects

Comparison of Body Temperatures Diff = Male – Female				Comparison of Heart Rates Diff = Male – Female			
Difference	–0.29	t Ratio	–2.29	Difference	–0.78	t Ratio	–0.63
Std Err Diff	0.13	DF	127.51	Std Err Diff	1.24	DF	116.70
Upper CL Diff	–0.04	Prob > |t|	0.0239	Upper CL Diff	1.67	Prob > |t|	0.5287
Lower CL Diff	–0.54	Prob > t	0.9880	Lower CL Diff	–3.24	Prob > t	0.7357
Confidence	0.95	Prob < t	0.0120	Confidence	0.95	Prob < t	0.2643

Shoemaker (1996)

in answering are: (1) Do mean body temperatures of men and women differ significantly? (2) Do mean heart rates of men and women differ significantly?

To answer the first question, we develop the following research hypothesis: "The mean body temperatures of men and women are different."

Comparison of body temperatures recorded for male and female participants (**Table 4-5**) shows the absolute difference of 0.29°F in the average male and female body temperatures, which is statistically significant (t-test, $p = 0.0239$). The data from this sample support the research hypothesis. In fact, on average, body temperature for male subjects is lower than that for female subjects by approximately 0.29°F.

To answer the second question, we develop the following research hypothesis: "The mean heart rates of men and women are different."

Comparison of heart rates recorded for male and female participants (see Table 4-5) shows that although female subjects have a higher heart rate by approximately 0.78 beats per minute (bpm) than male subjects, the difference is not statistically significant (t-test, $p = 0.5287$). The data from this sample do not support the research hypothesis. If, based on these data, the difference of 0.78 bpm is considered significant, there is a 53% likelihood that the conclusion is wrong. This is too high a chance of a wrong decision for any researcher.

Comparing More Than Two Population Means

For comparing means of more than two populations, a technique known as analysis of variance (ANOVA) is commonly used. When the assumptions underlying the ANOVA technique are not satisfied, the nonparametric technique, such as the Kruskal-Wallis test, is used as an alternative. Al-Obaidi, Wall, Mulekar, and Al-Mutairie (2011) developed a scale to assess self-confidence in patients reporting back pain and studied its reliability using data collected from 60 patients. The patients were classified by their occupation into three groups: full-time employee, retired, and housewife. The

Table 4-6 Results of ANOVA and Kruskal-Wallis Test

Analysis of Variance

Source	DF	Sum of Squares	Mean Square	F Ratio	Prob > F
Occupation	2	755.000	377.500	1.0802	0.3464
Error	57	19919.984	349.473		
C. total	59	20674.983			

Occupation	N	Mean	Std Dev
Full time	37	60.5405	19.8573
Retired	16	65.4375	15.2751
Housewife	7	53.1429	19.2564

Kruskal-Wallis tests (rank sums) Chi-square approximation

Chi-square	DF	Prob > Chi-Sq
2.1843	2	0.3355

low back pain level among participants was recorded using a visual analogue scale (VAS) that ranged from 0 to 100, with 0 indicating no pain and 100 the maximum pain. To compare the pain levels reported by patients in three groups, ANOVA or the Kruskal-Wallis test can be used, the results of which are shown in **Table 4-6**. The results, p-value > 0.05 for both tests (p-value $= 0.3464$ for an F-test from ANOVA and 0.3355 for Kruskal-Wallis test) indicate that the pain levels of patients did not differ significantly by their occupation.

Measuring Correlation Between Quantitative Data

The estimation and inference procedures discussed so far are for the univariate data, but often we are interested in the relation between two different sets of measurements; for example, the relationship between heights and weights of people or level of obesity and ethnicity. Scatterplots are good for identifying the nature of relation between two types of numerical data. The nature and strength of relation can be identified through a scatterplot. For example, a linear relation is one that can be described using a straight line (see Figure 4-6), and a nonlinear relation is one that needs models other than straight-line models to describe the behavior of data (see Figure 4-8). The relation between weight and height is positive because taller persons tend to weigh more. On the other hand, relation between heart rate and age of 0- to 12-month-old babies would be negative because the older babies tend to have lower heart rates than newborn babies. The relation between life expectancy and the number of persons per physician in a country (**Figure 4-9**) is nonlinear (U.S. Census Bureau, 2010). The lower life expectancy is observed for the countries with the higher number of persons per physician, but the rate of decrease is not

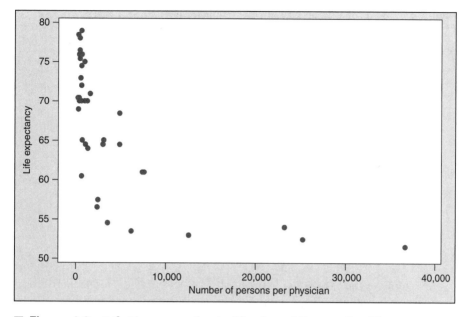

■ **Figure 4-9**   Life Expectancy by the Number of Persons Per Physician in Different Countries

constant. In fact, after a certain low level of life expectancy is reached (~52 years), further increase in the number of persons per physician does not really affect life expectancy much.

The strength and direction of a linear relation can be assessed using a Pearson's correlation coefficient. The correlation coefficient is a symmetrical measure (i.e., the correlation between X and Y is same as the correlation between Y and X) and takes values in the range $[-1, 1]$. Correlation coefficient values closer to zero indicate no relation between the two, whereas values closer to ± 1 indicate stronger relation. The negative values indicate negative relation (i.e., when one measurement increases, the other tends to decrease), and the positive values indicate the positive relation (i.e., both measurements tend to change in the same direction). The correlation coefficient of $r = 0.979$ indicates an extremely strong positive correlation between the out-of-pocket and insurance expenditure on health care—that is, as the out-of-pocket expense on health care increased, so did the insurance expenditure.

Measuring Association Between Quantitative Data

Chi-square test of independence is used to determine if there exists an association between quantitative data—for example, to study whether there is an association between the economic status and education of a person or if the obesity level of a person is associated with the person's ethnicity.

Table 4-7 Counts of Women Classified by Ethnicity and Obesity Level

Observed		Obesity Level						
Expected		*Underwt*	*Normal*	*Overwt*	*Obese-I*	*Obese-II*	*Obese-III*	*Total*
Ethnicity	AA	3	61	89	94	69	90	406
		5.02	83.63	108.71	86.13	58.54	63.97	
	Cau	8	129	160	105	67	61	530
		6.55	109.17	141.92	112.44	76.42	83.51	
	Other	1	10	11	7	4	2	35
		0.43	7.21	9.37	7.43	5.05	5.51	
Total		12	200	260	206	140	153	971

(Vincent et al., 2009)

To determine the association between obesity and ethnicity, researchers tested the following hypothesis: "The obesity level is associated with (or dependent on) ethnicity." The data collected from 971 women (Vincent et al., 2009) are classified into a 3 3 6 contingency table (**Table 4-7**). The first number in each cell shows the number of women from the sample classified into the categories associated with the corresponding row and column—that is, the observed count. The second number shows the number of women expected to meet those categories if obesity and ethnicity are independent—that is, if there is no association between ethnicity and obesity level. A comparison of observed and expected counts shows significant differences, leading to the conclusion that there is association between obesity level and ethnicity, or obesity level depends on ethnicity (chi-square test of independence, p-value < 0.0001).

Modeling Relation Between Variables

Once relation between two (or more) variables is established, *model-building techniques* are used to estimate the relation between them. For a known value of one variable, this estimated relation can be used to estimate or predict values of another variable. Analysis in which a relation is established to predict a quantitative variable using another quantitative variable is commonly referred to as *regression analysis*. In addition to a quantitative predictor variable, sometimes qualitative predictor variables redefined by assigning quantitative values such as male = 1 and female = 0 are also used in the regression analysis. For example, to help patients maintain their ideal weight, healthcare practitioners are interested in estimating the relation between weight and height of patients. Using such a relation, the ideal weight of a patient is determined for his or her height. Then, comparison of this expected weight with the actual weight measures can help healthcare professionals determine how much weight a patient needs to lose or gain to lead a healthy lifestyle.

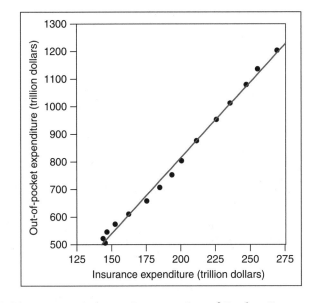

■ **Figure 4-10**   Linear Relation Between Out-of-Pocket Costs and Insurance Costs

A model development technique in which the likelihood of a qualitative variable is predicted using a quantitative variable is known as the *logistic regression*. Again, in addition to quantitative predictors, sometimes qualitative predictors are used—for example, a relation to determine the likelihood of survival of a baby as a function of gestational age and heartbeat.

Looking back at the healthcare costs of the last 15 years (see Figure 4-1), we notice a fairly linear relation between insurance cost and out-of-pocket cost that can be estimated using a linear relation (**Figure 4-10**), as:

Out-of-pocket expenses = –271.70 + 5.46 * Insurance Expenses.

This relation is indicated by the line drawn on the scatterplot. It indicates that over a 15-year period (1993–2007), for every dollar increase in the insurance expenses of healthcare cost, the out-of-pocket expenses have increased by $5.46 on average, a steep increase in expenditure for healthcare costs for consumers. On the other hand, a nonlinear relation (**Figure 4-11**) between life expectancy and number of persons per physician in a country shows that the life expectancy drops at a faster rate at first, as the number of persons per physician increases, but beyond approximately 5000 persons per physician, it drops at a much slower rate.

Alpert et al. (1997) studied congestive heart failure (CHF) among morbidly obese patients. **Figure 4-12** shows the relation between the likelihood of CHF and the duration of obesity, developed using logistic relation from data collected on 74 patients: 24

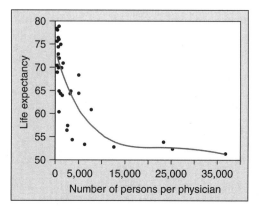

■ **Figure 4-11**   Nonlinear Relation Between Life Expectancy and Number of Persons Per Physician

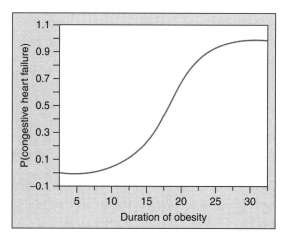

■ **Figure 4-12**   Logistic Relation Between the Likelihood of CHF and Duration of Obesity

with CHF and 50 without. The graph shows a sigmoidal relation and indicates that those who are obese for 12 years have only a 10% chance of suffering from CHF. However, for those who are obese for 22 to 24 years, the chance of CHF increases to 80 to 90%.

Concurrent Data Collection and Analysis

In qualitative projects involving interviews, as soon as the data sets are collected, the researcher prepares the data for analysis, leading to *concurrent data collection and analysis*. Such procedures are also known as *sequential* or *multistage procedures* (Wald, 1947). For example, the researcher prepares transcripts of recorded interviews and checks for accuracy (Morse & Field, 1995) and then begins the time- and labor-intensive process of data analysis. Concurrent data collection and analysis allows the researcher to determine if revision of subsequent data collection methods might increase clarity about the phenomena of inquiry. Such methods on average tend to require smaller sample sizes compared with the fixed-sample-size procedures (Ghosh, 1970). After analyzing a set of data, a researcher might choose to ask different questions, to vary the sample of participants, or to revisit previous participants and ask them to expand on their responses. The validity of the outcomes may be affected by changing the procedures and questions.

Pattern Recognition

One major aspect of data analysis is the pondering of and reflecting on data to fully understand their significance and meaning until one begins to recognize patterns and themes. *Patterns* are small units that contribute to themes, and *themes* are larger units of analyses that explain aspects of human behavior (Leininger, 1985). According to DeSantis and Ugarriza (2000, p. 362), *theme* is defined as an abstract entity that brings meaning and identity to a recurrent experience and its variant manifestations.

As such, a theme captures and unifies the nature or basis of the experience into a meaningful whole. Because themes are abstract, they are difficult to identify. In fact, themes often emerge from the data, but they do not spontaneously fall out or suddenly appear (DeSantis & Ugarriza, p. 355); rather, the researcher extracts them through careful reasoning and analysis. As Leininger (1985) noted:

> Much creative thought and analytical ability is needed to literally put the pieces together so that a theme or pattern of behavior is formulated that is congruent to the people being studied. Themes should be verified by the people, but the total gestalt or coherence of ideas rests with the analyst who has rigorously studied how different ideas or components fit together in a meaningful way when linked together. (p. 60)

■ Writing Research Findings

Writing the research findings is the final step of the analysis process. The written report reflects the quality of the analysis and bears witness to the goodness of the science. Having struggled to make sense out of collected data, the researcher is now confronted with yet another overwhelming task: clearly writing the findings so that others will read with interest and gain understanding of the phenomenon of inquiry.

In some instances, the organizational pattern of the report is predetermined by university or college standards, the funding agency requirements, or journal and book publishers' guidelines. However, even with preset guidelines, the researcher must choose how to develop each section, what to present, and how to present it, all the while ensuring the veracity of the process and the product in a manner that readily engages the reader. The researcher, who has maintained a passion for the topic throughout the arduous research process, may enjoy the writing process, for this is the opportunity to share one's passion with others.

Writing requires thoughtfulness and is seldom as easy as one anticipates. Reading successfully published work widely and attentively is basic to learning to write well. A good writer is a craftsman who has spent much time learning not only vocabulary but also the language of professional writing for a specific discipline and is prepared to write multiple drafts before a satisfactory product is developed.

Drafting a tentative outline facilitates the writing process and the writer's focus on the fundamental question of the research project. An outline also promotes an orderly approach to the writing task. Taking time to order his or her thoughts enables the writer to present the material in a logical manner that enhances the reader's understanding. Thinking about the entire report or manuscript can lead to a sense of being overwhelmed and result in writer's block. However, with an outline in place, the writer may focus on one section at a time without regard to the sequence as outlined. If ideas about other sections of the manuscript occur, the writer can easily scroll to the other section and jot down ideas. Technology has made it easy to move around different sections and add or change ideas. Using the correct format throughout the process and listing references as they are cited in the text helps immensely with the organization of the report.

■ Other Aspects of Data Analysis

In addition to the general principles described earlier, a researcher also needs to be aware of concepts of immersion, cognitive processes, and equal consideration of all data.

Being with the data intensely over a prolonged period can result in a researcher becoming intimate with and sensitive to the data, a process known as *immersion*. The researcher begins the process of data analysis by thoughtfully checking the data. The researcher becomes involved with the data as he or she listens to others' life stories, observes and writes field notes, reviews others' journals, or engages in other data collection methods. Through repeated reviews of the data, the researcher recognizes the patterns that can contribute to data analysis and interpretation.

All research methods require comprehending, synthesizing, and recontextualizing. The first task of the data analysis process is to comprehend, or to make sense of, the data. *Comprehension* occurs when the researcher identifies patterns of experience (Morse & Field, 1995). The researcher may use a variety of methods to facilitate comprehension. Van Manen (1990) suggested three general methods for examining texts: (a) the holistic reading approach, (b) the highlighting approach, and (c) the detailed reading approach.

For qualitative and quantitative data, before embarking on detailed analysis, the recommended first step is to generate summary statistics. They can help identify outliers, patterns, and trends in data, which is useful in selecting appropriate statistical analysis techniques.

For text data, comprehension is achieved when the researcher recognizes data redundancy and patterns within the text (Morse & Field, 1995; Van Manen, 1990).

Comparing participants' transcripts and sorting common categories across participants' transcripts facilitates *synthesis* (Morse & Field, 1995). This sifting process culminates in the researcher's ability to describe aggregate stories of participants' experiences and to cite specific participants' stories to support the generalization. *Recontextualizing* places findings within the context of established knowledge, clearly pointing out findings that support current knowledge or those that reveal new contributions to the body of knowledge (Morse & Field, 1995).

Equal Consideration of All Data

The researcher must give equal consideration to all data; no data should be discarded without investigation. At times, a researcher may find some data that do not fit with the remaining data; such data are known as *outliers*. Outliers should be investigated for possible measuring or recording errors. Outliers are important for developing a better understanding of the research project. For example, in a study of mothers launching children, Jezek (1993) noted that throughout the interview, one mother repeatedly stated, "He's not finished yet." Indeed, this child was not finished yet; he had joined the military, married, and had a child. But he was not finished because he was dishonorably discharged from military service, was unemployed, was divorced, and had relinquished support and care for his child to his mother. Among the participants, this mother was the only one with a child "not yet finished." However, other mothers had spoken about getting the child ready to leave home. Jezek (1993) finally concluded that a mother cannot launch a child who is "not yet finished."

■ Some Methodologies for Data Collected Through Interviews and Focus Groups

Over the past couple of decades, there has been a proliferation of methods for analyzing data collected through interviews and focus groups, such as phenomenology and ethnography.

Phenomenology

Phenomenology aims to understand lived experience. Van Manen (1984, p. 38) asserts that "Phenomenological research is the search for what it means to be human . . . a search for the fullness of living, for the ways . . . to possibly experience the world." According to Polkinghorne (1988, pp. 15–16), "locked within a personal existence: it transcends us as individuals as we communicate our personal thoughts and experiences to others, and as we, in turn, participate as hearers and viewers of their expressions."

Colaizzi (1978) proposed the following steps for analysis of data collected through interviews and focus groups:

1. Read the protocols (interview transcripts) to acquire a feel for them or to make sense of them.

2. Identify significant statements, phrases, or sentences that directly pertain to the investigated phenomenon.
3. Extract the significant statements from the protocols.
4. Formulate meanings for each significant statement.
5. Aggregate formulated meanings into theme clusters.
6. Formulate an exhaustive description of the phenomenon from the theme clusters.
7. Identify the fundamental structure of the phenomenon?

These steps should be used as a guideline and can be modified by researchers as needed (Colaizzi, 1978). Although the process may appear to be linear, it is more circular, moving back and forth among significant statements, formulated meanings, theme clusters, and the original transcripts. Theme clusters are subject to revision throughout data analysis. For example, Jezek (1993) studied mothers whose children were leaving home, and from among over 400 pages of 14 interview transcripts, identified 105 primary significant statements, formulated meanings for each, cluster formulated meanings into 21 theme categories, and merged them into an exhaustive description of "launching a child." **Table 4-8** illustrates one of those 21 themes in which he uses process of data analysis. The final step of analysis was identifying the

Table 4-8 Theme Cluster: College

Significant Statements	*Formulated Meanings*	*Exhaustive Description*
I just think it was a changing process that you go through.	The experience marks a changing process for the mother too.	Even though a mother has hopes and dreams for her child as he/she extends his/her boundaries beyond the family, it is a hard thing a mother must do to let him/her go. The experience marks a changing process for the mother too. Hopes and dreams don't always materialize and even a seemingly good launch can go awry.
And that was just really hard for me to drive off and leave him there with no friend in the world.	It is a hard thing a mother must do to let him/her go.	
A lot of the hopes and dreams that you have for your children sending them off to school don't always materialize the way you expect them.	A mother's hopes and dreams don't always materialize.	
And we felt like he was successfully launched and independent. Had a 3.98 average in college. . . . His junior year something happened. . . . Talked about dropping out of school. Didn't know what he wanted to do with his life. . . . . He didn't feel launched anymore. . . . And we took, not trying to, but seemed to take his responsibility back on us.	Even a seemingly good launch can go awry.	

Source: Jezek, K. (1993). *The meaning of launching a child: A mother's midlife as context for transition* (Unpublished doctoral dissertation). University of Texas at Austin.

Table 4-9 Fundamental Structure of Launching a Child

1. Mother's sense of connectedness with the child	Child as part of one's self
	Courageous mothering
2. Maturational imperative impels differentiation	Maternal mandate
	Child's maturation
	Mother's maturation
3. Mother's sense of loss	Family life as experienced
	Memories of past losses
	Anticipation of future losses
	Mourning/depression
4. Mother's self-reflection	Intergenerational ties
	Self as a reflection of one's mother
	Child as a reflection of one's self
5. Mother's sense of accomplishment	Sense of closure
6. Mother's letting go	Decision to accept the change
	Relinquishing control
7. Mother's metamorphosis	Sense of peace
	Sense of freedom to be one's self
	Valuing life
	Reaching to others as community

fundamental structure of the experience, which is shown in **Table 4-9**. The fundamental structure represents a synthesis of the 21 theme clusters.

In research involving diverse groups of human subjects, the *ethnographic* approach is used to understand other cultures and differences in their responses. Although it originated with the discipline of anthropology, nurses have used this type of approach to study culture and make sense of cultural beliefs, norms, values, functions, and structures and their effects on the study outcomes.

■ Conclusion

Nursing researchers need to carefully think through the research design when identifying the best method for data collection and analysis. Whether one chooses to collect qualitative, quantitative, or both types of data, the analysis methods need to be selected so that the best possible answers to the research questions are obtained.

The researcher for any project is charged with making sense of extensive, complex data and to do so in a manner that is accessible to the reader while maintaining the integrity of participants' stories (Dibley, 2011). Astute data analysis is a process of "making the invisible obvious" (Morse & Field, 1995, p. 126). The purpose of data analysis is to derive a description of the essential features of the experience investigated (Polkinghorne, 1989). Good research is more than description—it involves processes of synthesis, conceptualization, and abstraction (Morse, 1998, p. 443). Although some of these conclusions were discussed in the context of research involving qualitative data, they are equally applicable to research involving qualitative as well as mixed data.

REFLECTIVE ACTIVITIES

1. Read the article listed below. Discuss each article considering the following items: Chismark, E., & Evans, D. D. (2012). Adverse drug events in the emergency department: Why genetics matters in practice. *Advanced Emergency Nursing Journal, 34*(1), 3–9.
   a. What type of study was conducted?
   b. Describe the design of the study. Was this study well designed? Explain.
   c. What was the purpose of this study? Was it described clearly?
   d. What were the experimental units in which measurements were taken? Describe the measurements taken and the types.
   e. Describe the target population and the sampled population.
   f. Describe the sample taken and the method used to get that sample from the population.
   g. Describe any possible confounding effects that were controlled and any variables that should have been controlled.
   h. Was the statistical analysis used clearly stated in the article? If so, was it written in such a way that a person with a basic knowledge of statistics could understand results?
   i. Describe the results (conclusions) made in this study. Do you feel that the conclusion(s) were reasonable?
   j. Do you have any suggestions on how the study could be improved?
   k. Was the article write-up easy enough to follow?
2. Read the article listed below and answer the following questions: Love, R. A., Murphy, J. A., Lietz, T. E., & Jordan, K. S. (2012). The effectiveness of a provider in triage in the emergency department: A quality improvement initiative to improve patient flow. *Advanced Emergency Nursing Journal, 34*(1), 85–74.
   a. Describe the type of data collected by the investigators of this study.
   b. Refer to Figures 1 and 2 in the article. Identify the type of graph used. Describe the trend observed in the context of the study.
3. Read the article listed below and answer the following questions: Howard, P. K. (2010). Undiagnosed hypertension in the emergency department. *Advanced Emergency Nursing Journal, 32*(1), 3–6.
   a. Describe the type of study conducted.
   b. Discuss the limitations of this study in reference to the type of study.

4. Read the article listed below and answer the following questions: Odesina, V., Bellini, S., Leger, R., Bona, R., Delaney, C., Andemariam, B., . . . Tafas, C. (2010). Evidence-based sickle-cell pain management in the emergency department. *Advanced Emergency Nursing Journal, 32*(2), 102–111.
   a. Describe the type of study conducted.
   b. What type of conclusion will not be possible from this study?
   c. Refer to Figure 4-2 in this article. Describe the type of graph used. Compare in short the distributions of time to patient triage, time to placement in the treatment room, and time to evaluation by an MD.

REFERENCES

Alpert, M. A., Terry, B. E., Mulekar, M. S., Cohen, M. V., Massey, C. V., Fan, T. M., . . . Mukerji, V. (1997). Cardiac morphology and left ventricular function in normotensive morbidly obese patients with and without congestive heart failure, and effect of weight loss. *American Journal of Cardiology, 80,* 736–740.

Al-Obaidi, S., Wall, J. C., Mulekar, M. S., & Al-Mutairie, R. (2011). The reliability of prayer-based self-efficacy scale to assess self-confidence of Muslims with low back pain. *Physiotherapy Research International, 17*(2), 110–120.

Bailey, P. H. (1996). Assuring quality in narrative analysis. *Western Journal of Nursing Research, 18,* 186–194. Doi:10.1177/019394599601800206

Boutelle, K. N., Liney, H., Neumark-Sztainer, D., & Story, M. (2009). Weight control strategies of overweight adolescents who successfully lost weight. *Journal of the American Dietetic Association, 109*(12), 2029–2035.

Colaizzi, P. F. (1978). Psychological research as the phenomenologist views it. In R. S. Valle & M. King (Eds.), Existential phenomenological alternatives for psychology (pp. 48–71). New York, NY: Oxford University Press.

Dearmon, V., Buckner, E., Roussel, L., Mulekar, M. S., Mosley, A., Pomrenke, B., . . . Brown, S. (2013). Transforming care at bedside: Enhancing direct care and value-added care. *Journal of Nursing Management, 21,* 668–678.

DeSantis, L., & Ugarriza, D. N. (2000). The concept of theme as used in qualitative research. *Western Journal of Nursing Research, 22*(3), 351–372.

Dibley, L. (2011). Analyzing narrative data using McCormack's Lenses. *Nurse Researcher, 18*(3), 13–19.

Dirksen, S. R., & Epstein, D. R. (2008). Efficacy of an insomnia intervention on fatigue, mood and quality of life in breast cancer survivors. *Journal of Advanced Nursing, 61*(6), 664–675.

Fruh, S. M., Mulekar, M. S., Hall, H., Fulkerson, J. A., King, A., Jezek, K., & Roussel, L. (2012). Benefits of family meals with adolescents: Nurse practitioners' perspective. *Journal for Nurse Practitioners, 8*(4), 280–287.

Ghosh, B. K. (1970). *Sequential tests of statistical hypotheses.* Reading, MA: Addison-Wesley.

Gillis, A., & Jackson, W. (2002). *Research for nurses: Methods and interpretation.* Philadelphia, PA: F. A. Davis.

Hunt, M. R. (2010). "Active waiting": Habits and the practice of conducting qualitative research. *International Journal of Qualitative Methods, 9*(1), 69–76.

Jacelon, C. S., & O'Dell, K. K. (2005). Analyzing qualitative data. *Urology Nursing, 25*(3), 217–220.

Jezek, K. (1993). *The meaning of launching a child: A mother's midlife as context for transition* (Unpublished doctoral dissertation). University of Texas at Austin.

Leininger, M. M. (1985). *Qualitative research methods in nursing.* Philadelphia, PA: Grune & Stratton.

Lincoln, Y. S., & Guba, E. G. (1985). *Naturalistic inquiry.* Newbury Park, CA: Sage.

Morse, J. M. (1998). Validity by committee. *Qualitative Health Research, 8*(4), 443–445.

Morse, J. M., & Field, P. A. (1985). *Nursing research: The application of qualitative approaches.* Rockville, MD: Aspen Systems Corporation.

Morse, J. M., & Field, P. A. (1995). *Qualitative research methods for health professionals* (2nd ed.). Thousand Oaks, CA: Sage.

Polit, D., & Beck, C. T. (2006). *Nursing research: Generating and assessing evidence for nursing practice* (8th ed.). Philadelphia, PA: Lippincott Williams & Wilkins.

Polkinghorne, D. E. (1988). *Narrative knowing and the human sciences.* Albany: State University of New York Press.

Polkinghorne, D. E. (1989). Phenomenological research methods. In R. S. Valle & S. Halling (Eds.), *Existential-phenomenological perspectives in psychology* (pp. 41–60). New York, NY: Plenum Press.

Qi, B. B., Resnick, B., Smeltzer, S. C., & Bausell, B. (2011). Self-efficacy program to prevent osteoporosis among Chinese immigrants: A randomized controlled trial. *Nursing Research, 60*(6), 393–404.

Riemen, D. J. (1986). Noncaring and caring in the clinical setting: Patients' descriptions. *Topics in Clinical Nursing, 8*(2), 30–36.

Sharts-Hopko, N. C. (2002). Assessing rigor in qualitative research. *Journal of the Association of Nurses in AIDS Care, 13*(4), 84–86.

Shoemaker, A. L. (1996). What's normal? Temperature, gender, and heart rate. *Journal of Statistics Education, 4*(2). Retrieved from http://www.amstat.org/publications/jse/v4n2/datasets.shoemaker.html

Sully, J. L., Baltzan, M., Wolkove, N., & Demers, L. (2012). Development of a patient needs assessment model for pulmonary rehabilitation. *Qualitative Health Research, 22*(1), 76–88.

U.S. Census Bureau. (2010). *Statistical abstracts of the United States.* Retrieved from http://census.gov/library/publications/2010/compendia/statab/130ed.html

Van Manen, M. (1984). Practicing phenomenological writing. *Phenomenology and Pedagogy, 2*(1), 36–69.

Van Manen, M. (1990). *Researching lived experience: Human science for an action sensitive pedagogy* (2nd ed.). New York, NY: State University of New York Press.

Vincent, A., Mulekar, M. S., Porter, K. B., Armistead, C., Brooks, N., & Ringold, F. (2009). Relationship between percentage of desired weight loss and rate of pregnancy complications. *Abstracts of the ACOG.*

Wald, A. (1947). *Sequential Analysis.* New York, NY: Wiley.

CHAPTER 5

Navigating the Institutional Review Board

■ Ellen B. Buckner, Heather R. Hall, Linda A. Roussel, Carolynn T. Jones ■

■ Objectives:

- Explain the institutional review board (IRB) procedures to protect human subjects.
- Identify ethical principles that are foundational to the IRB process.
- Describe the link between research and quality improvement (QI) as they relate to the IRB process.
- Describe the types of IRB reviews.

■ Introduction

The purpose of this chapter is to establish insight into the IRB and describe the basic process of reviewing research in regard to the protection of human subjects and the necessity of connecting these with the safeguards and structures of an IRB application. Inherent in the processes of IRB review is the counterbalancing of the power differential that has been at the center of atrocities. Thus, the development of independent review has sought to have a single body to protect the rights and welfare of humans in this process (Tappen, 2011). The ethics of research are usually ensured through an IRB review. Most universities and healthcare agencies have their own IRB committees; however commercial IRBs also exist. Researchers must have their research projects (protocols) and informed consent forms reviewed by the requisite body, which may include both university and agency committees (Steneck, 2007).

Despite revelations of atrocities in clinical research that alarmed the international community during the post–World War II Nuremburg Trials, Dr. Henry K. Beecher brought to light multiple research violations in the United States scientific community in his publication "Ethics in Clinical Research" (1966). This publication led to the 1974 National Research Act and the 1974 Belmont Report. Federal regulations are established by Congress and are disseminated to the public as law in the Code of Federal Regulations (CFR). In 1991, the Federal Policy for the Protection of Human Subjects, or "Common Rule," was codified as 45 CFR part 46, subpart A. This required the establishment of IRBs to review all research in agencies receiving any federal funding. The Common Rule applies to all federally funded research conducted both intramurally and extramurally. The rule directs a research institution to assure the federal government that it will provide and enforce protections for the human subjects of research conducted under its auspices. These institutional assurances constitute the basic framework within which federal protections are affected. Local research institutions remain largely responsible for carrying out the specific directives of the Common Rule. They must assess research proposals in terms of their risks to subjects and their potential benefits, and they must see that the Common Rule's requirements for selecting subjects and obtaining informed consent are met (U.S. Department of Health & Human Services [DHHS], 2011b, 2012c).

Other parts of the Common Rule recognized the need for increased protections for vulnerable populations including children, pregnant women, and prisoners. The IRB has complete authority to review, approve, require modifications for, or disapprove of a study (DHHS, 2012c). See **Table 5-1** for a list of regulations pertaining to human subject research. These regulations may be obtained from the DHHS website ecfr.gov.

In the late 1990s, as human subject research expanded to international and low-resource countries, the U.S. Department of Health and Human Services, Office for Human Research Protections (OHRP) established requirements for federally funded institutions to register IRBs and to obtain a Federal-Wide Assurance (FWA) that ensures adherence to the Common Rule, Belmont, and the Declaration of Helsinki. Moreover, in another more recent example of the history of research ethics, the tragic death of Jesse Gelsinger in 1999, an investigator-initiated gene therapy

Table 5-1 U.S. Department of Health and Human Services and Food and Drug Administration Regulations

Regulation Topic	Citation
Common Rule (IRBs, Informed Consent, Vulnerable Subjects, Registration to clinicaltrials.gov)	45 CFR Part 46
Informed Consent	21 CFR Part 50
IRBs (and Registration to clinicaltrials.gov)	21 CFR Part 56
Conflict of Interest	21 CFR Part 54
Electronic Records and Signatures	21 CFR Part 11
Investigational New Drug Applications	21 CFR 312
Investigational Device Exemption	21 CFR 812

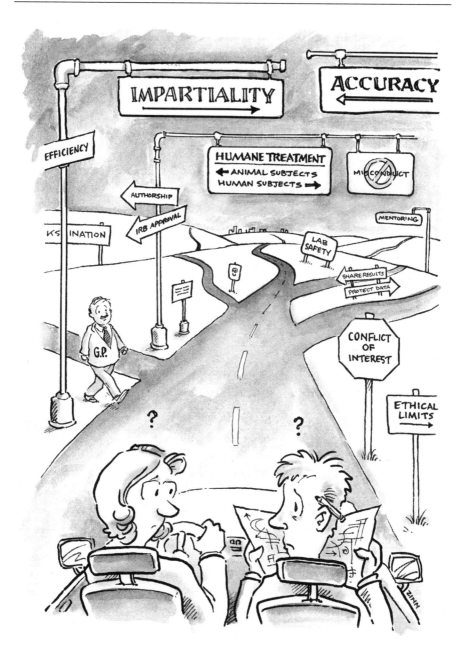

Setting Off on the Road to Responsible Conduct of Research

Source: Illustration by David Zinn, © 2011, www.zinnart.com

study, revealed the need for more extensive review in the areas of financial conflict of interest. Failure to disclose new findings could affect an IRB's willingness to consent to the study and also violates participants' true informed consent (Steinbrook, 2008). Current IRB procedures require review related to financial conflict of interest, stringent adverse event reporting, and disclosure of new research findings in the processes of protocol review and informed consent. In 2001, an accreditation process for IRBs was launched by the Association for Accreditation of Human Research Protection Programs (AAHRPP). This accreditation is now the accepted standard for IRBs regardless of funding sources. Additionally, clinical research regulations expanded requirements to include the registration of clinical trials (and soon, behavioral studies) into clinicaltrials.gov. The reason is to ensure that results of research are shared and that negative findings are not hidden or prohibited from being published.

Definition of Research

Research is defined as "a systematic investigation, including research development, testing and evaluation, designed to develop or contribute to generalizable knowledge" (DHHS, 2010a, 45 CFR 46.102[d]).

An investigation must meet certain principles to be classified as research. A research study involves an organized, logical investigation that can range from a scientific inquiry to a qualitative research study of a specified group. It may be local or multilocational. Research development, measurement, and assessment (e.g., literature review, pilot study, feasibility study, or preclinical study) must be included before a study is considered true research. Also, an investigator must design the protocol, data management plans, and data collection tools to collect reliable data or reduce threats to validity that will improve or supply generalizable information, experience, or understanding (Polit & Beck, 2012).

When an investigation meets the criteria for being defined as research with *human subjects,* the proposal and procedures require IRB review and approval. A *human subject* is defined as "a living individual about whom an investigator (whether professional or student) conducting research obtains" (DHHS, 2010a, 25 CFR 46.102(f). Examples of data from human subjects are (a) data either by involvement or interaction of any kind (e.g., email, observation), not necessarily face-to-face; or (b) data that distinguish one person from another (e.g., behaviors in specific places or times when the person is unaware; data collected for certain reasons when the participant counts on that data not becoming public). All human subject research requires IRB approval; however, procedures and activities that include contact with human participants and even data collection may not meet all the criteria for research that demand an IRB review. Some research activities, such as those designed as in-house QI, may be exempt from IRB review (Polit & Beck, 2012; Wilfond, 2013). It is important to consult with the IRB to determine the type of IRB review needed for a study.

Purpose of an Institutional Review Board

IRBs or ethics committees (ECs) are locally managed committees that are given the responsibility to assess research proposals that include human participation. The IRB has federal mandates if the research being reviewed is funded by a U.S. federal agency or is under the auspices of the Food and Drug Administration (FDA) (45 CFR 46.501, Subpart E; 21 CFR 56.106). Both the IRB process and the research involving human participants have received intensified examination by not only lawmakers, but also the general public because some participants have been harmed in the process of taking part in the research study (Beh, 2002; Oakes, 2002). This intensified inspection has had an impact on the IRB process and the IRB evaluators. Evaluators are now expected to know and understand both state and federal rules when assessing research procedures in *biomedical, behavioral, and social science* areas. IRB officials must train local evaluators and IRB members to such a level that the evaluators can even describe what many people might deem an insignificant risk to human participants. These new demands upon IRB members may cause conflict among the evaluators, their supervisors, and the researchers (Eissenburg et al., 2004).

Because the function of the IRB is to protect the public's health, IRB members include the representative public, in addition to scientific experts. The federal government set forth regulations in the Common Rule for determining membership criteria for an IRB (DHHS, 2012c). An IRB ordinarily involves persons from the following areas: (a) faculty who are not only associated with the institution but also represent multidisciplinary academic areas that are characteristically involved in research that includes human participants; (b) faculty who are associated with the institution but who would be classified as nonscientific faculty; (c) impartial delegates to represent the concerns of the community who have no official relationship with the institution but do live in the local area; and (d) local members whose primary responsibility would be to protect the rights of prisoners (e.g., lawyers or prisoner advocates), if the IRB examines research involving prisoners (DHHS, 2012b).

IRB members also must have a membership that includes adequate proficiency, or they must search for subject experts if members of the board are unfamiliar with a specified methodology or population being measured. Collectively, the IRB must have the knowledge, skill, and professional proficiency needed to accurately assess research activities often performed by their institution. Although IRBs serve their institutions, they do not represent the interests of their institutions. Federal regulations forbid institutional officials from overturning an IRB censure of a research proposal (DHHS, 2010a).

No research procedures, including screening for potential participants, may commence until the IRB has examined, evaluated, and agreed to approve the research. Even after the research process has begun, the investigator remains responsible for unceasingly safeguarding human participants; therefore, the IRB evaluates continuing research at least once per year. Also, if the investigator desires to make any changes in research procedures, the IRB must be notified and approve any modifications before the investigator executes the changes. The investigator can expect to receive immunity from this rule if a modification to an agreed-upon course of action was the result of an unforeseen danger to the human subject and the situation demanded an immediate response for the health and well-being of the participants. The IRB must immediately be made aware of any changes made in response to these circumstances; the investigator may not wait until the research is finished. Federal mandates give the IRB complete power to defer or completely withdraw all approval for research to be conducted if the IRB discovers the research procedures are not in accordance with their approved conditions or that some unforeseen harm may come to human subjects (DHHS, 2010b). Researchers must relate to IRBs and be both knowledgeable about and effective in their response. This demands an understanding of the history, principles, and procedures of the ethics review process (Polit & Beck, 2012).

Ethics and the Institutional Review Board

Beginning with the Declaration of Helsinki, the well-being of the individual research subject has been recognized as taking precedence over all other interests (World Medical Association, 2013).

The Belmont Report

The Belmont Report was written in 1979 and forms the conceptual background for the regulations governing research and scientific studies involving human participants. The Belmont Report identifies three primary principles: beneficence or nonmaleficence, respect for persons, and justice or equality of burden. The first principle, *beneficence*, ensures that the study benefits the participants and does not produce harm; although there may be some risks or inconvenience, precautions have been taken to minimize these. The second, *respect for persons*, ensures that a person's agreement to be part of a study is voluntary, based on a process of informed consent with a reasonable description of risks and benefits, and includes the right to withdraw; they are not a "means to an end." The third, *justice*, is reflected in the potential for all persons to be considered for inclusion—that no single group, especially a vulnerable population such as prisoners, is singled out to bear the burden or risks of participation, such as the testing of an experimental drug (Polit & Beck, 2012). In addition, The Belmont Report obligates the investigator to (a) acquire and give proof of informed consent; (b) ensure and value the privacy of human subjects; and (c) include further protection for human participants with inadequate self-sufficiency (The Commission, 1979).

The investigator must be aware of the ethical dichotomies in the research plan. In controlled (randomized) research studies, equipoise should exist, meaning that there is equality in the value of treatment A versus treatment B. IRBs will be called upon to evaluate this along with undue risks. Another issue is therapeutic misconception, which can occur when individuals believe that their participation will ensure a cure or health improvement, despite informed consent that does not support that belief. Research has shown that 40–80% of subjects showed basic misunderstandings of research trial design

(Appelbaum, Roth, & Lidz, 1987), and that as many as 70% have some sort of therapeutic misconception (Appelbaum, 2002). Moreover, the investigator must be aware that there are other human participants who may be subject to *coercion* (e.g., employees, students) or *undue influence* (e.g., low socioeconomic status) (Polit & Beck, 2012). For example, a grade should not be withheld or altered because of failure to participate in research. An alternative educational experience should be approved if the research participation is part of an academic course. An employee should not have to fear losing his or her job for failure to participate in an employer-sanctioned study. These situations often require additional protections. For example, a list of participants should not be shared with supervisors because that would affect voluntary participation. The investigator is obligated to endeavor to protect these at-risk participants (Polit & Beck, 2012).

To adhere to Belmont principles, the investigator is required to detail how beneficence will be ensured in the research procedures in the following five major areas:

- Procedures are being used that will cause minimal possibility of jeopardy or danger to human subjects even with responses to research questions.
- Data will be collected from present events or endeavors for any purposes unrelated to research.
- Any risk to human participants must be practical because it may correlate to any advantage to the participants and also to any anticipated research significance.
- Anonymity and privacy will be guaranteed and upheld.
- Data will be supervised to establish and ascertain participant privacy (The Commission, 1979).

Investigators navigating the IRB process must be certain that all human participants are equally considered for participation in the research, requiring honest and equitable treatment, without favoritism. Any research inconveniences and obligations must be distributed impartially. Moreover, investigators must plan research in a way that ensures that all human participants will share any advantages, help, or profit that arise from the research process. Investigators must explain how they will meet two primary conditions that are established on justice: (a) participants were chosen fairly and impartially, and (b) vulnerable human subjects or *population of convenience* were not taken advantage of or abused (The Commission, 1979).

Research Ethics Education

An investigator involved in research at any level will be required to complete basic training in the protection of human subjects. In this advanced, complex biomedical environment is not uncommon to care for or work with a patient who is also receiving experimental treatment. Therefore, today's healthcare provider must be aware of the principles of responsible conduct of research (RCR). With the breadth of scholarly work in health care, a clear understanding of these principles is mandatory for all professionals, regardless of whether they are working as a member of the research team (Polit & Beck, 2012). Basic training in the protection of human subjects may be obtained through the National Institutes of Health (NIH) or the Collaborative Institutional Training Initiative (CITI) modules (CITI, 2016; NIH, 2015).

Link Between Research and Quality Improvement Related to the Institutional Review Board Process

Multidisciplinary contexts demand that healthcare professionals understand the relationships among types of projects and innovations and the criteria for pursuing IRB approval. QI projects are those developed to test the efficiency and effectiveness of translating research into practice or evaluate the effects of intervention improvement (Polit & Beck, 2012). Confusion exists about which projects may or may not require IRB approval; regardless of professional opinions, IRBs reserve the right and the federally mandated responsibility to protect all human participants (The Commission, 1979).

Investigators who are conducting a QI project may have questions about their project meeting the definition applied to *research* and why they should submit their proposal to IRB for review. The DHHS (2010d) has responded to this concern. For example, an investigator wondered if his project could be classified as research, because there was an intention to publish a QI project. The answer from DHHS (2010c) was no. The plan to publish the project is not an adequate measure of establishing that a QI project involved research (DHHS, 2010d).

It is important for investigators to know that there are types of QI projects that do meet the definition of research; therefore, these projects are not exempt from IRB review and are held accountable to DHHS human subject rules (DHHS, 2010c). The DHHS gave an example of a QI project in which a clinical intervention is implemented untested. The purpose of the project was care improvement and data collection concerning patient effect to determine scientific confirmation about how the intervention accomplished its projected results. In this QI project example, the project met nonexempt human subjects research (DHHS, 2010c). The decision-points about clinical research versus QI studies have undergone bioethical debate (Wilfond, 2013).

QI can be both prospective and reflective. QI encourages healthcare clinicians to think out of the box and develop innovative ways to improve healthcare systems. It can be employed as a strategy to prevent errors or ensure that standards of care are being met (Duke University Medical Center, 2005). Because QI processes are significant contributors to the advancement of evidence-based practice (EBP), they may be disseminated through presentations and publications. These processes then become contributors to the general knowledge and now meet the criteria for review (McNett & Lawry, 2009).

Types of Institutional Review Board Reviews

The IRB is an independent body whose sole purpose is the protection of human subjects. In the IRB guidelines, this board is a local board with authority for approving or withholding approval (Fain, 2009). The IRB review is structured in three levels: (a) full board review, (b) expedited, and (c) exempt (Polit & Beck, 2012). Investigators need to know which type of review their research project requires.

Full review applications are evaluated by a convened board that includes scientific, nonscientific, and community members. Typically, a primary and secondary reviewer is designated for protocol review; however, all members read, consider, question, and vote to approve, modify, or disapprove the protocol. After IRB review and approval, responsibility of the conduct of research resides with the principal investigator (Polit & Beck, 2012). Full IRB review is usually reserved for studies with inherent risk, such as drug studies, studies on sensitive topics such as sexual behavior, and studies with vulnerable populations.

Expedited review is a lower IRB review level for research that poses nothing more than what is known as minimal risk to the participant. Minimal risk means that the participant can expect no more harm or accident to come to them than could be expected in just living everyday life. The research is entitled to an expedited review if it meets the minimal risk definition and all proposed activities meet the eligibility requirements as set forth in the Common Rule 45 CFR Part 46.1110 (Polit & Beck, 2012).

QI projects with minimal risks are often reviewed through *expedited* procedures. They are often reviewed by either the IRB chairperson or one or more individuals on the IRB designated by the IRB chairperson. Reviewers may deem the study as higher risk and require it be returned to the investigator for revision or submission as full review (Nerenz, 2009).

Finally, there is a category of *Exempt Review,* meaning the research does not involve human participants and human subjects are at no risk. This includes studies done in which the subjects cannot be identified, including the usual practice of education (educational tests), collecting existing data, observations of public behavior, and anonymous surveys (DHHS, 2010a).

The final determination of the type of IRB review required rests with the IRB chairperson and is not determined by the investigator.

Protection of Vulnerable Populations

Vulnerable populations are those with factors that would impair their ability to give voluntary consent. These include those with mental impairment, limitations of developmental status (children, developmentally disabled individuals), and special conditions, such as those incarcerated (prisoners). It also includes pregnant women because of the particular vulnerability of the developing fetus (45 CFR Part 46, Subparts B, C, and D, 2016).

The technical definition does not include other groups that could be considered vulnerable and susceptible to coercion, such as decision-impaired students or employees; however, studies or projects involving these groups may be required to include special safeguards, such as assurance that supervisors will not be notified of participation or answers and that grades will not be affected.

The special case of precautions and protections is that of child assent. For minors, parental consent is required, with the number of signatures depending on the level of risk. Higher risk may require both parents to sign. In addition, the evaluation of risk in children was redefined to be activities in the usual course of day-to-day living, or the "healthy child" criterion, meaning that investigators could not subject a child to higher level risk because the child's illness was life-threatening. In developing assent documents, a child-friendly language has been developed to read in ways understandable to a child aged 7–14 years. After age 14, a minor may be given an adult-type form for assent or a combined consent/assent form with signatures from both parent and child. The concept of emancipated minor may not apply to pregnant minors who do not have authority to consent for research even though they are legally able to give consent for care for themselves and their child. Thus, the parental standard for consent usually must be met or waived by the IRB (Polit & Beck, 2012).

Waiver of written informed consent may be approved if the creation of a signed consent document could link the participant to the study findings or individual data in ways that result in a loss of privacy. For example, if a woman is responding to a survey in a clinic treating sexually transmitted illnesses, a breach of confidentiality could cause psychosocial harm. This risk may argue for waiver of signed documentation of consent. It does not change the need for informed consent, and the investigator may prepare for this by drafting an information sheet for use in the consent process (DHHS, 2012b).

Another example of modifications for groups that do not technically meet the criterion of vulnerability but warrant special protections involves those with low literacy. The investigator may prepare low literacy consent (Flesch-Kincaid reading level of 7.0; see **Box 5-1**) and include a protocol provision to read the consent out loud. All protocols require an opportunity for the potential participant to ask questions and have them answered. Other modifications include large font size (14 or 16 points) for elders or those with lower visual acuity (Agency for Healthcare Research and Quality, 2009).

Protection of Human Rights

Human rights include privileges and demands and have been validated by the perceptiveness of a person or a group of persons. Human rights are applicable to all individuals involved in a research project, including (a) the team conducting the project, (b) the healthcare providers practicing in the project setting, and (c) the participants enrolled in the project. Prior to receiving approval to conduct a project, the human rights concerns must be resolved (Haber, 2010).

Elements of Institutional Review Board Application
Protocol Review and Consent

In preparing a protocol and IRB application for expedited or full review, there are key concepts of participant protection that must be ensured. Protocols may be submitted online through a program such as IRBNet, which is "a web based interface for the submission, correspondence, and monitoring of protocols" that makes the process paperless and also tracks the process through multiple review agencies and stages (see **Figure 5-1** IRBNet, 2012; University of South Alabama, 2011).

Box 5-1 Example of Flesch-Kincaid Reading Level of 7.0

Heart Health Study Information Sheet

You are invited to participate in a research study about your heart health. You may choose to be in the study or not. Dr. Linda Roussel is in charge of this study. She is a faculty member at the University of South Alabama (USA). She also runs Our Neighborhood Healthcare Clinic and outreach programs.

If you are in the study, you will be asked to answer questions from several surveys. We will take your blood pressure, height, weight, waist circumference, and basic laboratory values (such as cholesterol and blood sugar). These will be repeated approximately every 3–6 months. You have the right to skip any questions that you do not wish to answer. There are no known risks for you to participate in this study other than the usual risks of having your laboratory values and blood pressure taken. The laboratory values will be measured from a finger stick, which may cause slight discomfort and could cause a bruise.

There will be no payment, but healthy snacks will be given during the sessions. There will be no costs to you. You may benefit by receiving help from the outreach program. If you have *any* questions about the research, Dr. Linda Roussel or another member of the research team will be glad to answer these; her phone number is 251-609-1585. If you have questions about your rights or any complaints about the research, you may contact the staff at the Office of the USA IRB for Human Use at University Boulevard at 251-445-5678.

Your Personal Health Information (PHI) is protected by law. Under these laws, your health information cannot be used or given out to the research team without your permission. All records will be kept confidential. The results of this study might be published, but no information that identifies you will ever be given out. The following individuals will be able to see the research records to be sure the research is being done correctly—the research staff, the USA Research Compliance and Assurance Office, and the USA IRB. All information will be entered into a computer without names. Information stored on the computer will be password protected. Information stored in files will be stored in locked files.

Your permission does not run out. You may quit the study at any time. If you wish to quit, please contact any research team member or call Dr. Roussel at the number mentioned above. If you quit, you will be removed from the study. However, information already gathered may be used to complete the study.

You are not giving up any legal rights by agreeing to participate in this research. If you agree to be in the study, it means that you understand everything that has been explained to you. Feel free to ask about anything that is unclear at this time.

Thank you!

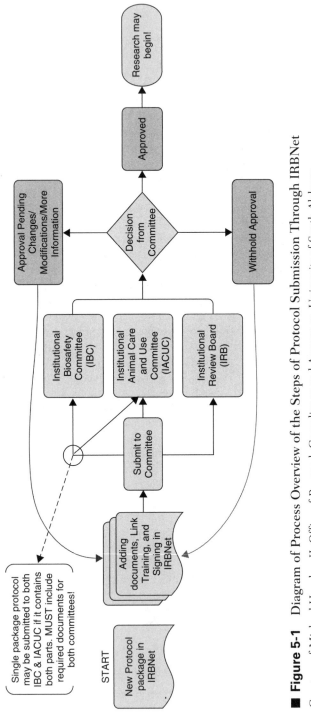

■ **Figure 5-1** Diagram of Process Overview of the Steps of Protocol Submission Through IRBNet

Courtesy of Michael Housley, II, Office of Research Compliance and Assurance, University of South Alabama.

Privacy, anonymity, and confidentiality refer to protections of identity. Consent and assent refer to basic willingness and voluntary participation. Data management includes understanding of the level of protection in different types of data collection as well as techniques for data to remain unidentifiable, cleaned, and stored. Procedures may be specified for screening and recruitment, and specific instructions may be developed for use of questionnaires, interviews or focus groups, obtaining physical data, or secondary analysis of clinical data records (Polit & Beck, 2012).

Key Elements of Informed Consent

Provision of informed consent is a process for participants in research or QI. It is an essential process that includes the conveying of information and the expectation of adequate understanding. There is increasing concern for low literacy and the need to keep the consent document at an appropriate reading level. In some cases, IRBs will approve low-literacy consent to be read aloud to potential participants. Sufficient time and opportunity for consideration of the decision and receiving input from others must be provided. To meet this requirement, some investigators mail consent forms to prospective subjects and review these prior to arrival at the study site. The participant may want to consult family, clergy, or other individual resources prior to agreeing. The provision of 24 hours for consent may be waived in minimal-risk studies but always should be a consideration as part of the process (DHHS, 2012b; Polit & Beck, 2012).

Many university IRB websites have provided comprehensive information on (1) how to submit studies for review and (2) regulatory requirements related to the Health Insurance Portability and Accountability Act (HIPAA), the Family Educational Rights and Privacy Act (FERPA), and the Genetic Information Nondiscrimination Act (GINA). In the consent process and through written informed consent, an individual may authorize the investigator's use of medical information or records. This is called a HIPAA authorization or waiver. Likewise, a student may authorize access to educational records protected by FERPA (DHHS, 2008; DHHS, 2012a).

■ The Consent Form

Human subjects should sign an informed consent form before participating in research. Even if the participant's only interaction with the investigator is an interview, the participant should sign a consent form. Often researchers employ checklists and comprehension checks for ensuring adequate informed consent (Kripalani, Bengtzen, Henderson, & Jacobson, 2008). Special methods can be used to enhance informed consent, including Patient Information Sheets, eConsent, Gamification, Video Consenting, and websites (Hoffner, et al., 2012; Tait, Voepel-Lewis, Levine, 2015). All materials and methods used for the informed consent form or process require IRB approval. Recruitment materials also must be IRB approved before implementing a study, including materials that use media, bulletin boards, fliers, posters, verbal scripts, letters, social media, email, or referrals. Ensuring the readability and comprehension of informed consent forms requires that scientific language and reading levels be reduced. Research on the informed consent process and documents often reveal issues in complexity in the informed consent document (Reinert et al., 2014). Documentation of the recruitment and informed consent process must be thorough, prior to commencing research and at all subsequent visits. The adage, *"if it is not documented, it was not done"* applies to informed consent as well as other clinical activities.

The IRB can determine to put aside the necessity for getting informed consent when (a) the risk to human subjects is negligible; (b) human participants' rights will not be harmfully influenced by not requiring participants to sign; (c) if performing the research without the waiver is not realistic; and (d) if significant, participants will be allowed to obtain more applicable information after they take part (DHHS, 2011a).

Before investigators submit to the IRB, the informed consent form should include the following:

- What the participants will be requested to do, who will ask them, and what the purpose is for doing what they will do
- Identification of the investigator and contact information for participants if they have questions they want answered
- Contact information of investigator and the IRB
- Advising participants of possible risks they may encounter if they participate in the research
- Alerting participants of their rights (e.g., right to examine data; right to abandon the research)
- Indicating if participants' names or any names will be used in the process or what substitutions for names will be made
- How the research results will be distributed and if participants will profit in any way from research participation
- That participants may withdraw from the research with no bias against them
- The understanding that a legal guardian must sign for a minor child to be able to participate
- Writing the consent form in the second person [e.g., *"You have the right . . ."*] (DHHS, 1998)

Investigators have the responsibility to acquaint the potential participants with any new findings that would affect their willingness to continue. Participants also must be given information on any alternative treatments they may consider in making their decision. A checklist of consent elements is presented in **Box 5-2** (DHHS, 1998). At the University of South Alabama, a subjects' bill of rights (see **Box 5-3**) accompanies the informed consent process (University of South Alabama, 2004).

Privacy refers to how one approaches the potential participant. It requires, in most cases, that the researcher not approach a person in any way that would identify the potential participant as having particular characteristics. It would also require some type of permission to contact a patient who could be eligible to participate. Privacy refers to the right of an individual to control what other people know about him or her.

Box 5-2 Informed Consent Checklist

Basic Elements

- A statement that the study involves research
- An explanation of the purposes of the research
- The expected duration of the subject's participation
- A description of the procedures to be followed
- Identification of any procedures that are experimental
- A description of any reasonably foreseeable risks or discomforts to the subject
- A description of any benefits to the subject or to others that may reasonably be expected from the research
- A disclosure of appropriate alternative procedures or courses of treatment, if any, that might be advantageous to the subject
- A statement describing the extent, if any, to which confidentiality of records identifying the subject will be maintained
- For research involving more than minimal risk, an explanation as to whether any compensation or medical treatments are available if injury occurs and, if so, what they consist of or where further information may be obtained
- An explanation of whom to contact for answers to pertinent questions about the research and research subjects' rights, and whom to contact in the event of a research-related injury to the subject
- A statement that participation is voluntary and that refusal to participate will involve no penalty or loss of benefits to which the subject is otherwise entitled, and the subject may discontinue participation at any time without penalty or loss of benefits to which the subject is otherwise entitled

Additional Elements as Appropriate

- A statement that the particular treatment or procedure may involve risks to the subject (or to the embryo or fetus if the subject is or may become pregnant) that are currently unforeseeable
- Anticipated circumstances under which the subject's participation may be terminated by the investigator without regard to the subject's consent
- Any additional costs to the subject that may result from participation in the research
- The consequences of a subject's decision to withdraw from the research and procedures for orderly termination of participation by the subject
- A statement that significant new findings developed during the course of the research, which may relate to the subject's willingness to continue participation, will be provided to the subject
- The approximate number of subjects involved in the study

Data from U.S. Department of Health & Human Services, http://www.hhs.gov/ohrp/policy/consentckls

---

Box 5-3 University of South Alabama Medical Research Subject's Bill of Rights

If you are invited to participate as a subject in a medical research study or are asked to consent on behalf of another, you have the right to:

1. Be informed of the purpose of the research.
2. Be given an explanation of the procedures to be followed in the research protocol and of any drug or device to be used.
3. Be given a description of any discomfort, risk, or potential medical complication that reasonably could be expected to occur as a consequence of participation in the research study.
4. Be advised of any potential benefits from your participation in the research, if applicable.
5. Be informed of any procedures, drugs, or devices that might be of help to you and provide an alternative to participation in the research.
6. Be informed of the process required to receive medical treatment promptly should complications arise as a result of your participation in the research.
7. Be given an opportunity to ask any questions concerning the research.
8. Be instructed that you may discontinue your participation in the research study at any time without jeopardizing the future medical care you receive at USA.
9. Be given a copy of a signed and dated written consent form, whenever written consent is required.
10. Be given the opportunity to decide freely and without undue pressure from others whether or not to participate in the research.

Data from University of South Alabama Office of Research Compliance and Assurance.

This right is limited in that no person can completely control what other people know about him or her if that knowledge is based on the individual's public speech, actions, or location. Informed consent is not required for research projects that monitor unidentified subjects' public behavior. However, when information that individuals would normally control is collected, informed consent indicates that the participant has voluntarily chosen to disclose certain information to investigators (Polit & Beck, 2012; University of Montana with Office of Research Integrity, 2002).

Anonymity is met if a study participant cannot be identified, such as by a survey with no names. A data set with matched Time 1 and Time 2 data is not anonymous because it has been collected in such a way as to be sure that the two times match; thus, at some point, the participant was identified. Anonymity is not the same as a de-identified data set and occurs only when there are no identifiers collected at all (Polit & Beck, 2012).

Confidentiality means that the identity of participants is not released and identity is protected. It can be maintained through code numbers on surveys and many precautions that ensure safe storage. Confidentiality is required in interviews in which the researcher clearly knows the participant. It can be encouraged but not ensured in focus groups. A breach of confidentiality is often considered a risk in any study, and some IRBs require all investigators to list it on the consent form. Any person engaged in research in which sensitive information is gathered from human subject participants (or any person who intends to engage in such research) may apply for a Certificate of Confidentiality (DHHS, 2011c; Office for Human Research Protections [OHRP], 2003; Polit & Beck, 2012). A Certificate of Confidentiality helps researchers protect the privacy of human research participants enrolled in biomedical, behavioral, clinical, and other forms of sensitive research. Certificates protect against compulsory legal demands, such as court orders and subpoenas, for identifying information or identifying characteristics of a research participant (OHRP, 2003; Polit & Beck, 2012).

Consent is agreeing to participate as an adult or providing permission for one's minor child to participate. It must be voluntary, obtained without coercion or undue influence, and follow a process of adequately informing the potential participant to make a reasoned decision whether to participate. Consent may be given by a guardian or a legally designated caregiver who is acting as a legal authorized representative for a participant (DHHS, 2010a; Polit & Beck, 2012).

Assent is agreement by a child, generally between the ages of 7 and 18, to participate in the research. Child assent must be accompanied by parental or guardian consent. Because children are not competent to give informed consent, informed consent of children's parents or legal guardians must be obtained. The age of majority varies from state to state, with most being 18 years but some being 19 or 21. Assent has been referred to as an affirmative agreement to participate (Polit & Beck, 2012).

Vulnerable populations refers to specific classes of persons who may be incapable of giving fully informed consent (e.g., developmentally delayed people) or may be at risk for unintended side effects because of their circumstance (e.g., fetuses, neonates, children, pregnant women, and prisoners) (DHHS, 2010a).

Incentives are reasonable compensations for participation. Most incentives provide for expenses to participate, such as travel, and may compensate someone for his or her time (Tomlinson, 2011). For the majority of the time, using incentives for recruitment and retention for research participants is innocuous. However, there are times when this is not the case. The responsibility related to ethics to advance health care must be balanced against the charge that participants are autonomous persons who deserve respect. Therefore, the ethical use of incentives can be significant in meeting that balance (Grant & Sugarman, 2004). Example incentives are a $25 gift card (adult), a movie pass or music download (adolescent), crayons (child), or discount coupons for baby supplies (pregnant woman, parent). Incentives must be given throughout the study, but a proportion may be reserved for study completion (Frederick, 2009).

Benefits refers to actual direct benefits the participant may expect to receive and the global benefits to society. A benefit could potentially be helpful to the participant (e.g., an intervention that may not be accessible to the participant otherwise, discussing their issue with an unbiased individual, and/or incentives). A risk-benefit assessment should be conducted (Polit & Beck, 2012).

Risks are included with every research study; however, risk can be minimal. *Minimal risk* is not larger than the risk an individual would come upon daily or during a routine procedure. If a risk is more than minimal, caution must be taken and a process must be followed to decrease risk and maximize the benefits. The possible risks to participating in the study should be shared with participants (e.g., physical harm, psychological distress, stigma, privacy, financial). The study should be restructured if the anticipated risks are greater than the anticipated study benefits (Polit & Beck, 2012).

Community-Based Participatory Research and Institutional Review Boards

Community-based participatory research is a research method that engages community and academic partnerships (Flicker, Travers, Guta, McDonald, & Meagher, 2007). Communities are recognized as more than a grouping of persons in a neighborhood. A better description of communities might be social networks that create subcultures with greater diversity. For example, people who reside in an urban center are likely to have higher rates of health and psychosocial problems compared to people living in rural areas (Flicker, Skinner, & Veinot, 2005). Community partners offer an opportunity to increase communication with academics using a research paradigm. Specific research questions can be created that reflect health issues of real concern to community partners. This collaboration would improve the researchers' ability to obtain informed consent and design a study to benefit the community (Minkler, 2005). New ethical concerns surface that traditional ethical review boards have not been required to consider in the past (Flicker et al., 2007). For example, how does the community interpret the research question(s)? Have community leaders contributed to the questions and design? This is particularly vital for the recruitment and retention of participants. IRB forms may favor traditional biomedical research methodology. This may unintentionally harm community-based research (Flicker et al., 2007). Members of the community should be included in all meetings related to research studies or QI initiatives. If these collaborative meetings do not occur, the perception might be lack of equality in terms of the cost-benefit of the scholarly work. The ethical component of all projects must be discussed before submitting the IRB application.

■ Conclusion

In any venue for dissemination—both presentations and publications—investigators are being asked to verify the review and approvals that were done with the initiation of the research. In an international survey of journal reviewers, Broome, Dougherty, Freda, Kearney, and Baggs (2010) found that the most commonly reported concern was inadequate protection of human research participants. Recently, some journals have required documentation of the IRB protocol number and approval date for submission of manuscripts to peer-reviewed journals. It is important that healthcare providers recognize this as a required element in the evaluation or critical appraisal of the work as they draw implications for practice. However, professionals are also in key positions to provide oversight for protection of human participants and patients who may be invited to participate or who may be involved without adequate attention to these safeguards. In many cases, whistleblowers have been individuals who identified serious omissions in these safety measures. Knowledge is power, and comprehension of the necessity of IRB and ethical review can only strengthen our multidisciplinary healthcare environments. In all of these, the focus is on issues of protection of human subjects and building structures and processes that strengthen relationships with the providers and public.

■ Case Studies in Institutional Review Board and Informed Consent Requirements

It is important to be able to apply the principles of human subject research protections as it relates to IRB approvals and informed consent. On initial review of these principles, it initially appears clear cut and intuitive. However, as human subject research opportunities present themselves, the lines related to regulatory requirements for studies can become blurred. Using the resources in this chapter, look at four examples or research to gain clarity about different types of requirements for IRB review and approval and for informed consenting.

Example 1

Cynthia is a nurse manager for a team of infusion nurses at an oncology practice that has two office locations. Each office location has an infusion team of four registered nurses (RNs). The physicians in the practice admit patients to two local hospitals that are designated as regional medical centers that have 400 and 620 beds, respectively. The oncology referral for breast cancer patients is robust, and the infusion clinic is busy. Cynthia and one of the physicians have learned about a novel new head-cooling device that is being developed by a local company. The "device" company (sponsor) representative has asked if the group would consider "trying it out" by participating in a small study of the device. The company has agreed to provide the device and instructions for the device (company generated study protocol) and is asking that it be studied in 15 cases of patients beginning initial chemotherapy treatment for stage 1 to 2 breast cancer. This oncology group does not have a clinical research staff, and Cynthia is navigating next steps.

It is important for nurses to understand the basics of clinical research regulations and human subject protections. Clinical trials take place in academic medical

(continues)

centers, private practices, and freestanding research companies. Nurses encounter varied opportunities to work on a clinical trial, either in a supportive role coordinating a study or in clinical role, caring for patients who happen to be enrolled in a study. Sometimes a clinical role can evolve into a study coordination role, either formally or ad hoc. Such opportunities, even unexpected ones, are more common than expected and present additional role requirements and role conflicts for nurses. Moreover, there renewed interest in clinical research ("moon-shot for cures for cancer") and those opportunities will continue to evolve. Moreover, nurses are key researchers on the process of clinical research, especially tool development and innovations in informed consenting.

In Example 1, the study is obviously a clinical trial of a device and would require full IRB review. While the study is an open-label study, which does not include a "comparator" device or double-blinding of the participant or research staff, it is still a clinical trial that is gathering safety and efficacy data on a new device. The company may or may not have submitted this study to the FDA as an investigational new device. Indeed, such a device may just as easily be an innovative product developed by a nurse! For now let's unpack what needs to be considered when moving ahead through the decision process of agreeing to participate in this project:

- What is the company's prior experience with this population and device?
- What does the "protocol" say?
- What is the specific population eligible for this study? New breast cancer, grade 1 to 2 is not specific enough. What if a relapsed patient wants to be in the study?
- What risks have been identified? How might the risks and benefits be articulated for potential participants and for the IRB?
- Which IRB will be used, because this is a private practice? What kind of IRB approval is needed?
- If the study is funded by a government agency, such as the NIH, what IRB requirements must be in place before it can review the study?
- Does the company provide an informed consent? How might the informed consent be reviewed and rewritten to conform to IRB policies and ensure it is in simple language? Are all of the elements of informed consent as described by regulations in place?
- The people will be participating in the study for multiple chemotherapy infusion visits. What are the implications for informed consent at each visit?
- How is informed consent documented? What if English is not a first language for some of the patients?
- Who will be listed as the investigator and sub-investigators?
- Is there a project contract and budget? What indemnifications will be in place? Will the product sponsor reimburse participants' if there is injury?
- What attendance is required by the IRB of the physician taking part in the study?
- What is the role of the nurse manager and staff in this study?

■ How will taking part in this study enhance the practice and care of patients in the practice?

■ Should this study be registered with clinicaltrials.gov?

Example 2

The community oncology practice described in Example 1 is using a new FDA-approved chilled cap to prevent hair loss in breast cancer patients on chemotherapy called Dignicaps®. The caps have circulating liquid that is kept at a steady cooling temperature (32°F) and are worn prior to, during, and after chemotherapy. Cynthia is considering several nursing research questions related to alopecia in chemotherapy patients as part of her Doctor of Nursing Practice (DNP) degree pursuits. Because the use of the caps prolongs the time requirement for patients to be in the infusion chairs (before and after infusion), Cynthia wants to use audioguided meditations and electric blankets to increase comfort and satisfaction of patients using this device. She also wants to include the use of a portable, disposable cooling cap to be worn home, because during the summer, a sharp contrast from cooling temperature to home transportation could possibly affect the efficacy of the cooling cap. What are the regulatory considerations for these study questions?

The use of cooling caps for the prevention of alopecia in chemotherapy patients existed in Europe prior to the United States and only gained FDA approval by Dignitana AB in 2013 (Dignicaps®). It is becoming incorporated as optimal care for avoiding alopecia for breast cancer chemotherapy patients; however, as with any newly approved device or medical treatment, third-party payers are slow to approve as standard of care and more readily and affordably accessible. Nursing care of patients using new treatments or medicines offer opportunities for innovative nursing research questions and quality improvement. In fact, nursing studies can enhance the case for third-party payer acceptance and policy decisions. In case Example 2, Cynthia is posing multiple questions and should focus a study plan that aims to measure comfort and satisfaction. Moreover, she is posing a new intervention that could measure efficacy.

■ *What classification of device is Dignicaps®? Does that matter?*

■ *Are these two different studies or one single study? Can those study questions be combined?*

■ *What tools will Cynthia use to measure comfort and satisfaction?*

■ *Will the guided meditations and electric blankets be standardized (same used for all?). What settings will be used for the electric blankets and when would the electric blanket be used and for how long?*

■ *What risks are associated with the use of electric blankets and in the satisfaction and comfort measurements?*

■ *What would be included in the informed consent form?*

■ *What kind of IRB approval is needed and which IRB will be used?*

(continues)

- *If Cynthia wants to introduce an alternative cooling system for the ride home, what is planned and how will that be standardized to ensure it is used similarly for all cases? What will this cost?*

Example 3

Cynthia determines that she does not have the resources available at the time to develop a portable cap to be used on the way home; however, she is going to investigate that for a later nursing research project. Moreover, she decides that she first needs to focus on piloting a tool to measure satisfaction and comfort for patients using cooling caps. Some patients already bring portable audio and blankets with them; and sometimes the clinic warmed blankets are available; however, those interventions are varied, and the use of comfort measures will be assessed generally in the survey as descriptive data, but will not be compared to satisfaction results. Cynthia is going to use existing tools (previously studied for reliability and validity) to measure patient comfort and satisfaction and has created a SurveyMonkey® survey (surveymonkey.com). Eligible patients will be asked to complete an anonymous survey using an Internet link generated by SurveyMonkey®. Patients without Internet connections will be allowed to complete the survey at subsequent clinic visits using a study iPad. No patient identifiers are collected in the study.

Because this study is measuring satisfaction and comfort, is anonymous, and poses no significant risk to the participants, full IRB review is not required; however, the study still requires IRB approval, but likely will only need expedited review. Consider these additional questions as you apply the principles in this chapter:

- *Who ultimately decides whether a study requires full review or expedited review?*
- *What will Cynthia need to do to prepare an expedited IRB submission?*
- *What elements will be required for the informed consent for this study? Is face-to-face informed consent required? Can survey URLs be sent out with an invitation letter and information sheet only? Who determines these requirements?*
- *Should Cynthia include patients in the development of the survey?*
- *How will Cynthia report findings to patients?*
- *How does SurveyMonkey® ensure privacy of participants?*
- *Will Cynthia disseminate her findings beyond the local clinic? Does this make a difference?*

Example 4

Cynthia notes that several patients are complaining that they are experiencing varied levels of alopecia despite the use of cooling caps at the clinic. After investigating these cases, it is difficult to ascertain the consistency of cooling cap usage, because of varied charting practices. Moreover, she also observes that during busy infusion days, some patients are not wearing the infusion caps long enough prior to the initiation of infusion, and, in some cases, there are more patients than cooling caps. She determines that a standard operating procedure (SOP) needs to be developed to improve the quality of care in patients using the cooling caps, as well as new training to ensure consistency in practice. She initiates a checklist and audit practice to instill quality control and quality assurance. Moreover, she uses staff and patient input when developing the SOP. After implementation, she will survey patients for their satisfaction and to measure if there are any improvements in rates of alopecia.

As presented in this chapter, the spirit of inquiry should be present for all levels of care and includes measuring quality indicators for patient care, safety, and satisfaction. There can be a fine line between quality improvement studies and research studies. What should be considered when developing research questions that are aimed at quality improvement?

- What kind of IRB approval is needed to measure the effectiveness of or adherence to a new SOP? Is Example 4 a research study or a quality improvement study?
- Is informed consent needed for this study?
- Should a study plan (study protocol) be developed for this QI study?
- Cynthia realizes that the SOP she developed could help other community cancer centers and submits an abstract of her results to a national nursing convention. She also plans to write a manuscript of her process, SOP, survey, and findings. Does this make a difference in categorizing this as research or quality improvement?

For Additional Information:

Bergenmar, M., Johansson, H., Wilking, N., Hatschek, T., & Brandberg, Y. (2014). Audio-recorded information to patients considering participation in cancer clinical trials: a randomized study. *Acta Oncologica, 53*(9), 1197–1204. doi:10.3109/0284186X.2014.921726

Cohn, E. G., Jia, H., Smith, W. C., Erwin, K., & Larson, E. L. (2011). Measuring the process and quality of informed consent for clinical research: development and testing. *Oncology Nursing Forum, 38*(4), 417–422. doi:10.1188/11.ONF.417-422

FDA (2015). Letter from FDA to target health. Retrieved from http://www.accessdata.fda.gov/cdrh_docs/pdf15/DEN150010.pdf

Griffith, K. S., Wright, L. S., Hackworth, J., & Gilheart, S. (2012). Editing research consent forms for lay readers. *AMWA Journal: American Medical Writers Association Journal, 27*(2), 51–54.

Hartnett, T. (2008). Quality improvement: when is it research that requires informed consent? *Research Practitioner, 9*(2), 36–42.

Lidz, C. W., Albert, K., Appelbaum, P., Dunn, L. B., Overton, E., & Pivovarova, E. (2015). Why is therapeutic misconception so prevalent? *Cambridge Quarterly Of Healthcare Ethics, 24*(2), 231–241. doi:10.1017/S096318011400053X

Komen, M. M. C., Breed, W. P. M., Smorenburg, C. H., van der Ploeg, T., Goey, S. H., van der Hoeven, J. J. M., . . . van den Hurk, C. J. G., (2016). Results of 20- versus 45-min post-infusion cap cooling time in the prevention of docetaxel-induced alopecia. *Supportive Care in Cancer,* 1–7. doi:10.1007/s00520-016-3084-7. Retrieved from link.springer.com/article/10.1007/s00520-016-3084-7

(continues)

U.S. Food and Drug Administration. (2015). Letter from FDA to Target Health. Located at http://www.accessdata.fda.gov/cdrh_docs/pdf15/DEN150010.pdf

Wilfond, B. S. (2013). Quality improvement ethics: lessons from the SUPPORT Study. *American Journal of Bioethics, 13*(12), 14–19. doi:10.1080/15265161.2013.851582

REFLECTIVE ACTIVITIES

1. Review an informed consent document and evaluate the elements.
2. Review a research proposal that has had a full review and justify the review by the IRB.
3. Describe three different populations considered to be vulnerable according to the descriptions in this chapter. What are the appropriate IRB procedures for protecting these human subjects?
4. Describe the differences between the elements of a research study proposal and a QI proposal in regard to the IRB.
5. Attend an IRB meeting or interview and IRB member.
6. Volunteer to participate in a research study.
7. Compare and contrast informed consent for a research study to informed consent for a medical procedure.
8. Obtain Human Subject Protections Certification from NIH or CITI

REFERENCES

Agency for Healthcare Research and Quality. (2009). *The AHRQ informed consent and authorization toolkit for minimal risk research.* Retrieved from http://www.ahrq.gov/fund/informedconsent/

Appelbaum, P. (2002). Clarifying the ethics of clinical research: A path toward avoiding the therapeutic misconception. *American Journal of Bioethics, 2*(2), 22–23.

Appelbaum, P. S., Roth, L. H., Lidz, C. W. (1987). False hopes and best data: Consent to research and the therapeutic misconception. *Hastings Center Report, 17*(2), 20–24.

Beecher, H. K. (1966). Ethics and clinical research. *New England Journal of Medicine, 274*(24), 1354–1360. doi:10.1056/NEJM196606162742405. (Reproduced in: Harkness, J., Lederer, S. E., & Wikler, D. (2001). Laying ethical foundations for clinical research, *Bulletin of the World Health Organization, 79*(4), 365–372. Ref. No.: 01-1218; PMCID: PMC2566401. Retrieved from http://www.ncbi.nlm.nih.gov/pmc/articles/PMC2566401/pdf/11368058.pdf)

Beh, H. G. (2002). The role of Institutional Review Boards in protecting human subjects: Are we really ready to fix a broken system? *Law and Psychology Review, 26*(1), 1–48. Retrieved from http://papers.ssrn.com/sol3/papers.cfm?abstract_id=1444616

Broome, M., Dougherty, M. C., Freda, M. C., Kearney, M. H., & Baggs, J. G. (2010). Ethical concerns of nursing reviewers: An international survey. *Nursing Ethics, 17*(6), 741–748. doi:10.1177/0969733010379177

Collaborative Institutional Training Initiative. (2011). *CITI course in the responsible conduct of research.* Retrieved from https://www.citiprogram.org/rcrpage.asp?language=english&affiliation=100

Duke University Medical Center. (2005). *What is quality improvement? Contrasting QI and QA.* Retrieved from http://patientsafetyed.duhs.duke.edu/module_a/introduction/contrasting_qi_qa.html

Eissenburg, T., Panicker, S., Berenbaum, S., Epley, N., Fendrich, M., Kelso, R., . . . Simmerling, M. (2004). *IRBs and psychological science: Ensuring a collaborative relationship.* American Psychological Association. Retrieved from https://www.apa.org/research/responsible/irbs-psych-science.pdf

Fain, J. A. (2009). *Reading, understanding, and applying nursing research* (3rd ed.). Philadelphia, PA: F. A. Davis.

Flicker, S., Skinner, H., & Veinot, T. (2005). Falling through the cracks of the big cities: Who is meeting the needs of young people with HIV? *Canadian Journal of Public Health, 96*(4), 308–312.

Flicker, S., Travers, R., Guta, A., McDonald, S., & Meagher, A. (2007). Ethical dilemmas in community-based participatory research: Recommendations for institutional review boards. *Journal of Urban Health: Bulletin of the New York Academy of Medicine, 84*(4), 478–493. doi:10.1007/s11524-007-9165-7

Frederick, M. (2009, November 19). *Offering incentives for research participation. WSIRB In-Service Training. DSHS Human Research Review Section.* Retrieved from http://www.dshs.wa.gov/pdf/ms/rda/hrrs/wsirbtraining/Incentives.pdf

Grady, C., Eckstein, L., Berkman, B., Brock, D., Cook-Deegan, R., Fullerton, S. M., & . . . Wendler, D. (2015). Broad consent for research with biological samples: Workshop conclusions. *American Journal of Bioethics, 15*(9), 34–42. doi:10.1080/15265161.2015.1062162

Grant, R. W., & Sugarman, J. (2004). Ethics in human subjects research: Do incentives matter? *Journal of Medicine and Philosophy, 29*(6), 717–738.

Haber, J. (2010). Legal and ethical issues. In G. LoBiondo-Wood & J. Haber (Eds.), *Nursing research: Methods and critical appraisal for evidence-based practice* (7th ed., pp. 246–267) St. Louis, MO: Mosby.

Hoffner, B., Bauer-Wu, S., Hitchcock-Bryan, S., Powell, M., Wolanski, A., & Joffe, S. (2012). "Entering a clinical trial: Is it right for you?": A randomized study of The Clinical Trials Video and its impact on the informed consent process. Cancer, 118(7), 1877–83. doi: 10.1002/cncr.26438.

IRBNet. (2012). *Innovative solutions for compliance and research management.* Retrieved from https://www.irbnet.org

Kripalani, S., Bengtzen, R., Henderson, L., & Jacobson, T. (2008). Clinical research in low-literacy populations: using teach-back to assess comprehension of informed consent and privacy information. *IRB: Ethics & Human Research, 30*(2), 13–19.

McNett, M., & Lawry, K. (2009). Research and quality improvement activities: When is institutional review board review needed? *Journal of Neuroscience Nursing, 41*(6), 344–347.

Minkler, M. (2005). Community-based research partnerships: Challenges and opportunities. *Journal of Urban Health: Bulletin of the New York Academy of Medicine, 82*(2, Suppl. 2), ii3–ii10. doi:10.1093/jurban/jti034

The National Commission for the Protection of Human Subjects of Biomedical and Behavioral Research. (1979). *The Belmont report: Ethical principles and guidelines for the protection of human subjects of research.* Retrieved from http://www.fda.gov/ohrms/dockets/ac/05/briefing/2005-4178b_09_02_Belmont%20Report.pdf

National Institutes of Health Office of Extramural Research. (2011). *Protecting human research participants.* Retrieved from http://phrp.nihtraining.com/users/login.php

Nerenz, D. R. (2009). Ethical issues in using data from quality management programs. *European Spine Journal, 18*(Suppl. 3), 321–330.

Oakes, J. M. (2002). Risks and wrongs in social science research: An evaluator's guide to the IRB. *Evaluation Review, 26*(5), 443–479. Retrieved from http://www.research.umn.edu/irb/download/EvaluatorsGuidetoIRB.pdf

Office for Human Research Protections. (2003). *Guidance on certificates of confidentiality.* Retrieved from http://www.hhs.gov/ohrp/policy/certconf.pdf

Polit, D. F., & Beck, C. T. (2012). *Nursing research: Generating and assessing evidence for nursing practice* (9th ed.). Philadelphia, PA: Lippincott Williams & Wilkins.

Reinert, C., Kremmler, L., Burock, S., Bogdahn, U., Wick, W., Gleiter, C. H., & . . . Hau, P. (2014). Quantitative and qualitative analysis of study-related patient information sheets in randomised neuro-oncology phase III-trials. *European Journal of Cancer, 50*(1), 150–158. doi:10.1016/j.ejca.2013.09.006

Steinbrook, R. (2008). The Gelsinger case. In E. J. Emanuel, C. Grady, R. A. Crouch, R. K. Lie, F. G. Miller, & D. Wendler (Eds.), *The Oxford textbook of clinical research ethics* (pp. 110–122). New York, NY: Oxford University Press.

Steneck, N. H. (2007). *ORI: Introduction to responsible conduct of research.* U.S. Department of Health & Human Services. Retrieved from http://www.ori.hhs.gov/publications/ori_intro_text.shtml

Tait, A. R., Voepel-Lewis, T., & Levine, R. (2015). Using digital multimedia to improve parents' and children's understanding of clinical trials. *Archives of Disease in Childhood, 100*(6), 589–593. doi:10.1136/archdischild-2014-308021

Tappen, R. M. (2011). *Advanced nursing research: From theory to practice.* Sudbury, MA: Jones & Bartlett Learning.

Tomlinson, T. (2011). When is it ethical to withhold a research incentive? *IRB: Ethics and Human Research, 33*(6), 14–16.

University of Montana with Office of Research Integrity. (2002). *Online research ethics course: Section six: Human participation in research.* Retrieved from http://ori.hhs.gov/education/products/montana_round1/human.html

University of South Alabama. (2004). *University of South Alabama medical research subjects' bill of rights.* Retrieved from http://www.southalabama.edu/researchcompliance/pdf/subjectsbillofrights.pdf

University of South Alabama. (2011). *Office of research compliance and assurance: IRBNet.* Retrieved from http://www.southalaba2ma.edu/researchcompliance/irbnet.html

U.S. Department of Health & Human Services. (1998). *Office for Human Research Protections: Informed consent checklist—basic and additional elements.* Retrieved from http://www.hhs.gov/ohrp/policy/consentckls.html/

U.S. Department of Health & Human Services. (2008). *Joint guidance on the application of the Family Educational Rights and Privacy Act (FERPA) and the Health Insurance Portability and Accountability Act of 1996 (HIPAA) to student health records.* Retrieved from http://www2.ed.gov/policy/gen/guid/fpco/doc/ferpa-hipaa-guidance.pdf

U.S. Department of Health & Human Services. (2010a). *Code of federal regulations.* Retrieved from http://www.hhs.gov/ohrp/humansubjects/guidance/45cfr46.html#46.102

U.S. Department of Health & Human Services. (2010b). *Guidance on IRB continuing review of research.* Retrieved from http://www.hhs.gov/ohrp/policy/continuingreview2010.html

U.S. Department of Health & Human Services. (2010c). *Human research protections frequent questions.* Retrieved from http://answers.hhs.gov/ohrp/questions/7285

U.S. Department of Health & Human Services. (2010d). *Human research protections frequent questions.* Retrieved from http://answers.hhs.gov/ohrp/questions/7286

U.S. Department of Health & Human Services. (2011a). *Human research protections frequent questions.* Retrieved from http://answers.hhs.gov/ohrp/questions/7289

U.S. Department of Health & Human Services. (2011b). *Information related to advanced notice of proposed rulemaking (ANPRM) for revisions to the Common Rule.* Retrieved from http://www.hhs.gov/ohrp/humansubjects/anprm2011page.html

U.S. Department of Health & Human Services. (2011c). *Frequently asked questions: Certificates of confidentiality.* Retrieved from http://grants.nih.gov/grants/policy/coc/faqs.htm#368

U.S. Department of Health & Human Services. (2012a). *Health information privacy: Summary of the HIPAA privacy rule.* Retrieved from http://www.hhs.gov/ocr/privacy/hipaa/understanding/summary/index.html

U.S. Department of Health & Human Services. (2012b). *Human research protections frequent questions.* Retrieved from http://answers.hhs.gov/ohrp/categories/1566

U.S. Department of Health & Human Services. (2012c). *The federal policy for human subject protections (The Common Rule).* Retrieved from http://www.hhs.gov/ohrp/humansubjects/commonrule/index.html

Wilfond, B. S. (2013). Quality improvement ethics: Lessons from the SUPPORT study. *American Journal of Bioethics, 13*(12), 14–19. doi:10.1080/15265161.2013.851582

World Medical Association. (2008). *World Medical Association Declaration of Helsinki: Ethical principles for medical research involving human subjects.* Retrieved from http://www.wma.net/en/30publications/10policies/b3/index.html

World Medical Association. (2013). Declaration of Helsinki: Ethical Principles for Medical Research Involving Human Subjects. Located at http://www.wma.net/en/30publications/10policies/b3/

CHAPTER 6

Critical Appraisal of Research-Based Evidence

■HEATHER R. HALL AND LINDA A. ROUSSEL■

■ Objectives:

- Define critical appraisal for quantitative research-based evidence.
- Define critical appraisal for qualitative research-based evidence.
- Identify critical appraisal tools.

■ Introduction

Critically appraising the evidence is an essential step in evidence-based practice (EBP) in response to a clinical question (Polit & Beck, 2012). The process of systematically evaluating research for its reliability, importance, and significance is critical appraisal. This process is a way to assess and understand research (Burl, 2009). The reader evaluates content for validity and applicability. Critical appraisal skills are necessary in considering whether the research was conducted appropriately. In addition, these skills are used to determine if the research results could be implemented in practice to improve patient outcomes. Essentially, the critical appraisal process is used to identify valuable information (National Council for Osteopathic Research, 2005).

Critical appraisal is foundational to translating research evidence into best practices. Healthcare providers must remember that neither value nor significance is guaranteed with the publication of a research report (Fain, 2009). Essential to the advancement and improvement of knowledge is the critical appraisal of research studies (Burns & Grove, 2009). The purpose of this chapter is to strengthen critical appraisal skills.

The critical appraisal process is vital to EBP, declaring decision-making on quality research evidence as an outcome. Critical appraisal integrates critical thinking, which involves the skill of drilling down events and explains the basis of situations (Brookfield, 1987). Critical thinking includes inductive and deductive reasoning, knowledge application, translation of research, validation of experience, innovation, and outcome evaluation (Oermann, 1991).

DiCenso, Guyatt, and Ciliska (2005) presented appropriate questions to determine the value of evidence: (a) Are the results valid? (b) What are the results? (c) How can I apply the results to patient care? Using questions as instruments—along with checklists, questionnaires, and surveys—allows one to present a focused, methodical approach to offer an in-depth understanding of the evidence-based research (DiCenso, Guyatt, & Ciliska, 2005).

A critique is a critical appraisal process that evaluates the content of a research report for scientific validity and application to the practice setting. Having knowledge of the topic, reading critically, and applying critique criteria are essential. The standards, guides, or questions used to critique an article are the criteria. The steps of the research process are evaluated, and questions are asked related to each step that meets the criteria. The process of critiquing can be compared to observing a finished puzzle. Does the puzzle form a complete picture, or is a piece in the wrong place (LoBiondo-Wood & Haber, 2010)?

A critique of the literature, also known as critical appraisal, evaluates a research study or group of studies in an approach that is organized and systematic. Established criteria are used for the critical appraisal of the evidence to establish its strength, value, and reliability in an objective manner. Applicability to research, education, or practice will be concluded with the appraisal (Fulton & Krainovich-Miller, 2010).

Multiple research textbooks include a set of questions and guidelines to assist readers with the critique of a research report (Burns & Grove, 2009; Fain, 2009; Polit & Beck, 2012). Fain (2009) stated that when evaluating research reports, one should reflect on specific guidelines during the critique process. The strengths and limitations of the research report are critical in making a determination related to the value of a study. However, some components of the report are considered to be consistently critical; these are vital in the critique process. Fain (2009) listed the following "critical components of the research process to be evaluated":

A. **Problem Statement:** Clarity of problem, Significance of problem for nursing, Purpose of study, Conceptual/Theoretical framework, Literature review, Hypotheses/research questions
B. **Research Methodology:** Research design, Sample/setting, Data collection procedures, Data collection instruments, Data analysis
C. **Results, Conclusions, and Interpretations:** Results of data analysis, Discussion of findings, and Recommendations/implications for further study in practice, education, and research. (p. 253, Table 13-2)

■ Appraisal of Quantitative Research-Based Evidence

Duffy (2005) maintained that there are relevant questions to be answered when evaluating quantitative research. The strengths and weaknesses of the study are identified, and the value of the study is suggested in these results. For the purpose of informing clinical decisions, the results of the appraisal are combined with the experience of the clinician, the professional's values, and the wishes of the patient.

Last, when evidence-based clinical decisions are made, the clinician evaluates them both on an individual basis and collectively to continually improve practice (Duffy, 2005). See **Table 6-1** for examples of critical appraisal tools for quantitative research.

A systematic review is a collection of studies related to a clinical question (Johnston, 2005). During the appraisal process of a systematic review, the clinician searches for explanation of the databases, strategies of searching, and terms used. The clinician evaluates studies included in and excluded from the systematic review. The statistical method used to acquire a single-effect measure of the summary of the results of all research in the review is the meta-analysis (Johnston, 2005). The Centre for Evidence-Based Medicine (CEBM) provides useful critical appraisal sheets that

Table 6-1   Critical Appraisal Tools for Quantitative Research

CONSORT Statement The CONSORT Group, Canada http://www.consort-statement.org/consort-statement/ CONSORT 2010 Statement: Updated guidelines for reporting parallel group randomized trials (Schulz, Altman, & Moher, CONSORT Group, 2010): http://www.consort-statement.org/Media/Default/Downloads/CONSORT%202010%20Statement/CONSORT%202010%20Statement%20-%20PLoS%20Medicine.pdf	The Consolidated Standards of Reporting Trials (CONSORT) statement is a thorough document that outlines an explanation and elaboration for reporting randomized controlled trials. It also includes the critical appraisal tool.
The TREND Statement Centers for Disease Control and Prevention (CDC), United States of America http://www.cdc.gov/trendstatement/ Improving the Reporting Quality of Nonrandomized Evaluations of Behavioral and Public Health Interventions: The TREND Statement (Des Jarlais, Lyles, Crepaz, & the TREND Group, 2004): http://www.cdc.gov/trendstatement/pdf/trendstatement_ajph_mar2004_trendstatement.pdf	The Transparent Reporting of Evaluations with Nonrandomized Designs (TREND) includes 22 items in a checklist format developed to direct constant report of nonrandomized controlled trials. The TREND report works well with the CONSORT statement developed for randomized controlled trials. This shared venture helps to encourage comprehensible reporting, producing research advancement and formulating evidence-based reports to improve practice and policy.
CASP: Randomised Controlled Trial (RCT) Checklist CASP UK, Better Value Healthcare Ltd http://media.wix.com/ugd/dded87_40b9ff0bf53840478331915a8ed8b2fb.pdf	Critical Appraisal Skills Program (CASP): RCT Tool is a checklist that provides critical guidelines necessary for randomized controlled trials.

Data from Division of Health Sciences International Center for Allied Health Evidence, 2011.

can readily be used to critique a variety of topics, including systematic reviews, diagnostics, randomized controlled trials (RCTs), and prognosis (CEBM, 2016). For example, using the systematic review appraisal sheet, the researcher can evaluate the merits of the work by asking questions that guide an intensive evaluation. Questions such as these are posed: Did the PICO (patient, intervention, comparator, outcomes) guide the systematic review? Were the studies included in the review sufficiently valid for the question asked? These topical questions go further by informing the researcher of what are considered best sources and where to find this information in the review. The researcher is then able to definitively report the quality of the review. This gives greater credence to systematic reviews that may be used to develop policies, procedures, and protocols that inform practice decisions for quality patient care (CEBM, 2012). Another useful critical appraisal resource is the PRISMA (preferred reporting items for systematic reviews and meta-analyses) statement evolving from the QUOROM (quality of reporting of meta-analysis). The PRISMA is a 27-item checklist and a four-phase flow diagram. The checklist provides a review of items that creates transparency of a systematic review (Liberati et al., 2009). See **Table 6-2** for CEBM critical appraisal sheets and the PRISMA.

Duffy (2005) described the critical appraisal process of quantitative research studies, including the following steps:

(1) Distinguish among the types of quantitative research. (2) Read the entire study and summarize the population characteristics, intervention/treatment, and results.

Table 6-2 Centre for Evidence-Based Medicine Critical Appraisal Sheets and the PRISMA

The Centre for Evidence-Based Medicine (CEBM): http://www.cebm.net/critical-appraisal/	The Systematic Review Critical Appraisal Sheet Diagnostic Critical Appraisal Sheet RCT Critical Appraisal Sheet Prognosis Critical Appraisal Sheet PICO Critical Appraisal Sheet Educational Prescription Critical Appraisal Sheet
The PRISMA Ottawa Hospital Research Institute, Canada The PRISMA Statement Checklist: http://www.prisma-statement.org/ Preferred Reporting Items for Systematic Reviews and Meta-Analyses: The PRISMA Statement Document (Moher et al. (2009)) http://journals.plos.org/plosmedicine/article?id=10.1371/journal.pmed.1000097	The PRISMA Statement includes evidence-based substance for explaining systematic assessments and meta-analyses as well as an amended addition of the QUOROM statement. The PRISMA Statement, with its checklist and flow diagram, is focused on randomized controlled trials; however, it can also provide a basis for producing organized appraisals of multiple types of research, particularly interventions.

(3) Choose and use an appropriate critical appraisal framework. (4) Evaluate the study. (5) Combine the results of the evaluation with clinical experience/expertise, professional values, and patients' preferences. (6) Use results to inform clinical decisions. (p. 283)

The researcher critically appraising quantitative research studies has multiple tools available to guide the process. The tools focused on quantitative methodology described in this chapter have been well designed, providing a variety of templates that add greater credence of the appraiser.

■ Appraisal of Qualitative Research-Based Evidence

Williamson (2009) stated that qualitative evidence addresses clinical questions related to the human health experience. A vital step in appraisal of qualitative research is to identify the best evidence for clinical practice. Appraisal of the evidence is important to ensure that the best field information is being applied in an economic, holistic, and efficient manner. The findings that have been critically appraised must be integrated with the clinician's abilities and patients' choices. It is a professional expectation for clinicians that they will use the process of EBP. This process includes appraisal of the evidence to establish whether the results are credible, usable, and trustworthy (Williamson, 2009).

Qualitative evidence must be used by clinicians to inform decisions in practice. A well-conducted meta-synthesis provides a precise representation of the experiences of the participants and is trustworthy (Williamson, 2009, p. 207). A meta-synthesis will give insight into the context of the circumstances, response of a human, and meaning for patients and will offer clinicians assistance in giving the best care to attain the best outcome (Williamson, 2009). See **Table 6-3** for an example of a critical appraisal tool for qualitative research.

■ Critique of A Systematic Review

Polit and Beck's (2012) guidelines for critiquing systematic reviews (pp. 674–675) were used to critique a systematic review by Ramdoss et al. (2011).

Article: Ramdoss, S., Lang, R., Mulloy, A., Franco, J., O'Reilly, M., Didden, R., & Lancioni, G. (2011). Use of computer-based interventions to teach communication

Table 6-3 Critical Appraisal Tool for Qualitative Research

CASP: Qualitative Checklist	Critical Appraisal Skills Programme (CASP): Qualitative Research is a checklist that provides values important to qualitative research methodology.
CASP UK, Better Value Healthcare Ltd	
http://media.wix.com/ugd/dded87_29c5b002d9 9342f788c6ac670e49f274.pdf	

Data from Division of Health Sciences International Center for Allied Health Evidence, 2011.

skills to children with autism spectrum disorders: A systematic review. *Journal of Behavioral Education, 20*(1), 55–76. doi:10.1007/s10864-010-9112-7

Purpose: The use of computer-based interventions (CBIs) to teach communication skills to children with autism spectrum disorders (ASD).

Aims:
1. To evaluate the evidence base regarding CBIs
2. To inform and guide practitioners interested in using CBIs
3. To stimulate and guide future research aimed at improving the efficiency and effectiveness of CBIs in communication for individuals with ASD

Conclusions:
1. CBI should not be considered a researched-based approach to teaching communication skills to individuals with ASD.
2. CBI does seem a promising practice that warrants future research to improve communication skills of children with mild to moderate ASD.

Introduction: Impairment in communication in ASD is described with relevant statistics and research to support the degree to which this is a problem area of concern. Several authors were cited relative to the degree of the problem, including children with total absence of communication and limited or unusual ways of communicating. Confounding these problems are limited school and community involvement as well as the communication impairments that span the individual's lifetime. Additional communication techniques are described, which are often complex and may present logistical obstacles to the implementation of communication interventions within the variety of settings where children find themselves (e.g., group homes, schools, or children's homes). The use of technology is also described as being a possible way to provide interventions and deliver instructions, particularly given that these methods have been used as instructional tools for children without disabilities. The cost-benefit regarding software programming specifically related to clear routines and expectations, reducing distractions, and providing additional controls for the influence of autism-specific characteristics was also highlighted as a potential positive for CBI. The review purpose and aims were also restated in the introduction of the systematic review.

Method: The researchers clearly identified the method used to conduct the systematic review. The Method section described inclusion predetermined criteria: (a) participant characteristics, (b) communication skills targeted, (c) details regarding the CBI, (d) outcomes of the intervention, and (e) certainty of evidence. Search procedures were clearly revealed and included the use of four electronic databases: Education Resources Information Center (ERIC), MEDLINE, Psychology and Behavioral Sciences Collection, and PsycINFO. Peer-reviewed studies written only in English were reviewed, and keyword searches within the preceding databases were conducted to find appropriate, valid, and reliable research evidence. Terms such as *ASD* or *development disability* or *pervasive developmental disorder; computer* or *computer-assisted* or *computer-based* or *computer-aided software;* and *language* or *communication* or *speech* or *social* were used for the keyword search. From the search, 222 study abstracts were reviewed to identify studies for possible inclusion (using the inclusion and exclusion criteria stated in the article). The time span for the hand searches was January to June 2010. The search of the databases, journals, and reference list took place during June and July 2010.

The Method section contained a well-organized discussion of how data were extracted from each identified study using the inclusion and exclusion criteria. The researchers indicated a variety of procedural aspects of extraction, including setting, experimental design, and interobserver agreement (IOA). Each of the individual study outcomes of CBI on communication skills was summarized to determine if both communication skills and other skills (e.g., education) were targeted and relevant in data analysis. A detailed description of statistical procedures, including the nonoverlap of all pairs (NAP) and relevant calculations, was provided that specifically related to effect size and group and single-study design studies. The researchers discussed the use of guidelines recommended by Parker and Vannest (2009), which used NAP scores between 0 to 0.65 classified as *weak effects*, 0.66 to 0.92 as *medium effects*, and 0.92 to 1.0 as *strong effects*. The terms *suggestive, preponderance,* and *conclusive* were introduced to refer to the level of certainty of evidence in each study evaluated and rated. Suggestive, considered the lowest level of certainty, does not involve a true experimental design and may include intervention-only studies. Preponderance of certainty includes studies that used an experimental design and adequate IOA and treatment fidelity. Dependent variables were also operationally defined, and specific detail was included to replicate the study. Conclusive certainty of evidence was described as having all the preponderance level and at least some control of alterative explanations for any treatment gains.

Ramdoss et al. (2001) thoroughly discussed reliability of the search process and interrater agreement by revealing that two authors individually applied inclusion and exclusion criteria to determine the final list of 18 studies from the original 222 abstracts. The 10 research studies that incorporated the inclusion criteria were approved. Using the 10 studies, the authors independently extracted information to develop an initial summary. These were checked by the remaining coauthors. Coauthors used a checklist composed of the original study summary and particular questions about definitive aspects of the research study. Involving the coauthors, the study and summaries were reviewed and the checklist completed and edited for accuracy if the summary was deemed inaccurate. The procedure persisted until coauthors reached 100% consensus of the correctness of the summaries. A detailed table (Table 1) offered a summary of participant characteristics, communication skills, details of the CBI, outcomes, and certainty of evidence. Using Table 1: Summary and Analysis of Reviewed Studies, Ramdoss et al. provided descriptive explanations of the results. The table includes the following information: citation, participant characteristics, communication skill(s) targeted, CBI, and results and certainty of evidence. An additional table (Table 2: Summary of Software Characteristics) was included that detailed the type of software, capabilities of the software, availability and price, minimum system requirements, and citations. The Outcomes section (within the Results section) synthesized the overall individual study findings with a leading statement: all studies noted that CBI was associated with participant improvement on communication-related dependent variables. A section on certainty of evidence was included that summarized the overall certainty. A total of 6 of the 10 studies were rated as suggestive because of the use of nonexperimental designs or deficiency of experimental control relating to enhancement of the dependent variable, communication skill. Specific reasons for each study's certainty of evidence rating were clearly and comprehensively described.

Discussion: The Discussion section details the overall summary and analysis of the 10 studies reviewed. Ramdoss et al. noted that research results disclosed that the literature foundation presented an incomplete review when one recognized the inclusive extent of existing research literature. They described a scarce number of studies ($n = 10$) and a limited number of participants ($n = 70$). Procedural value was also determined to be limited because some of the research studies had designs that offered merely an indicative level of confidence regarding the capability of CBI to provide consequential progress for children with ASD in the area of communication. To be clear, all studies did report some improvement in communication. Ramdoss et al. concluded that although using CBI to enhance communication of children with ASD should not currently be regarded as a research-based strategy, there remains hope in using this strategy in research studies of children with ASD.

The Discussion section also described important considerations for practitioners to be aware of, specifically that software programs had limited peer review, and thus quality could not be determined. With this in mind, the success of the intervention may be largely dependent on the extent to which the system is able to implement the technique. Ramdoss et al. stated that CBI programs should be generalizable and involve natural settings that provide natural consequences associated with clearly identified communication behaviors in those settings. This was not the case in the studies reviewed. Because this was a systematic review and not a meta-analysis, individual results of the studies were not expressed in a standard way. There was no mention of relative risk, odds ratio, or mean difference between the groups; thus, results were not displayed in a forest plot.

Overall Strengths: Overall, the strength of the systematic review was that it showed promise that using CBI to teach communication skills to children with ASD warranted future research. Specifically, outcomes revealed that all studies reported that CBI was noted to have participant improvement on communication-related dependent variables. Inclusion and exclusion criteria were clearly identified with specific search strategies, database study extraction, and the IOA described in detail.

Overall Weaknesses: The weaknesses of the study related to the limited number of studies and participants. Additionally, methodological issues were reported, with most studies revealing a suggestive certainty of evidence. As stated, Ramdoss et al. noted that the studies revealed that the existing literature base was limited with respect to the overall scope of the existing research. The authors described an inadequate number of studies ($n = 10$) and a limited number of participants ($n = 70$). Methodological quality was determined to be limited because a number of the studies' research designs provided only a suggestive level of assurance that using CBI would prove to show meaningful improvement in communication skills of children with ASD.

Implications for Nursing: Nurses who are aware of CBI technology and the idea of using computer programming as an intervention for children with mild to moderate ASD can share contact information with families. By giving parents this option, nurses are bringing the latest intervention strategy to parents. Because computers are often accessible in educational settings and in most homes, parents and children with ASD may find that their nurse has given them the idea of a new intervention strategy they had never thought would be possible. Because nurses often find themselves as the first line of support for parents of a child with ASD, they need access to the latest research for these families. Nurses need to have information such as names and contact numbers for local support network leaders, special education coordinators, and school nurses, as well as Internet information. Nurses have the opportunity to guide parents toward the support their family needs.

Implication for Future Research: Future research is required to (a) find ways to use CBI with children diagnosed with all levels of ASD from mild to severe and (b) compare and contrast achievement levels (academics and behaviors) of children with ASD participating in various interventions led by a person versus CBI.

■ Conclusion

Basic guidelines are associated with the process of critically appraising quantitative and qualitative research. These guidelines stress the importance of examining the expertise of the authors; reviewing the entire study; addressing the study's strengths, weaknesses, and logical links; and evaluating the contribution of the study to practice (Burns & Grove, 2009).

As nursing advances secondary to research and EBP, the skill of critical appraisal is necessary for nurses. Critical appraisal tools for research-based evidence can be used by doctoral students, faculty, and nurses in the practice setting to increase their understanding related to the process. It is a requirement for students enrolled in research and EBP courses to evaluate quantitative research related to value (Duffy, 2005).

The critical appraisal tool links in this chapter offer trustworthy information essential for EBP. Nurses in the clinical setting may find the links to be useful for searches through multiple tools for the critical appraisal process. In addition, faculty teaching research and EBP courses may find the links useful to relate the appraisal process to EBP (Duffy, 2005).

Necessary components to apply the best evidence into practice include (a) levels of evidence, (b) quantitative and qualitative research methods, and (c) questions to appraise the evidence. Formulating conclusions and making a judgment related to the evidence are essential to the process of EBP and clinical decision making (Melnyk & Fineout-Overholt, 2005).

■ **Exemplar One: Critical Appraisal: From Class Room to Practice**

David James

In response to various Institute of Medicine (IOM) reports and other seminal works outlining the need for a greater focus on safety and quality in health care (Winters & Echeverri, 2012), the Quality and Safety Education for Nurses (QSEN) competencies have been incorporated in academic programs of Nursing (Cronenwett et al., 2007). The QSEN initiative represents a new paradigm in education for nurses. The QSEN competencies include knowledge, skills, and attitudes (KSAs) related to EBP for both pre-licensure students and graduate students (QSEN Institute, 2014). Although these EBP competencies have been incorporated into academic programs across the nation, the EBP KSAs are often lacking in education provided to practicing RNs.

Indeed, Pravikoff, Tanner, and Pierce (2005) identified that practicing nurses did not value the role of research in their clinical practice. This identified lack of value was compounded by other barriers to utilizing EBP, including a lack of understanding research articles and inability to critique research articles (Pravikoff et al. 2005). To help address these barriers, many organizations implement EBP committees. These committees take many structures; however, most provide an opportunity for nurses to meet regularly for networking, education, and mentorship. In addition, the committees often provide oversight for the structure and processes of evidence-based nursing practice in the organization. Despite these committees, nursing leaders struggle to address the gap between the identified QSEN EBP competencies addressed in nursing curriculum and the reality of EBP competencies present in practicing staff.

The following illustrates one strategy used by a Magnet designated hospital. Similar to other organizations, the hospital has a standing monthly *Evidence-Based Practice and Research Council*; the council is open to any interested member of nursing services, however, the council membership targets direct care staff RNs. The council serves as a resource for nurses by providing networking, mentoring, and educational offerings. During one of the scheduled monthly council meetings, participants utilized a team-based journal club critique teaching strategy described by Nadleson, S., and Nadelson, L. (2014) and adapted in a Doctor of Nursing Practice (DNP) program, to implement a team-based journal club critique. To encourage attendance, continuing education credits were provided. The team-based critique hinges on the utilization of a standardized critical appraisal tool (Nadleson and Nadleson, 2014). The continuing educational offering began with a brief introduction of the objectives and timeline for the class. The first 10 minutes of the class was spent reviewing definitions and steps of EBP—highlighting the need to critically appraise the evidence. In addition to broad overview of EBP, students were introduced to the Critical Appraisal Skills Programme (CASP) website. The CASP website provides links to various critical appraisal tools and resources. In particular, the CASP checklists provide a manageable set of questions, which can be answered as "yes," "no," or "can't tell" to address the validity, reliability, and applicability of the reviewed article.

After this introduction, participants were divided into groups of three to five. Each group was provided with a copy of a quantitative research article related to pressure ulcer prevention and the appropriate CASP checklist for the quantitative research. Participants were given 20 minutes to read the article and individually answer the check list questions as they read. The groups were then given 10 minutes to discuss their answers. They were encouraged to focus on areas of disagreement in their appraisals. The final 10 minutes of the continuing education consisted of selected team report outs. These report outs focused on scholarly dialogue within the group and highlighted variations in evaluation of the article. Facilitators focused on encouraging scholarly dialogue and clarifying questions related to methodology and statistical analysis.

As a formal continuing education offering, evaluations were completed. Institutional review board (IRB) approval was obtained from the local IRB office to use aggregate data for both internal and external dissemination. Overall scores were very positive, and comments reflected active engagement. Participants liked the structure of the CASP tool provided and the ability to engage in scholarly dialogue. Although some did request the article in advance, based on previous experience the council chair was unsure how many would actually read the article prior to the educational offering. The exercise proved to be an engaging way for staff to develop the skills for critical appraisal and see the value of evidence based practice by exploring a clinically relevant research article. The process has been shared with the hospital's shared governance council as a tool to help them identify the best evidence for proposed practice changes. Future applications include the use of a virtual medium for the group critique journal club format.

References

Cronenwett L., Sherwood G., Barnsteiner J., Disch J., Johnson J., Mitchell P., . . . Warren J. (2007). Quality and safety education for nurses. *Nurse Outlook, 55*(3), 122–131.

Nadelson, S., & Nadelson, L. S. (2014). Evidence-based practice article reviews using CASP tools: A method for teaching EBP. *Worldviews on Evidence-Based Nursing, 11*(5), 344–346. doi:10.1111/wvn.12059

Pravikoff, D., Tanner, A., & Pierce, S. (2005). Readiness of U.S. nurses for evidence-based practice: Many don't understand or value research and have had little or no training to help them find evidence on which to base their practice. *American Journal of Nursing, 105*(9), 40–52.

QSEN Institute. (2014). QSEN. http://qsen.org. Accessed January 20, 2016.

Winters, C. A., & Echeverri, R. (2012). Academic education: Teaching strategies to support evidence-based practice. *Critical Care Nurse, 32*(3), 49–54. doi:10.4037/ccn2012159

▪ **Exemplar Two: How to Use Qualitative Methods for Process Improvement: Observation, Interviews, and Documentation**

Sallie Shipman

Qualitative methods often seem intimidating to practicing nurses, but in reality they are used in practice every day and also serve as an excellent tool for process improvement. Process improvement is trying to make things better or examining process to increase effectiveness (American Society for Quality, 1996; Cambridge Dictionaries Online, 1996). The use of qualitative methods at the beginning or combined with a quantitative approach in mixed methods can guide the direction of process improvement. In more than 20 years as a nurse, I have witnessed implementation of new protocols in which the individuals who developed the protocol were far removed and never sought input from those affected by the protocol. Qualitative methods provide a wealth of information and can help bridge the gap between frontline practice and administration. The purpose of this exemplar is to demonstrate how to use qualitative methods for process improvement and provide an association between practice and qualitative terminology. Examples from my personal experiences as a clinical nurse leader (CNL) and nurse educator will help demonstrate how observation, interviews, and documents can be used for process improvement.

Observation

Observation is a core skill for a nurse performing a patient assessment, but also can prove a useful tool with process improvement. However, when using observation as a method for process improvement, the nurse must take a step back and make a conscious effort to observe purposefully. When conducting an observation, the nurse can take the role of participant, observer, or both participant and observer (ATSDR, 2011; CDC, 2008; Creswell 2007, 2009; Marshall & Rossman, 2011). Observation can guide to the recognition of issues or problems not previously known. Below are circumstances in which observation may help in process improvement (CDC, 2008, p. 2):

- When you are trying to understand an ongoing process or situation
- When you are gathering data on individual behaviors or interactions between people
- When you need to know about a physical setting
- When data collection from individuals is not a realistic option.

Nurses must observe to identify and solve problems, but not at the expense of those who are being observed. Observation can be overt (participant is aware of the observation) or covert (participant is not aware of the observation). Ethical issues must be considered, and individuals who are observed always must be protected (ATSDR, 2011; CDC, 2008; Creswell 2007, 2009; Marshall & Rossman, 2011). Some questions to ask before observing: Are the participants aware they are being observed? Are the participants agreeable to being part of a process improvement project? Are you planning to publish your project? If you plan on publishing your project, IRB approval must be secured first. Nursing faculty also can help guide you through ethical considerations.

Application of Observation

Observation was used for process improvement when teaching fundamentals to undergraduate nursing students. The students were complaining about lecture in the clinical practice laboratory. Observation helped to understand the issues and why the students were unhappy. Based on direct observations, a recommendation was made reserving a room for content requiring an extended amount of lecture time, which led to increased student satisfaction.

Interviews

Nurses use the skill of interviewing each time they obtain a patient history. Like observation, interviews can help guide you to the issues/problems for a process improvement. Interviews can be conducted in-depth (one-on-one) or as focus groups.

In-Depth

There are several types of in-depth interviews: structured, semi-structured, unstructured, and informal (Cohen & Crabtree 2006; Creswell, 2007). Structured interviews are conducted using specific questions with little room for variation (e.g., telephone interviews). The interviewer follows a guide during semi-structured interviews but may explore relevant topics brought up by the participant for further clarification (e.g., interview with nurses who responded during a disaster). During unstructured interviews the participants tell their story (e.g., ethnographic unstructured interviews—oral history). Talking to people without a guide would constitute an informal interview (e.g., observing a social setting of interest).

Application of In-Depth Interview. Semi-structured interviews were used during dissertation research. The author explored the lived experiences of first-time nurse responders during disaster (Shipman et al., 2016). The in-depth interview processes provide a wealth of information; however, time constraints must be considered when using this method for process improvement. For example, each of the hour-long interviews yielded approximately 25 pages of data to analyze.

Focus Groups

Focus groups usually include 8 to 12 participants per session and last approximately 1.5 to 2 hours (Iowa State University – University Extension, 2004). The participants can be selected or have similar characteristics. The data collected are the words from the participants through audiotape or notes taken during the forum. The data are analyzed for consistent themes.

(continues)

Application of Focus Group. A CNL organized focus groups when tasked with the process improvement project of evaluating our department's pandemic influenza planning. The public health areas were using a pandemic influenza planning tool based on Centers for Disease Control and Prevention grant guidance. During the evaluation process, focus groups were conducted with the staff in each area. A comprehensive report was developed, including the successes, challenges, recommendations, and lessons learned that helped the department move from pandemic influenza planning toward an all-hazards planning approach.

Documentation and Audiovisual Materials

The final forms of qualitative data for potential use in process improvement are documentation and audiovisual materials. When the nurse examines written words (e.g., chart review) qualitative methods are used. Creswell (2007) provides some other examples that fall into this category: Researcher journaling of observations, Participant journaling, Personal letters, Public documents, Autobiographies and biographies, Photos or videotapes, Conducting chart audits, Reviewing medical records, Email or electronic messages, Phone text messages, and Examination of personal possessions or ritual objects.

Application of Documentation

In addition to the focus groups held during the pandemic influenza process improvement project, documentation collected from the pandemic influenza planning tool report for each area prior to conducting the focus groups were reviewed. Those data led to the questions that were asked in each of the areas during the focus group sessions.

Currently, a study is being conducted using pilot data collected from undergraduate and social work students who participated in a poverty simulation. The students wrote a one-page narrative answering specific questions about their perception of poverty after the simulation experience. These data are being analyzed, and themes are emerging while examining the learning outcomes related to poverty.

References

Agency for Toxic Substances and Disease Registry. (2011). Evaluation methods. *Principles of Community Engagement* (2nd. ed.). Retrieved from http://www.atsdr.cdc.gov/communityengagement/pce_program_methods.html

American Society for Quality. (1996). *Handbook for basic process improvement.* Retrieved from http://rube.asq.org/gov/handbook-for-basic-process-improvement.pdf

Cambridge Dictionaries Online. (2016). *Process improvement.* Retrieved from http://dictionary.cambridge.org/us/dictionary/english/process-improvement

Centers for Disease Control and Prevention. (2008). *Data collection methods for program evaluation: Observation.* Retrieved from http://www.cdc.gov/healthyYouth/evaluation/pdf/brief16.pdf

Cohen D., & Crabtree B. (2006). *Qualitative research guidelines project*. Retrieved from http://www
.qualres.org/HomeInte-3595.html

Creswell, J. (2007). *Qualitative inquiry and research design: Choosing among five approaches*
(2nd ed.). Thousand Oaks, CA: Sage Publications.

Creswell, J. (2009). *Research design: Qualitative, quantitative, and mixed method approaches*
(3rd ed.). Thousand Oaks, CA: Sage Publications.

Iowa State University – University Extension. (2004). Focus group fundamentals. *Methodology
Brief*. Retrieved from https://store.extension.iastate.edu/Product/pm1969b-pdf

Marshall, C., & Rossman, G. B. (2011). *Designing qualitative research* (5th ed.). Thousand Oaks,
CA: Sage Publications.

Shipman, S., Stanton, M., Tomlinson, S., Olivet, L., Graves, A., McKnight, D., & Speck, P. (2016).
Qualitative analysis of the lived-experience of first-time nurse responders in disaster. *Journal
of Continuing Education in Nursing, 47*(2), 61–71.

University of Minnesota. (2011). *Reflection in service-learning classes*. Retrieved from http://www
.servicelearning.umn.edu/info/reflection.html

■ Exemplar Three: Exemplar: Using Qualitative Approaches for Process Improvement

Sallie Shipman

The study of words or qualitative research can provide insight to process problems and the need for improvement changes. However, reviewing qualitative studies can be a challenge (Jeanfreau & Jack, 2010), especially when you try to look through a quantitative lens. Improving quality care requires attention to both methods. The purpose of this exemplar is to provide a brief explanation of approaches used in qualitative research and provide questions to guide the reader through the evaluation of these methods.

Narrative Inquiry

Narrative Inquiry is an approach used to explore the life and stories of lived experience of an individual or individuals with similar experiences (Creswell, 2007, 2009; Marshall & Rossman, 2011). Data collection is conducted through interviews and documents. The experiences are then analyzed to develop themes and retell the stories in a chronological order. The end result is a narrative of the individuals' experience or common themes from the combined experience.

Phenomenology

Phenomenology is an approach that focuses on the understanding of the lived experience or phenomenon (Creswell, 2007, 2009; Marshall & Rossman, 2011).

(continues)

The researcher interviews, observes, and/or analyzes documents from several individuals who have shared an experience. Data are analyzed for significant statements, meaning units, textural and structural description, and a description of the "essence" (Creswell, 2007, p. 157). The written report describes the essence of the experience.

Grounded Theory

Grounded theory is an approach in which the researcher develops a theory grounded from data collected from the field (Creswell, 2007, 2009; Marshall & Rossman, 2011). The data must lead to the development of the theory and is based on the views of the participants. The analysis of a process action or interaction involving many individuals leads to the developed theory. Interviews are the primary data collection method and should include large samples of 20 to 60 individuals (Creswell, 2007). Data are analyzed through open coding, axial coding, and selective coding. The end result is the development of a theory often illustrated in a figure and written report.

Ethnography

Ethnography is an approach used to describe and interpret a group of a similar culture and the shared experiences of the group members (Creswell, 2007, 2009; Marshall & Rossman, 2011). The researcher spends extended time in the field collecting data. Observations, interviews, and document reviews are the primary methods used in ethnographical studies. Data are analyzed to develop themes about the group, along with creating a narrative of the group's culture.

Case Study

The case study is an approach using a case or multiple cases to describe and analyze an in-depth account of a particular situation, program, activity, or event (Creswell, 2007, 2009; Marshall & Rossman, 2011). Data are collected through observations, interviews, documents, or artifacts. The thematic analysis leads to a description of the case or cases along with a description of established themes and cross themes.

Critically Appraising Qualitative Research

Below are the suggested first questions to ask when evaluating qualitative literature:

1. "Was there a clear statement of the aims of the research?" (CASP, n.d., p. 2)
2. "Is a qualitative methodology appropriate?" (CASP, n.d., p. 2)

Some examples answering the first two questions include the following:

Example of Narrative Inquiry with a Phenomenological Analysis

Shipman, S., Stanton, M., Tomlinson, S., Olivet, L., Graves, A., McKnight, D., & Speck, P. (2016). Qualitative analysis of the lived-experience of first-time nurse responders in disaster. *Journal of Continuing Education in Nursing, 47*(2), 61–71.

- ▪ **Focus:** Nurses who responded in disaster only one time
- ▪ **Unit of analysis:** Ten nurses who have responded to only disaster
- ▪ **Data collection:** In-depth interviews
- ▪ **Data analysis:** Narrative stories and phenomenological analysis for themes

Example of Ethnography and Grounded Theory

Fothergill, A. (2004). *Heads above water.* Albany, NY: State University of New York Press.

- ▪ **Focus:** In-depth look into the women's role during and after the Red river flood that occurred on April 11, 1997
- ▪ **Unit of analysis:** Feminist theory in her ethnography and appears to be directly involved with the subjects because of the personal nature of her beliefs of the disparities of women
- ▪ **Data collection:** 60 interviews—mixed method studies of the disaster victims (female and male), utilizing interpretivist or poststructural theoretical framework
- ▪ **Data analysis:** Themes (e.g., the coping mechanisms of women with their societal "downward mobility" due to the loss of their material possessions; p. 13). Many of the women had never experienced poverty until they lost everything in the flood, leading to a newfound understanding or empathy for those who receive assistance.

Example of a Case Study

Shipman, S., Stanton, M., Hankins, J., Odom-Bartel, R. (2013). Incorporation of the clinical nurse leader in public health practice. *Journal of Professional Nursing, 29*(1), 4–10.

- ▪ **Focus:** Focus on the role of the CNL in public health
- ▪ **Unit of analysis:** The role of the CNL was used to provide evaluation while promoting progress and improvement of planning efforts with the performance improvement planning microsystem
- ▪ **Data collection:** Interviews, observations, documents, program implementation
- ▪ **Data analysis:** Aspects of the CNL and how they were implemented

After the first two questions are asked, the next question could be, "Is it worth continuing?" (CASP, n.d., p. 2). If the answer is yes, then complete the assessment by answering the following questions:

1. "Was the research design appropriate to address the aims of the research?" (CASP, n.d., p. 3).
2. "Was the recruitment strategy appropriate to the aims of the research?" (CASP, n.d., p. 3).

(continues)

3. "Was the data collected in a way that addressed the research issue?" (CASP, n.d., p. 4).
4. "Has the relationship between researcher and participants been adequately considered?" (CASP, n.d., p. 4).
5. "Have ethical issues been taken into consideration?" (CASP, n.d., p. 5).
6. "Was the data analysis sufficiently rigorous?" (CASP, n.d., p. 5).
7. "Is there a clear statement of findings?" (CASP, n.d., p. 6).
8. "How valuable is the research?" (CASP, n.d., p. 6).

References

Creswell, J. (2007). *Qualitative inquiry and research design: Choosing among five approaches* (2nd ed.). Thousand Oaks, CA: Sage Publications.

Creswell, J. (2009). *Research design: Qualitative, quantitative, and mixed method approaches* (3rd ed.). Thousand Oaks, CA: Sage Publications.

Critical Appraisal Skills Programme. (n.d.). 10 questions to help you make sense of qualitative research. *Qualitative Research Checklist 31.05.13.* Retrieved from http://www.systematicreviewsjournal.com/content/supplementary/2046-4053-3-139-s8.pdf

Fothergill, A. (2004). *Heads above water.* Albany, NY: State University of New York Press.

Jeanfreau, S., & Jack, L. (2010). Appraising qualitative research in health education: Guidelines for public health educators. *Health Promotion Practice, 11*(5): 612–617. doi:10.1177/1524839910363537

Marshall, C., & Rossman, G. B. (2011). *Designing qualitative research* (5th ed.). Thousand Oaks, CA: Sage Publications.

Shipman, S., Stanton, M., Hankins, J., & Odom-Bartel, R. (2013). Incorporation of the clinical nurse leader in public health practice. *Journal of Professional Nursing, 29*(1), 4–10.

Shipman, S., Stanton, M., Tomlinson, S., Olivet, L., Graves, A., McKnight, D., & Speck, P. (2016). Qualitative analysis of the lived-experience of first-time nurse responders in disaster. *Journal of Continuing Education in Nursing, 47*(2), 61–71.

REFLECTIVE ACTIVITIES

1. Using the following resource from Table 2: The Centre for Evidence-Based Medicine (CEBM), critically appraise the following systematic review:
   Liao, W., Huang, C., Huang, T., & Hwang, S. (2011). A systematic review of sleep patterns and factors that disturb sleep after heart surgery. *Journal of Nursing Research, 19*(4), 275–288. doi:10.1097/JNR.0b013e318236cf68

2. Using the following resource from Table 2: PRISMA, critically appraise the following meta-analysis:
   Conn, V. S., Hafdahl, A. R., & Brown, L. M. (2009). Meta-analysis of quality of life outcomes from physical activity interventions. *Nursing Research, 58*(3), 175–183. doi:10.1097/NNR.0b013e318199b53a

REFERENCES

Brookfield, S. (1987). *Developing critical thinkers: Challenging adults to explore alternative ways of thinking and acting.* Milton Keynes, England: Open University Press.

Burl, A. (2009). *What is critical appraisal* (2nd ed.)? Hayward Group. Retrieved from http://www
.medicine.ox.ac.uk/bandolier/painres/download/whatis/What_is_critical_appraisal.pdf

Burns, N., & Grove, S. K. (2009). *The practice of nursing research: Appraisal, synthesis, and generation of evidence* (6th ed.). St. Louis, MO: Saunders.

Centre for Evidence-Based Medicine. (2016). Critical Appraisal Tools. Retrieved from http://www.cebm
.net/critical-appraisal/

Des Jarlais, D. C., Lyles, C., Crepaz, N., & the TREND Group. (2004). Improving the reporting quality of nonrandomized evaluations of behavioral and public health interventions: The TREND statement. *American Journal of Public Health, 94*(3), 361–366.

DiCenso, A., Guyatt, G., & Ciliska, D. (2005). *Evidence-based nursing: A guide to clinical practice.* St. Louis, MO: Mosby.

Division of Health Sciences International Center for Allied Health Evidence. (2014). *Critical appraisal tools.* Retrieved from http://www.unisa.edu.au/Research/Sansom-Institute-for-Health-Research/Research/Allied-Health-Evidence/Resources/CAT/

Duffy, J. R. (2005). Critically appraising quantitative research. *Nursing & Health Sciences, 7,* 281–283.

Fain, J. A. (2009). Critiquing research reports. In J. A. Fain (Ed.), *Reading, understanding, and applying nursing research* (3rd ed., pp. 251–270). Philadelphia, PA: F. A. Davis.

Fulton, S., & Krainovich-Miller, B. (2010). Gathering and appraising the literature. In G. LoBiondo-Wood & J. Haber (Eds.), *Nursing research: Methods and critical appraisal for evidence-based practice* (7th ed., pp. 56–80). St. Louis, MO: Mosby.

Johnston, L. (2005). Critically appraising quantitative evidence. In B. M. Melnyk & E. Fineout-Overholt (Eds.), *Evidence-based practice in nursing and healthcare: A guide to best practice* (pp. 79–125). Philadelphia, PA: Lippincott Williams & Wilkins.

Liberati, A., Altman, D. G., Tetzlaff, J., Mulrow, C., Gotzsche, P. C., Ioannidis, J. P. A., . . . Moher, D. (2009). The PRISMA statement for reporting systematic reviews and meta-analyses of studies that evaluate healthcare interventions: Explanation and elaboration. *BMJ, 339*(b2700). Retrieved from http://www.bmj.com/content/339/bmj.b2700 doi: 10.1136/bmj.b2700

LoBiondo-Wood, G., & Haber, J. (2010). Integrating the processes of research and evidence-based practice. In G. LoBiondo-Wood & J. Haber (Eds.), *Nursing research: Methods and critical appraisal for evidence-based practice* (7th ed., pp. 5–26). St. Louis, MO: Mosby.

Melnyk, B. M., & Fineout-Overholt, E. (2005). Making the case for evidence-based practice. In B. M. Melnyk & E. Fineout-Overholt (Eds.), *Evidence-based practice in nursing and healthcare: A guide to best practice* (pp. 3–24). Philadelphia, PA: Lippincott Williams & Wilkins.

Moher D., Liberati A., Tetzlaff J., Altman D.G., & The PRISMA Group. (2009). Preferred reporting items for systematic reviews and meta-analyses: The PRISMA statement. *PLoS Med 6*(7), e1000097. doi:10.1371/journal.pmed.1000097

National Council for Osteopathic Research, University of Brighton. (2005). *Evidence-based practice-tutorial: Critical appraisal skills.* Retrieved from http://www.brighton.ac.uk/ncor/tutorials/EBP_Tutorial_intro_Critical_Appraisal_Skills.pdf

Oermann, M. (1991). *Professional nursing practice: A conceptual approach.* Philadelphia, PA: Lippincott Williams & Wilkins.

Parker, R. I., & Vanest, K. (2009). An improved effect size for single-case research: Nonoverlap of all pairs. *Behavior Therapy, 40,* 357–367.

Polit, D. F., & Beck, C. T. (2012). *Nursing research: Generating and assessing evidence for nursing practice* (9th ed.). Philadelphia, PA: Lippincott Williams & Wilkins.

Ramdoss, S., Lang, R., Mulloy, A., Franco, J., O'Reilly, M., Didden, R., & Lancioni, G. (2011). Use of computer-based interventions to teach communication skills to children with autism spectrum disorders: A systematic review. Journal of Behavioral Education, 20(1), 55–76. doi:10.1007/s10864-010-9112-7

Schulz K. F., Altman D. G., Moher D., & CONSORT Group. (2010). CONSORT 2010 statement: Updated guidelines for reporting parallel group randomised trials. *PLoS Med 7*(3), e1000251. doi:10.1371/journal.pmed.1000251

Williamson, K. M. (2009). Evidence-based practice: Critical appraisal of qualitative evidence. *Journal of the American Psychiatric Nurses Association, 15*(3), 202–207. doi:10.1177/1078390309338733

PART II

Scholarship of Administrative Practice

CHAPTER 7

Evidence-Based Leadership Practices

▪ VALORIE DEARMON ▪

■ Objectives:

- Identify the evidence base for leadership practices.
- Describe the link between leadership theory and evidence-based (EB) leadership practices.
- Identify leadership models as a conceptual framework for scholarly administrative practice.
- Assess a model of the interrelationship of leadership, environments, and outcomes for nurse executives (MILE ONE).

■ Introduction

Leadership is crucial to meeting the challenges of the healthcare industry. Rising costs, access to care, quality, and safety are at the forefront of healthcare concerns. More than a decade has passed since the release of the Institute of Medicine's (IOM's) landmark report, *To Err is Human,* which publicly reported significant medical errors resulting from healthcare system failures (Kohn, Corrigan, & Donaldson, 2000). Subsequent IOM reports have followed recommending sweeping redesign of broken systems (Eden, Wheatley, McNeil, & Sox, 2008; IOM, 2011; Page, 2003). Concerned government, public, and private sectors have joined together in response to concerns, demanding unprecedented transformation and accountability. In 2010, the Affordable Care Act was passed into US law for the purpose of improving healthcare quality, accessibility, and control costs. Despite passage of the law, the legislation remains highly controversial. Although the verdict is still out in respect to long-term results, early indicators suggest the law has contributed to a significant drop in the rate of uninsured, 17% reduction in hospital-acquired conditions, 1.3 million fewer medical errors, and over $10 billion in cost savings (Agency for Healthcare Research and Quality [AQRH], 2015). The job to repair the many flawed aspects of health care has begun, but the road is long and performance improvement is never ending (AQRH, 2015; Classen et al., 2011; Thomas & Classen, 2014). As frontline providers and the largest body of healthcare professionals, nurses are called to carry on the efforts of forerunners and to *lead* research, process redesign, and practice improvements (IOM, 2011). Healthcare improvement opportunities are far too many for historical top-down leadership alone, calling for leadership from all levels of the organization (Porter O'Grady & Malloch, 2016; Ryan, Harris, Mattox, Camp, & Shirey, 2015). The unparalleled petition for change mandates leadership at its best. The question is: Are nurses prepared for this challenge?

Leadership is a valued commodity that scholars and business leaders have sought to understand for centuries. Businesses in all industries, including health care, need innovative leaders to find solutions to vexing problems. The concept of leadership is multidimensional and commonly oversimplified in popular leadership books. Applied to the performance of individuals, groups, processes, and organizations (Lynham & Chermack, 2006; Northouse, 2016), leadership has a variety of meanings; thus, there exists no *one* agreed-upon definition (Stogdill, 1974). Early attempts at understanding leadership focused more on the individual and defining the characteristics of a leader. Recent theories recognize leadership as a complex phenomenon consisting of relationships between leaders and followers, roles, situational context, and even timing of events.

The call for unprecedented healthcare reform requires leadership from *all* nurses whether practicing in an administrative, managerial, academic, advanced practice, or clinical role. The role of the leader is to bring others together and gain commitment for the work to be done. Engagement and stakeholder ownership of transformative processes is paramount to recalibrate the healthcare delivery system. Maxwell (1998) suggested, "Leadership is influence—nothing more, nothing less" (p. 17), and "true leadership cannot be awarded, appointed, or assigned" (p. 14). If leadership is, in essence, the ability to influence, where is the road map that shows nurse leaders how to best *influence* the sweeping changes required in health care today? The purpose of this chapter is to explore the existing body of leadership evidence and underscore emerging best leadership practices.

■ Environmental Context

The face of health care has changed dramatically over the past two decades. For years, healthcare outcomes were shielded from the scrutiny of the public eye. Today, we live in a "value-driven age" in which accountability lies not in the work itself but in whether the work makes a difference (Porter-O'Grady & Malloch, 2016). Contemporary times entail of a public that asks difficult questions and seeks answers substantiated by proof: What am I getting for my healthcare dollar? How safe is the care? Why should I choose you for my healthcare provider?

The economic climate is a significant driver of healthcare transformation. Healthcare expenses consume a substantial percentage of the gross domestic product

(GDP). In 2012, the US spent two and a half times more on health care than other developed countries, or an average of $8915 per person, accounting for 17.2% of the GDP (Centers for Medicare and Medicaid Services [CMS], 2013). Yet, higher healthcare expenditures have failed to produce a healthier population. The US lags behind other industrialized countries in specific healthcare indicators such as life expectancy, cardiovascular disease, cancer, obesity, and alcohol use (Organisation for Economic Co-operation and Development [OECD], 2014). Furthermore, patients using the flawed healthcare system continue to experience preventable injury and death (IOM, 2001; Classen, 2011; Thomas & Clausen, 2014). Organizations such as the AHRQ, the Joint Commission, and the Institute for Healthcare Improvement, among others, are leading the charge to improve quality and safety within health care. To that end, accrediting agencies and payers are establishing benchmarks challenging and even mandating providers to demonstrate quality through measures of success. In recent years the CMS began linking payment to quality performance such as hospital-acquired conditions (CMS, 2013). Early reports indicate that reimbursement linked to quality performance results in cost savings reduced mortality (AHRQ, 2015). Pressure mounts for leaders as mandates increase for public reporting of quality and safety outcomes, reimbursement is decreased, and penalties are applied.

The demand for large-scale transformation and cost containment comes during an era characterized by chaos, complexity, and a shrinking world. Information technology has exploded, blurring the boundaries of institutions and growing the availability of data exponentially. The knowledge upsurge has narrowed the power gaps found between providers and healthcare consumers, administrators and staff, and physicians and nurses. The rapid execution of cost-cutting strategies such as restructuring, mergers, acquisitions, and hospital-physician realignments has altered organizational structure and operations. In the midst of chaos, demands have increased for quality, transparency, and accountability. Effective leadership is required to redesign systems and processes for positive clinical outcomes (National Center for Healthcare Leadership [NCHL], 2010). Contemporary leaders are forced to confront traditional practices and implement worthwhile innovations. Moreover, leaders are challenged to rethink what leadership looks like. Transformation of health care begins with the transformation of leadership practices in which the power base is shared between the leader and followers (Kellerman, 2012) in pursuit of quality and safety. Effective leaders of today value the capabilities of frontline staff and leverage the strengths of the team to improve systems and practices.

Strong leadership is cited as the most significant determinant for excellence in patient care (American Organization of Nurse Executives [AONE], 2015; Anderson & Garman, 2014); conversely, the lack of effective leadership is considered an impediment to safe care (Buerhaus, 2004; Sammer, Lykens, Singh, Mains, & Lackan, 2010). The profession is challenged by shortages of well-prepared nursing leaders (MacMillan-Finlayson, 2010) workforce shortages, high attrition rates, and the call to lead transformative changes. The changing landscape of health care requires leaders to forge new paths. Yet, without a roadmap, how does one proceed? What is the new paradigm for contemporary leaders? Is there evidence to guide future direction?

■ Evidence-Base for Leadership Practice

Evidence-based practice (EBP) is founded on empirical evidence from research, supported by scientific principles, and expert opinion. If sufficient evidence exists, the practice guided by the evidence promotes positive predictable outcomes. Despite man's long-time interest in leadership, research in this area is scant, limiting the body of existing knowledge. The lack of evidence to validate best practices is not surprising given the multidimensional phenomenon of leadership that is confounded by human factors and applied in an ever-changing world. To further complicate the quest for EB leadership, times leadership and management literature is interlaced.

Although the management and leadership concepts have similarities, the two are distinctively different. Management is associated with budgeting, organizing, staffing, measurements, controls, and smart problem-solving techniques when plans go awry. Conversely, leadership is about vision and gaining support for the vision generally through various methods of communication. It is about innovation, in which leaders inspire others to look at situations differently, behave differently, and ultimately produce different outcomes. According to John Kotter (2012), both management and leadership are important, one no more important than the other. Historically, healthcare organizations have been built upon strong management practices with defined processes, rules, and compliance incentives and leadership often has been seen as the responsibility of executives and managers. These traditional leadership and management practices for employees, managers, and executives have been well rehearsed and are firmly embedded into organizational cultures. Therefore, many frontline workers have been socialized into roles of compliance and complacency rather than to be energized by creativity, innovation, and engagement. Executives and managers feel the weight of the responsibility to "fix" the problems. Today, the world is moving so fast that the balance between organizational leadership and management has to change for timely and effective response. Leaders are called for from all levels of the organization. Yet, for leaders to emerge throughout the organization, a major paradigm shift is required by all to change organizational cultures deeply influenced by traditional leadership and management practices.

"Best" leadership practices have evolved over time, though not always based on science. There continues to be a litany of blockbuster books written about leadership. However, most publications offer strategies for quick success based on experiential knowledge or personal philosophy rather than EB inquiry. It is rare to find a well-researched leadership book aimed at explaining and directing practice among the best-sellers. The dearth of leadership EB inquiry extends to the nursing profession, as well. Most of what is known about leadership has been unearthed by other disciplines and applied to nursing. Scholarly knowledge is necessary to guide leadership practice. Yet, few studies have successfully linked leadership practices to measurable outcomes (Lynham & Chermack, 2006). Effective leaders critically review professional literature in search of EBPs (Kovner & Rundall, 2006; Rousseau, 2006). Nursing leaders can contribute to the evidentiary foundation for leadership practice by collaborating with researchers to scientifically test leadership practices.

▪ Leadership Theory

A plethora of leadership theories and approaches have emerged over the years, changing paradigms and shaping beliefs about leadership practices. The notion that leaders are born not made was prevalent in the early 1900s and continues to be a point of debate. The early years of the 20th century defined leadership as a process of domination in which leaders forced others to obey (Moore, 1927). By the 1930s, attempts to understand leadership focused predominantly on defining the traits of leaders. Despite recurring efforts, researchers have yet to agree on a specific set of leadership traits (Bass, 1985). Trait theory focused solely on the leader and failed to recognize the importance of situational context or followers. Leadership theories in the 1940s began to see leadership as a process greater than the leader and entertained the idea that leaders persuaded groups rather than coerced change. Hersey, Blanchard, & Johnson (1996) introduced situational leadership, suggesting leaders emerge based on the circumstances and, therefore, vary across given situations. Contemporary theories negate the conviction that leadership is an individualized phenomenon and describe leadership as a reciprocal process consisting of the leader and followers (Kellerman, 2012). The significance of followers to successful change cannot be underestimated. In this context, followers are not described as passive or subservient, but rather individuals who partner with the leader for a common purpose.

Despite an abundance of diverse and opposing leadership approaches (e.g., trait, situational, behavioral, relational, transformational), there have been limited attempts at integrating leadership models. Lynham and Chermack (2006) were the first to propose an integrated theoretical framework as a guide for leadership practices. The conceptual model, based on general systems theory (Senge, 1990), presents the phenomenon of leadership as a subsystem operating in a larger performance system acted on by external environmental elements. The conceptual framework represents an initial attempt to understand leadership within the context of a system (Burns, 2001; James, 2010).

▪ Leadership Models

Quantum Leadership

Porter-O'Grady and Malloch (2008) were among the first to offer an EB framework for nursing leadership, placing clinical practice at the center of an organization.

The framework underpins the importance of managing infrastructure, processes, and behaviors (Upenieks, 2003). Porter-O'Grady and Malloch (2008) described five key elements for EBP leadership: physical environment, caregiver demographics, operational structures, technology, and culture. EB leadership recognizes the many intersections and relationships found in complex systems calling for leaders to remove barriers, reshaping both conversations and relationships. Consistent with others' beliefs (Meredith, Cohen, & Raia, 2010; Nelson, Batalden, & Godfrey, 2007), EBP leadership redefines organizational relationships and appreciates the value of engaged point-of-care workers configured in existing and supportive infrastructure. Porter-O'Grady & Malloch (2008) contend there is no lack of talent or capacity to innovate; there is only the need to coordinate, integrate, and facilitate change initiatives within a social and organizational context. Critical skills of the new leader include the ability to innovate, think, plan, and implement. Measures of success are determined by patient, caregiver, organizational, and financial outcomes (Porter-O'Grady & Malloch, 2008).

Model of the Interrelationship of Leadership, Environments, and Outcomes for Nurse Executives

The Model of the Interrelationship of Leadership, Environments, and Outcomes for Nurse Executives (MILE ONE) is an EB framework based on the American Nurses Association (ANA) Scope and Standards for Nurse Administrators and the AONE Nurse Executive Competencies. The model's aim is to operationalize chief nurse executives' (CNEs') influence, identify measures of CNE success, and explicate patient, workforce, and organizational improvement (Adams & Ives Erickson, 2011; Adams, Erickson, Jones, & Paulo, 2009). The model suggests a paradigm of the dynamic interrelationship of the nurse executive, professional practice/work environments (PPWEs), and patient and organizational outcomes. Adams et al. suggested that CNEs experience role conflict and patient care is mired in the absence of universally adopted CNE measures of success. The MILE ONE shifts the evaluation of CNE success from a focus on standard patient outcomes to an emphasis on the improvement of the PPWE exhibited through practices such as staff engagement and empowerment. The model emphasizes three EB concepts:

- Nurse executives influence the PPWE.
- PPWEs influence patient and organizational outcomes.
- Patient and organizational outcomes influence nurse executives.

The model has been studied and is useful when applied as the framework for exemplar quality initiatives focused on improving documentation (Adams, Denham, & Ramirez Neumeister, 2010). Findings suggest that when the CNE focuses on PPWE, staff become increasingly engaged and assume ownership of practice. A dynamic cycle is sustained through staff engagement and successful achievement of organizational goals; the CNE, valuing the process and results, continues to enhance the PPWE.

Evidence-Based Management

Debate continues about whether leadership and management are distinct processes. Many similarities exist, such as being goal directed, working through people, and exercising influence. Kotter (2012) contends that leadership and management are markedly different. He argues that the primary function of managers is to bring order to organizational chaos through planning, organizing, staffing, and controlling, whereas the primary function of leadership is to thrive in chaos and promote change and movement.

EB management is defined as "the systematic application of the best available evidence to business processes, strategic decisions, and the evaluation of managerial practices" (Kovner, Fine, & D'Aquila, 2009, p. 1). In essence, EB management refers to doing the right things right (Kovner & McAlearney, 2013). Kovner and McAlearney argues that data managers often make decisions based on intuition or best judgment rather than gathering data to support the decision. For instance, to increase patient throughput in the emergency department, one may increase the size of the patient transport department, yet later learn that increasing the number of transporters failed to have an impact on patient throughput. Basic employee and organizational performance data are needed for EB management application (Kovner et al., 2009). Kovner and Rundall (2006) have offered a model of EB management that consists of a five-step process for decision-making that includes:

1. Formulating the research question
2. Searching for relevant research findings and other evidence
3. Determining the validity, quality, and applicability of the evidence
4. Presenting the data in a manner to promote use of evidence in decision-making
5. Applying the evidence in decision-making

The EB management model has elements similar to those of the clinical practice EBP models and includes the fundamental steps of process improvement. EB management is distinguished from other quality improvement processes such as the Shewhart's Plan-Do-Check-Act (PDCA) cycle related to the use of *evidence* in the process. Kovner and Rundall's (2006) EB management model was specifically designed to address three categories of management questions: (a) business transaction management, (b) operational management, and (c) strategic management.

Despite the abundance of available evidence, the use of EB management practices remains weak. Pfeffer and Sutton (2006) suggest that too much information in the area of management may overwhelm users. There is a volume of how-to and quick-fix advice for managers. These management teachings are frequently presented as authoritative. However, a closer look reveals that the most popular management strategies originate from anecdotal reports or implied findings rather than from rigor and scholarship. Few companies are considered "great companies" in which the organizational culture encourages and supports EBP (Rousseau, 2006). Lack of facts (preferably research-based evidence) for decision-making drives managers to rely on "experience, formal power, incentives, and threats" (Rousseau, 2006, p. 262). By using a shared body of knowledge as the basis for management practices, valid learning and continuous improvements occur (Kovner & Rundall, 2006; Pfeffer & Sutton, 2006; Rousseau, 2006). EB management provides a framework to replace the trial-by-error decision-making approach used by most managers (Rousseau, 2006). Even when evidence exists, managers typically do not use it. For example, in a 2005 study by Kovner, 68 managers throughout the country were interviewed to assess their use of research in decision-making. Study findings indicated that none of the managers used research-based evidence for decision-making (Kovner & Rundall, 2006). Pfeffer and Sutton purported that leaders can diffuse EB management within their organization by requesting sound evidence for proposed changes, reviewing the logic behind the evidence, and encouraging pilot programs before dissemination.

Good to Great Company Leaders

Collins (2001) conducted a 15-year study of practices that transformed good companies into great companies. The study revealed unexpected findings about leaders of great companies. Leaders who converted good companies into great companies were found to be "self-effacing, quiet, reserved, and even shy" (Collins, 2001, p. 12) rather than the stereotypical image of a powerhouse. Collins characterized these top or *Level* 5 leaders as a blend of personal humility (shying away from personal acclaim) and professional will. Level 5 leaders were noted to have unrelenting resolve directed toward company success and to do whatever it takes to meet the goals of the organization. Furthermore, leaders of great companies recognized that having *the right people* on the bus is important to organizational success. With the right people in place, employees charter the organizational course and drive success, negating the need for leaders to coax or prod employees toward organizational goals.

■ Antecedents of Leadership

Leadership is a complex phenomenon with broad meaning and a wide range of applications. Reflecting on the antecedents of an abstract idea can provide insight into the phenomenon. An antecedent is an experience that precedes other concepts (Chinn & Kramer, 2008). Antecedents may be viewed as either causal or influential to the concept. Although a blueprint for leadership success is not clearly outlined in the literature, evidence of recurring antecedents does exist for present day healthcare leaders.

Effective leaders:

- Relate the principles of complexity science to the healthcare system, noting the dynamic subsystems and relational components (Nelson et al., 2007; Porter-O'Grady & Malloch, 2016; Wheatley, 2006).
- Identify traditional hierarchical and individual locus of control leadership styles as obsolete in multifaceted, dynamic enterprises (Singer et al., 2009; Wheatley, 2006).

- Appreciate the knowledge, talents, diversity, and contributions of workers from all spheres of the organization as they apply to process improvement (Kabcenell, Nolan, Martin, & Gill, 2010; NCHL, 2010; Swensen, Pugh, McMullan, & Kabcenell, 2013).
- Recognize the importance of staff engagement in promoting commitment (Simpson, 2009a, 2009b; Strumwasser & Virkstis, 2015), ownership (Rutherford et al., 2008), and sustainability of process change (Kabcenell et al., 2010).
- Value the importance of positive work environments and their link to nurse satisfaction (Laschinger & Leiter, 2006; Simpson, 2009a, 2009b; Tourangeau, Cranley, Laschinger, & Pachis, 2010) and clinical outcomes (Lake & Friese, 2006; McGillis-Hall et al., 2003; McClure, Poulin, Sovie, & Wandelt, 1983).
- Understand the significance of staff empowerment to satisfaction in the workplace and intent to leave (Armellino, Quinn-Griffin, & Fitzpatrick, 2010; Richardson & Storr, 2010; Spence Laschinger, Wilk, Cho, & Greco, 2009; Ulrich, Buerhaus, Donelan, Norman, & Dittus, 2005).
- Appreciate the importance of relationships, effective communication, collaboration, and teamwork as they apply to promotion of patient safety (Kalisch, Curley, Stefanov, 2007; Wheelan, Burchill, & Tilin, 2003) and a positive work environment (Jain, Miller, Belt, King, & Berwick, 2006; Joint Commission, 2008; Leonard, Graham, & Bonacum, 2004).

It is not enough to know the precursors for effective leadership. The successful nurse leader must earnestly contemplate each and carefully deliberate how to translate what is known into practice.

■ Leadership Competencies

Leadership is required at all levels of the organization, in professional circles, and for public health policy development. Professional organizations identify leadership as an essential competency for all advanced practice nurses. There are more than 250,000 advanced practice registered nurses (APRNs) who have masters or doctoral degrees. The APRN consensus model defined APRNs as certified registered nurse anesthetists, certified nurse-midwives, clinical nurse specialists, and certified nurse practitioners (National Organization of Nurse Practitioner Faculties, 2008). However, advanced nursing degrees extend beyond the scope of the APRN definition and include degrees in areas such as advanced public health, nursing informatics, clinical nurse leadership, and nursing administration. Each specialty area has a designated professional organization; all recognize the importance of leadership for advanced practitioners, and some specify core leadership competencies for the role. AONE and the ANA define national competencies for nurse managers and nurse executives. AONE and the American Nurses Credentialing Center (ANCC) offer national certification examinations to midlevel managers and nurse executives desiring to distinguish themselves (ANA, 2009; ANCC, 2012; AONE, 2015). Furthermore,

The Essentials of Doctoral Education for Advanced Nursing Practice considers an in-depth knowledge of organizational and administration leadership and healthcare policy as the basis for leadership competencies of doctor of nursing practice graduates (American Association of Colleges of Nursing, 2006).

Leadership within the dynamic healthcare system is not limited to formal leadership positions. Ninety percent of decisions and actions within organizations occur at the point of service (Porter-O'Grady & Malloch, 2016). Informed clinical leaders recognize the value of establishing collaborative teams to generate and sustain innovative solutions. To that end, effective leaders cultivate relationships that are fair, inclusive, respectful, and transparent and that carefully attend to what has *heart* and *meaning* to those doing the work (Kritek, 2011).

▪ Leadership Essentials

Personal Leadership

According to Bennis (2009), evolution of a leader is a personal journey. Leadership probably cannot be taught from a textbook, but it can be learned (Bennis, 2009; NCHL, 2010). To become an effective leader in contemporary times requires considerable work, self-reflection, and a willing spirit to grow. *The Seven Habits of Highly Effective People* by Stephen Covey (1989) discusses the importance of personal leadership. Personal leadership that is principle-centered is a prerequisite for effectively leading others. Covey (1992) proposes principle-centered leaders gain the trust of others through their own trustworthiness.

Covey stresses that our self-paradigm affects how we relate to the world and suggests that when we change our self-talk, we change the view of ourselves. He reminds us that proactive people focus energy on improving themselves, whereas reactive people waste time being concerned about things they cannot change. Covey contends that focusing on one's self allows the person to enlarge his or her circle of influence.

Commitment to change is not solely limited to one's self; courage is required to challenge the status quo and lead people on different paths when evidence points to a new direction (Kritek, 2011; Porter-O'Grady & Malloch, 2008). Kritek asserted that conflict engagement is a moral imperative in health care; patients suffer when providers lack the courage to speak up. Patterson, Grenny, McMillan, and Switzler (2002) discussed the importance of having *crucial conversations* and described artful confrontation as a blend of both intellectual and emotional intelligence (EI).

Emotional Intelligence

The phenomenon of EI is described as one's ability to be aware of, understand, and control one's emotions. According to Goldman (2006), EI is defined by four competencies: self-awareness, self-management, social awareness, and relationship management. Research suggests that EI is more important than intellectual intelligence (IQ) for leadership success (Goldman, 2006; Bradberry & Greaves, 2009). In a study by Bradberry and Greaves, most top performers scored high in EI whereas bottom performers scored low. A study by Mayer, Roberts, and Barsade (2008) indicates that emotions stimulate thinking; therefore, awareness of ones' emotions provides the opportunity to select and direct thoughtful responses. EI has been proposed as an expression of transformational leaders (Akerjordet & Severinsson, 2010). For example, when leaders exercise self-control during criticism, are not threatened by innovative thinking, and respect the knowledge of others, creativity of the team is enhanced (Akerjordet & Severinsson, 2010). Unlike IQ, emotional competence can be developed through self-reflection, knowledge, and effort (Goldman, 2006). Although some researchers purport that EI is the most important driver of leadership and personal excellence, to date, all scientists are not overwhelmingly convinced (Akerjordet & Severinsson, 2010; Herbert & Edgar, 2004). EI may very well be an underlying construct of leadership theory (Morrison, 2008; Stichler, 2006); however, there remains little evidence linking EI to nursing leadership (Akerjordet & Severinsson, 2010).

Personal Integrity, Credibility, and Authenticity

Trust is an essential ingredient for leadership. A 3-year study by Gallup indicated that staff engagement is much more likely to occur when staff trust their leader (Rath & Conchie, 2008). Findings suggested that only 1 in 12 employees engage at work when a leader is not trusted (Rath & Conchie, 2008). Trust takes time to develop and is engendered when leaders remain authentic, follow through, and demonstrate honesty, integrity, and respect (Rath & Conchie, 2008). Credibility occurs from demonstrating knowledge and consistency in core values. Transparency, another essential element of effective leadership (Kerfoot, 2006), was defined by Milton (2009) as the "intentional, ethical choice to be clear, plain, forthright and above board" (p. 23). Choosing to apologize and admit errors is a form of transparency that demonstrates integrity and garners confidence and trust (Milton, 2009).

Authenticity is emerging as a leadership concept. Authenticity refers to the genuineness of the leader. Authentic leaders are true to themselves, not others. However, authentic leadership is not about self; it is about the genuine relations formed between the leader and others. These relationships are dynamic and evolving. *Authenticity* is a term commonly used to describe the transformative leader known for valuing the strengths of others and promoting empowerment. Avolio and Gardner (2005) describe authentic leaders as based in strong ethical values and positive psychological capital; they suggest four constituents of authentic leadership: self-awareness, internalized moral perspective, balanced processing, and relational transparency.

The importance of relationships between leader and followers cannot be underestimated; when more than 10,000 people were asked what the most influential leader in their life contributed to their well-being, the following key themes emerged: hope, compassion, trust, and stability (security) (Rath & Conchie, 2008). However, relational leadership is not solely dependent on the leader; followers also have a role in the reciprocal process (Eagly, 2005).

Maximizing Potential

Accepting that one person cannot possess excellence in every skill, self-reflective leaders inventory natural strengths and develop a personal plan to maximize a person's potential (Rath & Conchie, 2008). If a leader recognizes personal strengths to be strategic thinking and execution of a plan and weaknesses to be the ability to influence and build relationships, the leader learns how to effectively use hidden potential. A leader carefully surrounds himself or herself with the "right people" to balance the essential elements for success (Collins, 2001; Rath & Conchie, 2008). Leaders who utilize employees' strengths can significantly increase staff engagement (Rath & Conchie, 2008, p. 2). Facilitating change and embedding safe practices require staff involvement and engagement (Botwinick, Bisognano, & Haraden, 2006; Sammer et al., 2010). Evidence suggests that staff engaged in their work have a positive impact on organizational outcomes (Laschinger & Leiter, 2006; Schaufeli & Bakker, 2004; Spence Laschinger et al., 2009; Tourangeau et al., 2010). Empowerment, defined as "feelings of effectiveness to do meaningful work" (Spence Laschinger et al., 2009, p. 637), is a precursor to employee engagement. Studies suggest that environments promoting empowerment improve nurses' perceptions of work effectiveness (Spence Laschinger et al., 2009; Tourangeau et al., 2010) and nurse satisfaction (Laschinger, Finegan, Shamian, & Wilk, 2004; Tourangeau et al., 2010). Servant leadership is a style of leadership that demonstrates respect for others and promotes empowerment, staff satisfaction, and quality of care (Neill & Saunders, 2008). According to Upenieks (2002, 2003), an empowered environment augments leadership success.

■ Transformational Leaders

Transformational leaders' actions are founded on knowledge and understanding of complexity science. Transformational leaders recognize health care as a system with dynamic and relational parts that are changing at nanosecond speed. Unpredictable outcomes related to ever-changing parts are a distinguishing feature of complexity theory (Institute of Medicine, 2004). Transformational leaders recognize that systematic change is far from the reach of any one individual, but instead lies in the hands of those closest to point of care. Salanova, Lorente, Chambel, and Martínez (2011) reported a direct link between transformational leadership and work engagement.

Burns (1978) described transformational leadership as complex, with both leader and followers heightening one another's motivation and morality. Transformational leaders inspire followers to move beyond their own self-interests and work toward a collective goal (Burns, 1978). Bass (1985) suggested that transformational leaders gain trust and esteem from their followers. Transformational leadership is cited as the form of leadership used most frequently in organizations with magnet status (Upenieks, 2003).

Contemporary leaders must be visionary, embrace change, and be able to "adapt and predict" transformation. Creativity and innovation are crucial attributes of a transformational leader. In the midst of chaos and uncertainty, leaders must find hope and meaning in their work and engender the same in others (Porter-O'Grady & Malloch, 2008).

Transformational change is not limited to changes in structure and processes such as those created by quality improvement initiatives but extends to reshaping organizational culture and values (Institute of Medicine, 2004). Lukas et al. (2007) proposed a model for transformation that embeds reliable systemwide EBP improvements to patient care. The model identifies five relational factors critical to successful transformation of patient care:

- Incentive to transform
- Commitment of leadership to quality
- Active engagement of staff in meaningful improvement activities
- Resource allocation to meet organization goals
- Integration and alignment of the organization (breaking down silos, creating a shared vision, obtaining commitment, and changing processes throughout the system to accommodate and sustain the changes in a microsystem)

These factors insidiously transform complex organizations through incremental changes in vision, culture, operational functions and processes, information technology infrastructure, and human resources (Lukas et al., 2007).

Transformational Change Exemplar

Leadership is vital in large complex systems to achieve excellent clinical care and eliminate preventable injuries and deaths. Success stories inspire, offer hope, and provide direction to leaders responsible for organizational and system change. Ascension Health, a 65-hospital healthcare system, reported significant success in improving clinical care and decreasing mortality rates within the institutions following a commitment to patient care excellence (Hendrich et al., 2007). Ann Hendrich, nurse executive for Ascension Health, in partnership with other chief executives, provided system leadership that engaged members throughout the large complex healthcare ministry. Excellence in leadership led to system reductions in falls (Lancaster et al., 2007), perioperative adverse events (Ewing, Bruder, Baroco, Hill, & Sparkman, 2007), birth trauma (Mazza et al., 2007), nosocomial infections (Berriel-Cass, Adkins, Jones, & Fakih, 2006), and facility-acquired pressure ulcers (Gibbons, Shanks, Kleinhelter, & Jones, 2006). Hendrich recognized the importance of identifying key stakeholders and engaging those closest to the problems. Systemwide summits were held to bring the stakeholders together, to create a shared vision of safe care, to gain commitment, and to rapidly disseminate organizational knowledge (Hendrich et al., 2007). Hendrich was successful in arguing for the resources required for patient safety and quality. Collaborating with finance, nursing built a value proposition and business case that led to a $60 million commitment in capital dollars for systemwide replacement of beds. Acquiring expensive beds with advanced technology required a commitment to the following:

- Decrease the number of work-related injuries
- Reduce the incidence of pressure ulcers
- Reduce the incidence of ventilator-acquired pneumonia
- Decrease rental costs for beds

Nursing leadership is accountable to develop highly reliable, patient-safe organizations (Riley, 2009; Sammer et al., 2010). The Ascension story is evidence of one nursing leader's contribution to a journey to excellence.

Exemplar of Leadership at the Microsystem Level

The IOM aims (safe, effective, efficient, equitable, timely, patient-centered) for quality cannot be achieved without the mobilization of providers at all levels of the organization. It is within clinical microsystems (subsystems buried within the larger macrosystem) that the essence of health care is provided. Leaders within these smaller subsets serve as change agents facilitating improved processes, safety, and patient care. Susan Wilkinson, a clinical nurse leader (CNL) of a 24-bed unit just outside of Birmingham, Alabama, is an exemplar of a leader making a difference at the heart of patient care. Through her leadership of quality improvement initiatives, the unit has cut average wait time of the discharge process in half, reduced use of urinary catheters and hospital-acquired urinary tract infections, and increased compliance with mandatory core measures. Patient satisfaction with care on the unit soared to an all-time high. The patient care innovations on the unit serve as examples for change initiatives for other units within the hospital. Wilkinson leads by example and uses leadership skills to coach, mentor, teach, and engage staff. The CNL works with members of the staff in promoting teamwork, communication, empowerment, and positive staff morale. Participation of staff in improvement initiatives wins the support and ownership of staff. Positive outcomes from the clinical microsystem have rippling effects throughout the organization as innovative approaches spread among other units (S. Wilkinson, personal communication, July 10, 2011).

■ Conclusion

Nurses are crucial to the success of healthcare transformation. Immersed in the patient care experience, nurses are well positioned to lead system redesign that enhances access, quality, and patient safety. Present times characterized by complexity, chaos, and increasing technology challenge traditional leadership practices and call for a new paradigm of leadership. Identification of best practices in leadership is complicated by the complexity of the subject and the volumes and varied forms of knowledge on the matter. Little effort has been made to evaluate and synthesize the research into a meaningful whole. However, common themes are beginning to surface from the literature. Experts agree that to transform systems, leadership must shift from the traditional power-base model to a relationship model of leadership. Present times call for leaders who are comfortable sharing the locus of control with members throughout the organization, with a focus on actualizing the potential in both self and others rather than dominating or forcing the change. The research is clear that collaboration and teamwork are vital to confronting the overwhelming challenges of health care; thus, leaders of today must be capable of creating a shared vision, effectively communicating, and strengthening the relationships among staff. Furthermore, research suggests that engagement and commitment to quality improvement occur when leaders value, respect, and empower frontline workers.

Appreciating the diversity and wisdom of those doing the work contributes to leadership success. Nurses must seek to translate and integrate the best evidence into practice related to leadership and at the same time advance the state of leadership science.

REFLECTIVE ACTIVITIES

1. Using the model of EB management offered by Kovner and Rundall (2006), consider a decision in your organizational system and/or practice using the five-step process for decision-making.
2. Consider your own EI in light of your own leadership style.

REFERENCES

Adams J. M., & Ives Erickson J. (2011). Applying the Adams Influence Model (AIM) in nurse executive practice. *Journal of Nursing Administration, 41*(4), 186–192.

Adams, J. M., Denham, D., & Ramirez Neumeister, I. R. (2010). Applying the model of the interrelationship of leadership environments and outcomes for nurse executives: A community hospital's exemplar in developing staff nurse engagement through documentation improvement initiatives. *Nursing Administration Quarterly, 34,* 201–207.

Adams, J. M., Erickson, J. I., Jones, D. A., & Paulo, L. (2009). An evidence-based structure for transformative nurse executive practice: The model of the interrelationship of leadership, environment, and outcomes for nurse executives (MILE ONE). *Nursing Administration Quarterly, 33,* 280–287.

Agency for Healthcare Research and Quality. (2015). 2014 National Healthcare Quality & Disparities Report (NIH Publication No. 150007). Retrieved from http://www.ahrq.gov/sites/default/files/wysi wyg/research/findings/nhqrdr/nhqdr14/2014nhqdr.pdf

Akerjordet, K., & Severinsson, E. (2010). The state of the science of emotional intelligence related to nursing leadership? An integrative review. *Journal of Nursing Management, 18,* 233–382. doi:10.1111 /j.1365-2834.2010.0187

American Association of Colleges of Nursing. (2006). *The essentials of doctoral education for advanced nursing practice.* Retrieved from http://www.aacn.nche.edu/DNP/pdf/Essentials.pdf

American Nurses Association. (2009). *Nursing administration: Scope and standards of practice.* Silver Spring, MD: Nursesbook.org

American Nurses Credentialing Center. (2012). *Certification.* Retrieved from http://www.nursecreden tialing.org

American Organization of Nurse Executives. (2015). *AONE nurse executive competencies*. Retrieved from http://www.aone.org/

Anderson, M. M., & Garman, A. M. (2014). *Leadership development in healthcare systems: Towards an evidenced-based approach*. Chicago, IL: National Center for Healthcare Leadership. Retrieved from http://nchl.org/Documents/Ctrl_Hyperlink/NCHL_Leadership_Survey_White_Paper_Final_05.14_uid6232014300422.pdf

Armellino, D., Quinn-Griffin, M. T., & Fitzpatrick, J. J. (2010). Structural empowerment and patient safety culture among registered nurses working in adult critical care units. *Journal of Nursing Management, 18*, 796–803.

Avolio, B. J., & Gardner, W. L. (2005). Authentic leadership development: Getting to the root of positive forms of leadership. *Leadership Quarterly, 16*, 315–338.

Bass, B. M. (1985). *Leadership and performance*. New York, NY: Free Press.

Bennis, W. (2009). *On becoming a leader*. New York, NY: Basic Books.

Berriel-Cass, D., Adkins, F. W., Jones, P., & Fakih, M. G. (2006). Eliminating nosocomial infections at Ascension Health. *Joint Commission Journal on Quality and Patient Safety, 32*, 612–620.

Botwinick, L., Bisognano, M., & Haraden, C. (2006). *Leadership guide to patient safety* (IHI white paper). Cambridge, MA: Institute for Healthcare Improvement. Retrieved from http://www.IHI.org

Bradberry, T., & Greaves, J. (2009). *Emotional Intelligence 2.0*. San Diego, CA: TalentSmart.

Buerhaus, P. (2004). Lucian Leape on patient safety in U.S. hospitals. *Journal of Nursing Scholarship, 34*, 366–370. doi:10.1111/j.1547-5069.2004.04065.x

Burns, J. M. (1978). *Leadership*. New York, NY: Harper & Row.

Burns, J. P. (2001). Complexity science and leadership in healthcare. *Journal of Nursing Administration, 31*, 474–482.

Centers for Medicare and Medicaid Services. (2013). National health expenditure data. Retrieved from https://www.cms.gov/research-statistics-data-and-systems/statistics-trends-and-reports/nationalhealthexpenddata/nationalhealthaccountshistorical.html

Chinn, P. L., & Kramer, M. K. (2008). *Integrated theory and knowledge development in nursing* (7th ed.). St. Louis, MO: Mosby.

Classen, D. C., Resar, R., Griffin, F., Federico, F., Frankel, T., Kimmel, N., … James, B. C. (2011). 'Global Trigger Tool' Shows That Adverse Events In Hospitals May Be Ten Times Greater Than Previously MeasuredGreater Than Previously Measured. *Health Affairs, 30*(4), 581–589.

Collins, J. (2001). *Good to great*. New York, NY: HarperCollins.

Covey, S. R. (1989). *The seven habits of highly effective people*. New York, NY: Fireside Books.

Covey, S. R. (1992). *Principle-centered leadership*. New York, NY: Fireside Books.

Eagly, A. H. (2005). Achieving relational authenticity in leadership: Does gender matter? *Leadership Quarterly, 16*, 459–474.

Eden, J., Wheatley, B., McNeil, B., & Sox, H. (Eds.). (2008). *Knowing what works in health care: A road map for the nation*. Retrieved from http://books.nap.edu/openbook.php?record_id=12038

Ewing, H., Bruder, G., Baroco, P., Hill, M., & Sparkman, L. P. (2007). Eliminating perioperative adverse events at Ascension Health. *Joint Commission Journal on Quality and Patient Safety, 3*, 256–266.

Gibbons, W., Shanks, H. T., Kleinhelter, P., & Jones, P. (2006). Eliminating facility-acquired pressure ulcers at Ascension Health. *Joint Commission Journal on Quality and Patient Safety, 32*, 488–496.

Goldman, D. (2006). *Emotional intelligence: Why it can matter more than IQ* (10th ed.). New York, NY: Bantam Books.

Hendrich, A., Tersigni, A. R., Jeffocat, S., Barnett, C. J., Brideau, L. P., & Pryor, D. (2007). The Ascension Health journey to zero: Lessons learned and leadership perspectives. *Joint Commission Journal on Quality and Patient Safety, 33*, 739–749.

Herbert, R., & Edgar, L. (2004). Emotional intelligence: A primal dimension of nursing leadership. *Nursing Leadership, 17*, 56–63.

Hersey, H., Blanchard, R. H., & Johnson, D. E. (1996). *Management of organizational behavior: Utilizing human resources*. Upper Saddle River, NJ: Prentice Hall College Division.

Institute of Medicine. (2004). *Transformational leadership and evidence-based management*. In A. Page (Ed.), Keeping patients safe: Transforming the work environment of nurses (pp. 4–160). Washington, DC: The National Academies Press.

Institute of Medicine. (2011). *The future of nursing: Leading change, advancing health.* Retrieved from http://books.nap.edu/openbook.php?record_id=12956

Jain, M., Miller, L., Belt, D., King, D., & Berwick D. M. (2006). Decline in ICU adverse events, nosocomial infections and cost through a quality improvement initiative focusing on teamwork and culture change. *Quality and Safety in Health Care, 15,* 235–239. doi:10.1136/qshc.2005.016576

James, K. M. (2010). Incorporating complexity science theory into nursing curricula. *Creative Nursing, 16,* 137–142.

Joint Commission. (2008). *Behaviors that undermine a culture of safety.* Sentinel Event Alert, Issue 40. Retrieved from http://www.jointcommission.org/assets/1/18/SEA_40.PDF

Kabcenell, A., Nolan, T., Martin, L., & Gill, Y. (2010). *The pursuing perfection initiative: Lessons on transforming health care* (IHI white paper). Cambridge, MA: Institute for Healthcare Improvement. Retrieved from http://www.IHI.org

Kalisch, B., Curley, M., & Stefanov, S. (2007). An intervention to enhance nursing staff teamwork and engagement. *Journal of Nursing Administration, 37,* 77–84.

Kellerman, B. (2012). The end of leadership. New York, NY: HarperCollins.

Kerfoot, K. (2006). The transparent organization: Leadership is an open organization. *Urologic Nursing, 26,* 409–410.

Kohn, L. T., Corrigan, J. M., & Donaldson, M. S. (Eds.). (2000). *To err is human: Building a safer health system.* Institute of Medicine. Washington, DC: National Academies Press.

Kotter, J. P. (2012). *Leading change.* Boston, MA: Harvard Business Review Publisher Press.

Kovner, A. R., & McAlearney, A. S. (2013). *Health services management: Cases, readings, and commentary.* Chicago, IL: Health Administration Press

Kovner, A. R., Fine, D. J., & D'Aquila, R. (2009). *Evidence-based management in healthcare.* Chicago, IL: Health Administration Press.

Kovner, A. R., & Rundall, T. G. (2006). Evidence-based management reconsidered. *Frontier of Health Services Management, 22,* 3–33.

Kritek, P. B. (2011, June). *Getting from heat to light: Conflict skills in this world of change.* Improvement Science Summit conducted at the meeting of University of Texas Academic Center for Evidence-Based Practice, San Antonio, TX.

Lake, E. T., & Friese, C. R. (2006). Variations in nursing practice environments: Relation to staffing and hospital characteristics. *Nursing Research, 55*(1), 1–9.

Lancaster, A. D., Ayers, A., Belbot, B., Goldner, V., Kress, L., Stanton, D., . . . Sparkman, L. (2007). Preventing falls and eliminating injury at Ascension Health. *Joint Commission Journal on Quality and Patient Safety, 33,* 367–375.

Laschinger, H. K., Finegan, J., Shamian, J., & Wilk, P. (2004). A longitudinal analysis of the impact of workplace empowerment on work satisfaction. *Journal of Organizational Behavior, 25,* 527–545.

Laschinger, H., & Leiter, M. (2006). The impact of nursing work environments on patient safety outcomes: The mediating role of burnout/engagement. *Journal of Nursing Administration, 36,* 259–267.

Leonard, M., Graham, S., & Bonacum, J. D. (2004). The human factor: The critical importance of effective teamwork and communication in providing safe care. *Quality and Safety in Health Care, 13*(Suppl. 1), i85–i90. doi:10.1136/qshc.2004.010033

Lukas, C., Holmes, S., Cohen, A., Restuccia, J., Cramer, I., Shwartz, M., & Charns, M. (2007). Transformational change in health care systems: An organizational model. *Health Care Management Review, 32,* 309–320.

Lynham, S. A., & Chermack, T. J. (2006). Responsible leadership for performance: A theoretical model and hypotheses. *Journal of Leadership & Organizational Studies, 12,* 73–88.

MacMillan-Finlayson, S. (2010). Competency development for nurse executives: Meeting the challenge (Executive Development). *Journal of Nursing Administration, 40,* 254–257.

Mateo, M. A., & Kirchhoff, K. T. (2009). *Research for advanced practice nurses: From evidence to practice.* New York, NY: Springer.

Maxwell, J. C. (1998). *The 21 irrefutable laws of leadership.* Nashville, TN: Thomas Nelson.

Mayer, J. D., Roberts, R. D., & Barsade, S. G. (2008). Human abilities: Emotional intelligence. *Annual Review of Psychology, 59,* 507–536.

Mazza, F., Kitchens, J., Kerr, S., Markovich, A., Best, M., & Sparkman, L. P. (2007). Eliminating birth trauma at Ascension Health. *Joint Commission Journal on Quality and Patient Safety, 3,* 15–24.

McClure, M. L., Poulin, M. A., Sovie, M. D., & Wandelt, M. A. (1983). *Magnet hospitals: Attraction and retention of professional nurses.* Washington, DC: American Academy of Nursing.

McGillis-Hall, L., Doran, D., Baker, G. R., Pink, G., Sidani, S., O'Brien-Pallas, L., & Donner, G. J. (2003). Nurse staffing models as predictors of patient outcomes. *Medical Care, 41,* 1096–1109.

Meredith, E., Cohen, E., & Raia, L. (2010). Transformational leadership: Application of Magnet's new empiric outcomes. *Nursing Clinics of North America, 45*(1), 49–64. doi:10.1016/j.cnur.2009.10.007

Milton, C. L. (2009). Transparency in nursing leadership: A chosen ethic. *Nursing Science Quarterly, 22,* 23–26. doi:101177/0894318408329159

Moore, B. V. (1927). The May conference on leadership. *Personnel Journal, 6,* 124–128.

Morrison, J. (2008). The relationship between emotional intelligence competencies and preferred conflict-handling styles. *Journal of Management, 16,* 974–983.

National Center for Healthcare Leadership. (2010). *Best practices in healthcare leadership academies* (White paper). Retrieved from http://www.nchl.org

National Organization of Nurse Practitioner Faculties. (2008). *Consensus model for APRN regulation: Licensure, accreditation, certification & education.* Retrieved from http://c.ymcdn.com/sites/www.nonpf.org/resource/resmgr/docs/indepenpracpprfinal2013.pdf

Neill, M. W., & Saunders, N. S. (2008). Servant leadership: Enhancing quality of care and staff satisfaction. *Journal of Nursing Administration, 38,* 395–400. Doi:10.1097/01.NNA.0000323958.52415.cf

Nelson, E. C., Batalden, P. B., & Godfrey, M. M. (2007). *Quality by design: A clinical microsystem approach.* San Francisco, CA: Jossey-Bass.

Northouse, P. G. (2016). *Leadership: Theory and Practice* (7th ed.). Thousand Oaks, CA: SAGE publications.

Organisation for Economic Co-operation and Development. (2014). OECD Health Statistics 2014. Retrieved from http://www.oecd.org/els/health-systems/oecd-health-statistics-2014-frequently-requested-data.htm

Page, A. (Ed.). (2003). *Keeping patients safe: Transforming the work environment of nurses.* Retrieved from http://www.institute.nhs.uk/delivering_through_improvement/general/our_vision.html

Patterson, K., Grenny, J., McMillan, R., & Switzler, A. (2002). *Crucial conversations: Tools for talking when stakes are high.* New York, NY: McGraw-Hill.

Pfeffer, J., & Sutton, R. J. (2006). Evidence-based management. *Harvard Business Review, 84*(1), 63–74.

Porter-O'Grady, T., & Malloch, K. (2008). Beyond myth and magic: The future of evidence-based leadership. *Nursing Administration Quarterly, 32,* 176–187.

Porter-O'Grady, T., & Malloch, K. (2016). *Leadership in nursing practice: Changing the landscape of health care* (2nd ed.). Sudbury, MA: Jones and Bartlett.

Rath, T., & Conchie, B. (2008). *Strength based leadership: Great leaders, teams, and why people follow.* New York, NY: Gallup Press.

Richardson, A., & Storr, J. (2010). Patient safety: A literature review on the impact of nursing empowerment, leadership and collaboration. *International Nursing Review, 57,* 12–21.

Riley, W. (2009). High reliability and implications for nursing leaders. *Journal of Nursing Management, 17,* 238–246. doi:10.1111/j.1365- 2834.2009.00971x

Rousseau, D. M. (2006). Is there such a thing as "evidence-based management"? *Academy of Management Review, 31,* 256–269.

Rutherford, P., Phillips, J., Coughlan, P., Lee, B., Moen, R., Peck, C., & Taylor, J. (2008). *Transforming care at the bedside how-to guide: Engaging front-line staff in innovation and quality improvement.* Cambridge, MA: Institute for Healthcare Improvement. Retrieved from http://www.IHI.org

Ryan, R. W., Harris, K. K., Mattox, L. Singh, O., Camp, M., & Shirey, M. R. (2015). Nursing leader collaboration to drive quality improvement and implementation science. *Nursing Administration Quarterly, 39*(3), 229–238.

Salanova, M., Lorente, L., Chambel, M. J., & Martínez, I. M. (2011). Linking transformational leadership to nurses' extra-role performance: The mediating role of self-efficacy and work engagement. *Journal of Advanced Nursing, 11*(10), 2256–2266. doi:10.1111/j.1365-2648.2011.05652.x

Sammer, C., Lykens, K., Singh, K., Mains, D., & Lackan, N. (2010). What is patient safety culture? A review of the literature. *Journal of Nursing Scholarship, 42,* 156–165. Doi:10.1111/j.1547-5069.2009.01330.x

Schaufeli, W., & Bakker, A. (2004). Job demands, job resources and their relationship with burnout and engagement: A multi-sample study. *Journal of Organizational Behavior, 25,* 293–315.

Senge, P. (1990). *The fifth discipline: The art and practice of the learning organization.* New York, NY: Doubleday Currency.

Simpson, M. R. (2009a). Engagement at work: A review of the literature. *International Journal of Nursing Studies, 46,* 1012–1024.

Simpson, M. R. (2009b). Predictors of work engagement among medical-surgical registered nurses. *Western Journal of Nursing Research, 31,* 44–65. doi:10.1177/0193945908319993

Singer, S., Falwell, A., Gaba, D., Meterko, M., Rosen, A., Hartmann, C., & Baker, L. (2009). Identifying organizational cultures that promote patient safety. *Health Care Management Review, 34,* 300–311.

Spence Laschinger, H., Wilk, P., Cho, J., & Greco, P. (2009). Empowerment, engagement and perceived effectiveness in nursing work environments: Does experience matter? *Journal of Nursing Management, 17,* 636–646. doi:10.1111/j.1365.2834.2008.00907.x

Stichler, J. F. (2006). Emotional intelligence: A critical leadership quality for the nurse executive. *AWHONN Lifelines, 10,* 422–425.

Stogdill, R. M. (1974). *Handbook of leadership: A survey of theory and research.* New York, NY: Free Press.

Strumwasser, S., & Virkstis, K. (2015). Meaningfully incorporating staff input to enhance frontline engagement. *Journal of Nursing Administration, 45*(4), 179–182.

Swensen, S., Pugh, M., McMullan, C., & Kabcenell, A. (2013). High-impact leadership: Improve care, improve the health of populations, and reduce costs (IHI White Paper). Cambridge, MA: Institute for Healthcare Improvement.

Thomas, E. J., & Classen, D. C. (2014). Patient safety: Let's measure what matters. *Annals of Internal Medicine, 160*(9), 642–643.

Tourangeau, A., Cranley, L., Laschinger, H., & Pachis, J. (2010). Relationships among leadership practices, work environments, staff communication and outcomes in long-term care. *Journal of Nursing Management, 18,* 1060–1072. doi:10.1111/j.1365-2834.2010.01125.x

Ulrich, B., Buerhaus, P., Donelan, K., Norman, L., & Dittus, R. (2005). How RNs view the work environment: Results of a national survey of registered nurses. *Journal of Nursing Administration, 35*(9), 389–396.

Upenieks, V. (2002). What constitutes successful nurse leadership? A qualitative approach utilizing Kanter's theory of organizational behavior. *Journal of Nursing Administration, 32,* 622–632.

Upenieks, V. (2003). Nurse leaders' perceptions of what compromises successful leadership in today's acute inpatient environments. *Nursing Administration Quarterly, 27,* 140–152.

Wheatley, M. (2006). *Leadership and new science: Discovering order in a chaotic world* (3rd ed.). San Francisco, CA: Berrett-Koehler Publishers.

Wheelan, S. A., Burchill, C., & Tilin, F. (2003). The link between teamwork and patients' outcomes in intensive care units. *American Journal of Critical Care, 12,* 527–534.

CHAPTER 8

Evaluating Organizational Frameworks for Systems Change

■ Patricia L. Thomas ■

■ Objectives:

- Examine dimensions of organizational behavior and systems that align with success in contemporary healthcare organizations.
- Explore critical elements of culture to promote safety, empowerment, and action.
- Describe strategies that promote organizational effectiveness and safety grounded in evidence.

■ Introduction

Schein (1997) described how culture and leadership are two sides of the same coin. In his view, leaders create cultures by creating groups and are then responsible for determining who will lead the groups. A unique function of leaders is to perceive the functional and dysfunctional aspects of a culture and then manage the change and evolution of it to support survival of the group in a changing environment (Schein, 1997, p. 15). Given this, the interwoven nature of leadership and organizations becomes readily apparent. Although much has been written about the importance of leaders in organizations, an underlying assumption within organizations is that leaders and followers create a space in which organizational goals are attained through collective effort. This space is often described as the culture, and the tone and tenor of the relationships are referred to as climate (Arnold, 2013; Schein, 1997; Yang, Wang, Chang, Guo, & Huang, 2009).

Changes in healthcare organizations often mirror societal change, influenced by shared experiences, values, norms, perceptions, economics, and political pressures of a given time. Scanning the landscape of health care, it is clear that society is calling for transformational change in healthcare delivery outcomes, cost reductions, safety, improved care experiences, and greater involvement in decisions by patients, families, and staff to bring about radical and revolutionary change and improvements in our care delivery system.

The work of Donabedian and his framework of structure, process, and outcomes have been described as foundational to organizational work. Likewise, leadership competencies and attributes have been highlighted to outline the evidence, actions, and characteristics of healthcare leaders with the purpose of embracing an interdependence of thought, action, and measurement in an attempt to evaluate the effectiveness and efficacy of contemporary organizations. Although both are important, neither is sufficient to explain the purpose and functioning of organizations. This chapter will explore the existing body of evidence on the subject of organizations—specifically, concepts of systems and systems thinking, structural empowerment, and organizational learning—through an operational lens influenced by organization theory to call attention to culture and climate and their resulting influence on best practices as they are known today.

■ Organizational Culture Theory

Contemporary organizations have invested human and financial resources in training programs and organizational problem analysis defined by quality structures and improvement methodologies. Development of total quality management programs and organizational culture assessments, perceptions of safety, and demonstrations of effectiveness supported by tenets of human resource or human relations schools of organization theory provide the justification for these expenses. It is believed that employee participation and involvement in decision-making leads to improvements in productivity, quality, and organizational performance (Abdelhandi & Drach-Zahavy, 2012; Ammouri, Tailakh, Muliira, Geethakrishnan, & Al-Kindi, 2015; Krive, 2013; Laschinger, Read, Wilk, & Fiegan, 2014; Rundquist & Givens, 2013; Squires, Tourangeau, Laschinger, & Doran, 2010). In an attempt to support effective coping mechanisms when faced with accelerated change, leaders and managers are looking for new ways to view individuals, organizations, and group behaviors to facilitate adaptation (Barden, Griffin, Donahue, & Fitzpatrick, 2011).

Although the concept of organizational culture can be difficult to define, analyze, measure, and manage, organizational culture is recognized as a critical link in understanding how organizations change and learn. Leaders have shown great interest in understanding the concept of organizational culture as a means to explain organizational phenomena, with the intent of manipulating the phenomena to create more effective organizations (Schein, 1997). Schein defined the culture of a group as a pattern of shared basic assumptions that the group learned as it solved its problem of external adaptation and internal integration that has worked well enough to be considered valid and, therefore, to be taught to new members as the correct way to perceive, think, and feel in relation to those problems (p. 12).

For a culture to exist, a group must have stable membership with a history of shared learning. Culture, as a concept, is most useful to help explain incomprehensible or irrational behaviors of groups and organizations. Because group behavior is predicated on patterns of shared beliefs and taken-for-granted assumptions, which allow one to fully comprehend organizational culture examination, evaluation of both is required (Schein, 1997). Aside from the values, beliefs, norms, and expectations shared by organizational members, behavioral norms and expectations are displayed through the roles and relationships established and supported within an organization (Schein, 1997).

Leadership and Organizational Culture

As organizations have changed, so have the roles, responsibilities, and expectations of employees and managers. Managerial innovations designed to empower employees require leaders to discard beliefs of hierarchical control and reactive blind obedience. These innovations embrace the commitment to establish cultures of learned willingness and individual accountability (Barden et al., 2011; Jacques, 1996; Linnen & Rowley, 2014; Porter-O'Grady, 2012, 2015).

Many leaders hold a cursory or casual definition of organizational culture that includes the climate, practices, and values that managers attempt to infuse into their organizations. This implies a one-size-fits-all approach and a "right," strong, or "quality" culture, or a "wrong," weak, or ineffective culture. Schein (1997) saw these definitions as superficial and simplistic. Elements of organizational culture are often the most stable and difficult aspects to influence in group behavior. Perceptions related to complex group learning are only partly influenced by leader behavior. Schein proposed the utilization of anthropological models as a mechanism to critically examine deep and complex structures of organizational cultures. The anthropological models allow deliberate examination of the context and deeper meaning displayed in social and role behaviors that comprise organizational culture analysis (Schein, 1997).

Social and behavior scientists debate the value in differentiating organizational climate from organizational culture. It is agreed that both are concerned with sense making, filtering, and the attachment of meaning in organizational experiences (Bellot, 2011; Greenslade, & Jimmieson, 2011; Ross, 2011; Schein, 1997; Weick, Sutcliffe, & Obstfeld, 1999). Disagreement lies in whether organizational climate and culture are the same and whether differentiation of the variables contributes to greater understanding of an organization's culture. Bellot (2011) and Greenslade and Jimmieson (2011) speculated that unit or organizational climate represents shared perceptions among employees within work units regarding which formal and informal policies, practices, events, and procedures contribute to the sense-making process that employees undertake to understand what is expected and rewarded. In this regard, organizational climate is a discrete social context that has the potential to capture the social environment and its influence on organizational effectiveness. Others dismiss organizational climate as a transient tone or setting mood and draw a direct connection between climate and culture (Ashanasy, Wilderom, & Peterson, 2011). What is agreed is that both climate and culture influence safety, quality, and outcomes, although the relationships are complex and not readily understood (Ross, 2011).

Appreciation that changes to organizational culture typically start with a focus on strategy, structure, work processes, roles, and accountabilities is only a small part of the change. Full and complete change requires changes in people's behavior that include their values, the climate, informal operating systems, rituals, and communication patterns within the organization. It is through shared leadership insights experienced during discontinuous change that the modification of concrete signals, actions, norms, and practices occurs, leading to a shared sense of purpose and meaning in work (Ashanasy, Wilderom, & Peterson, 2011; Christian, Bradley, Wallace, & Burke, 2009; Schein, 1997). These are pivotal elements in organizational change that require time and are often overlooked.

■ Systems Thinking

Discussion of organizations would be incomplete without discernment found in systems theory and organizational learning. Irrespective of professional discipline, systems theory provides a framework to appreciate the complexity of organizations underscored by the predictability of systems. Ludwig von Bertalanffy (1969) theorized that principles exist that apply to all systems regardless of their specific elements and goals (Senge, 1990). In his view, the characteristics of systems—namely, wholeness, differentiation, progression, centralization, hierarchical order, finality, and equifinality—are present in all systems regardless of a distinction between professional disciplines and orientation. General systems theory enables specialists and professionals from varied backgrounds to share insights and discoveries within a context and language found in systems theory to explain and expand one another's discoveries. It provides a unifying framework to examine content from different disciplines into a comprehensive body of knowledge that can be applied to biological and social systems because of the dependence and interrelationships between the parts and the whole (Senge, 1990; Senge, Kleiner, Roberts, Ross, & Smith, 1994; von Bertalanffy, 1969). These principles are central to discussions about organizations: the inputs, throughputs, and outcomes of patient care; the professionals who interact within the system; and results (whether desired or undesired) based on the process and structures endorsed by the participants. In simple terms, a system can be thought of as an aggregate of elements (human and material) organized to accomplish goals (North, 2012; Porter-O'Grady, 2015; Williams, 2015).

Recognizing contemporary issues in healthcare organizations, the social context and behaviors described in culture—such as respect, appreciation, participation, and communication—overlie the principles of systems thinking and serve as a lever in organizational learning and sustainable change. Systems thinking focuses on the interrelatedness of relationships in a system. It recognizes that an action or event in one part of the whole affects all the other parts (North, 2015; Williams, 2015; Senge, 1990). It includes an organization's hierarchy and process flows but also embraces attitudes, perceptions, quality of products, and customer service. Each of these areas is displayed in healthcare organizations, with the latter gaining greater attention as customer satisfaction, employee satisfaction, safety, and outcomes are taking center stage in healthcare delivery, competitive advantage, and employee recruitment and retention.

■ Kanter's Structural Theory of Organizational Behavior

In corporations generally and nursing specifically, the work of Kanter's structural theory of organization has been a theoretical cornerstone to guide research that aims to understand power and behaviors in organizations. In recent years, systems thinking, organizational learning, and shared governance have been added to the repertoire of theoretically driven application studies in an effort to build knowledge regarding organizational effectiveness on sound empirical evidence.

Kanter's work, initially published in 1977 in *Men and Women of the Corporation,* described how power in an organization is derived from structural conditions, not personal characteristics or socialization effects (Kanter, 1977). Kanter asserted that work environments provide access to information, resources, and support, and opportunities to learn, thus empowering staff. Within this environment, employees act on their expertise, knowledge, and judgment, thereby accomplishing the work of the organization with greater ease and satisfaction, which produces higher quality work. As a result, employees have higher organizational commitment, stronger and healthier relationships with management that are built on trust and respect, and greater overall satisfaction with the contributions made.

Concepts and elements of Kanter's model have been utilized in middle-range nursing research to establish a body of knowledge that has contributed to understanding leadership, teams, individual nursing roles, and the organizational impact of empowered work environments. This has extended the evidence-based understanding of the perceptions of empowerment and the role of the leader and follower, with resultant impacts to operational outcomes and satisfaction (Dahinten, et al., 2014; Laschinger & Fida, 2015; Laschinger, Nosko, Wilk, & Finegan, 2014; MacPhee, et al., 2014).

■ Shared Governance and Distributed Leadership

In review of the literature regarding nursing governance, much has been learned over the last 30 years. Although there is general belief that staff ownership and support for changes in organizations are most effective when decentralized decision-making is in place and represent the preferred model, healthcare organizations across the country have had varied success in implementing shared leadership and decision-making models (Bamford-Wade & Moss 2010; Barden et al., 2011; Beglinger, 2015; Clavelle, Porter-O'Grady, & Drenkard, 2013; Dearmon, Riley, Mestas, & Buckner, 2015; Fray, 2011; Hess, 2011; Shepard, Harris, Chung, & Himes, 2014).

Shared governance is a structured model of empowerment gleaned from organizational development experts. Initially introduced to nursing in the 1970s by Christman

(1976) and Cleland (1978), it has been further developed by clinical leaders over the last 30 years. Further support for elements of empowerment was developed by Kanter's structural empowerment theory (Kanter, 1977, 1997), which recognizes that staff are empowered; this recognition results in actions that can be attributed in part to access to resources, opportunity, and information, which leads to greater satisfaction and professional development (Porter-O'Grady, 2015; Clavelle, Porter-O'Grady, & Drenkard, 2013).

In their seminal work on shared governance, Porter-O'Grady and Finnigan (1984) defined shared governance as a collaborative structure in which managers and clinicians partner to make decisions about clinical and operational practices. Shared governance affords direct care clinicians responsibility for decisions related to their practice and is grounded in professional values and principles of autonomy, shared decision-making, and participation. Simply stated, shared governance models put ownership of the organization's work on those who provide the services (Barden et al., 2011; Clavelle, Porter-O'Grady, & Drenkard, 2013; Dearmon, et al., 2015; Fray, 2011; Hess, 2011; Hoying & Allen, 2011; Porter-O'Grady & Finnigan, 1984; Shepard, Harris, Chung, & Himes, 2014).

Shared governance aligns nursing standards and decision-making to foster professional autonomy and accountability. These are the same environmental elements encompassed by the American Nurses Credentialing Center's (ANCC's) Magnet Recognition Program criteria, to which many organizations aspire (Beglinger, 2015; Buckman, Sellers, & Batchellar, 2012; Shepard, et al., 2014). Shared governance models have been implemented throughout the world, the shared beliefs being that authority over and involvement in decision-making lead to staff autonomy, enhanced perceptions of control over practice, and, ultimately, greater job satisfaction and staff retention (Crow, Nguyen, & DeBourgh, 2014; Hoying & Allen, 2011; George & Sovering, 2013). In support of these findings, The Institute of Medicine report *Keeping Patients Safe: Transforming the Work Environment of Nurses* (2004) contended that employees must be empowered and engaged to achieve the needed level of quality in patient care in the current healthcare environment. Fundamental to this transformation are nonhierarchical communication systems and nonhierarchical decision-making (Hoying & Allen, 2011). Control over nursing practice has been identified as a structure that eliminates traditional hierarchal models to engage team members in decisions that influence organizational outcomes (Bamford-Wade, & Moss 2010; Barden et al., 2011; Beglinger, 2015; Clavelle, Porter-O'Grady, & Drenkard, 2013; Dearmon, et al., 2015; Fray, 2011; Hess, 2011; Shepard, et al., 2014).

Magnet Organizations

Presently, organizations nationally and internationally are working toward earning Magnet designation, a recognition of excellence in nursing practice demonstrated through evidence that highlights an organization's commitment to exemplary professional practice, strong nursing leadership, and quality outcomes grounded in evidence-based practices (EBPs) and nursing research (American Nurses Credentialing Center (ANCC), 2015b; Messmer & Turkel, 2010). Magnet designation has been accomplished by approximately 7% of all registered hospitals in the United States and is awarded by the ANCC, a separate arm of the American Nurses Association (ANA; AHA FastFacts on U.S. Hospitals, 2011, as cited by ANCC, 2015b). Heralded as the gold standard for demonstration of exceptional nursing practice that recognizes quality patient care and nursing excellence, Magnet recognition provides consumers a benchmark to measure the quality of care they can expect to receive in an organization. As an extension of this, it elevates the standards of the profession overall (ANCC, 2015b; Messmer & Turkel, 2010).

What many do not realize is the history of the Magnet program and its grounding in nursing research. In 1983, the American Academy of Nurses (AAN) Taskforce on Nursing Practice in Hospitals conducted a study in 163 hospitals nationwide to examine the attributes that attracted and retained well-qualified nurses and promoted high-quality patient care. Forty-one hospitals were described as "Magnet" hospitals based on their ability to attract and retain professional nurses. The common attributes in these organizations were analyzed, categorized, and deemed the "14 Forces of Magnetism" based on characteristics that distinguished these organizations from others. It is important to note that the nation was experiencing a nursing shortage (not dissimilar to the current state), and there was great interest in understanding why some organizations were thriving while others were struggling, often within the same communities (ANCC, 2015b; Messmer & Turkel, 2010).

Since 1982, research grounded in the conceptual framework of Magnet has been conducted that highlights the nursing benefits of a positive practice environment. Research findings have consistently emphasized that professional nursing practice situated in organizations with adequate staffing, supportive managers, collaborative interdisciplinary relationships, opportunities for professional growth, autonomy, participation in decision-making, and practice supported by EBPs and research yields lower staff turnover, higher staff satisfaction, and subsequent recruitment and retention of talented staff (ANCC, 2015c; Barden et al., 2011). Although there are clear gains for nurses in Magnet organizations, there are also measurable positive impacts to an organization in both clinical and financial outcomes (Drenkard, 2010; Higdon, Clickner, Gray, Woody, & Shirey, 2013; Jayawardhana, Welton, & Lindrooth, 2014; Joanna Briggs Institute, 2010).

For the past 20 years, Magnet hospital research has framed characteristics of hospital environments such as shared governance, participatory management, expectations of professional nursing practice and autonomy, professional development and advancement opportunities, and strong interdisciplinary relationships (Grant, Colello, Riehle, & Dende, 2010; Gonzalez, Zedreck, Wolf, Ddujak, & Jordan, 2015; Hess, DesRoches, Donelan, Norman, & Buerhaus, 2011; McHugh, Lesley, Smith, Wu, Vanak, & Aiken, 2013; Shepard, et al., 2014;). It is also recognized that these organizational characteristics do not naturally occur, but rather are created by nurse leaders who support professionalism and nursing excellence (Hess, DesRoches, et al., 2011; Kelly, McHugh, & Aiken, 2011).

In 2007, the ANCC undertook a statistical analysis of the Magnet appraisal team scores, which resulted in 30 clusters for the sources of evidence that led to an empirical model for the Magnet Recognition Program. In 2008, the Commission on Magnet introduced the new conceptual model that grouped the original 14 Forces of Magnetism into five components: transformational leadership; structural empowerment; exemplary nursing practice; new knowledge, innovation, and improvements; and empirical outcomes (ANCC, 2015c; Grant et al., 2010; Messmer & Turkel, 2010; Wolf, Triolo, & Ponte, 2008). In addition to streamlining the standards and sources of evidence into five domains or components, the new model places emphasis on empirical outcomes and on the creation of new knowledge and innovations, and it anticipates an agile organization poised to consider interrelated concepts of transformational leadership, collaboration, and organizational outcomes (ANCC, 2015c; Wolf et al., 2008). The release of the 2014 ANCC Magnet Manual streamlined and simplified the documentation needed for Magnet designation application submission (*2014 Magnet Application Manual,* 2013).

Recognizing a need and expressed interest across the globe regarding means to address quality of nursing practice and healthcare delivery, the ANCC broadened the Magnet orientation and identity by establishing international credentialing in 1999. Based on a combination of socioeconomic, political, and professional forces that includes globalization, deregulation, healthcare restructuring, and nursing shortages, the ANCC responded by acknowledging that universal needs exist, and evidence supporting Magnet designation can be applied to health services and institutions throughout the world (ANCC, 2015d). Once thought of as a hospital recognition, Magnet designation encompasses hospitals, skilled nursing facilities in long-term care, and international hospitals, most recently incorporating metrics and measures for ambulatory care settings (ANCC, 2015b).

Pathway to Excellence

The Pathway to Excellence program evolved from the Texas Nurses Association's (TNA's) Texas Nurse Friendly Hospital initiative that began in 2003. The ANCC assumed ownership in 2007 when TNA sought transfer of the program for sustainability. A total of 51 hospitals earned the Nurse Friendly Hospital distinction in meeting the 12 practice standards to improve the work environment and nurse retention under the TNA and were subsequently grandfathered as ANCC Pathway designees (Stringer, 2010; Wood, 2009).

Pathway to Excellence is a new organizational credential that recognizes facilities, including hospitals and nursing homes, that have positive work environments in which nurses flourish. High retention, nurse satisfaction, interdisciplinary collaboration, and patient satisfaction are the cornerstones of the designation (Swartwout, 2012).

Although Pathway and Magnet designations are distinct, many organizations use Pathway to Excellence as a bridge or first step toward Magnet designation (ANCC, 2015a; Swartwout, 2012; Stringer, 2010; Wood, 2009).

Pathway to Excellence is suitable for facilities, clinics, and critical access hospitals of all sizes, as well as hospitals and long-term care facilities (Swartwout, 2012). Many Pathway organizations recognize that they need time and resources to accomplish the research and outcomes requirements for Magnet designation and choose to use Pathway to Excellence as the starting point in establishing a strong work environment for nursing practice.

In 2008 and 2009, the ANCC made minor revisions to the TNA standards so they could apply to national and international audiences. The current Pathway to Excellence practice standards include:

- Control of nursing practice
- Safety of the work environment
- Systems to address patient care concerns
- A solid nurse orientation
- A chief nursing officer involved at all levels of the organization
- Professional development opportunities
- Competitive wages
- Nurse recognition
- Balanced lifestyle
- Exemplary interdisciplinary collaboration
- Leadership accountability
- Quality initiatives (ANCC, 2015a; Stringer, 2010; Wood, 2009).

Hospitals that seek Pathway to Excellence designation submit a written application that describes how their organization meets the 12 standards. After a three-panel nurse review process, a determination is made as to whether the organization can proceed to the second phase, which includes an ANCC online survey to confirm that the application document reflects the nurses' perceptions of the organization. At least 51% of the facility's nurses must fill out the form, and 75% of the results must be favorable (ANCC, 2015a; Wood, 2009).

As a point of application, many organizations have used the framework and essential elements of the Magnet and Pathway to Excellence designations to establish a strategic plan with the purpose of garnering organizational support to improve the work environment and retention of nurses. The testimonials of chief nursing officers and staff alike highlight the importance of clarity, focus, and commitment to defined outcomes as levers to achieving improvement in clinical, financial, and satisfaction outcomes and translating the research and evidence into action. In shifting attention to the value and import of contributions of nurses within the organization, coupled with elevating their practice, other disciplines and departments experience higher performance. Testimonials demonstrating organizational outcomes that emphasize improved quality, staff satisfaction and retention, advancement of the profession, collaboration, appreciation for standards of care, and safety outcomes can be found on the ANCC website (http://nursecredentialing.org/Pathway/AboutPathway/Pathway DefiningMoments).

Malcolm Baldrige National Quality Award

The Malcolm Baldrige National Quality Award was established in 1987 to recognize business, healthcare, education, and nonprofit sectors for performance excellence. Administered by the Baldrige Performance Excellence Program and managed by the National Institute of Standards and Technology through the U.S. Department of Commerce, the award is bestowed on up to 18 organizations annually that promote awareness of performance excellence. These organizations serve as role models of continual improvement and efficient and effective operations as a way of engaging and responding to customers and stakeholder expectations. These efforts are demonstrated through innovation, improvement, visionary leadership, and organizational learning (Arnold, Goodson, & Duarte, 2015; Baldrige, 1995, 2015, Burke, & Hellwig, 2011; Duarte, Goodson, & Arnold, 2013).

In 1999, Baldrige Award criteria were developed for healthcare organizations (Arnold, Goodson, & Duarte, 2015; Baldrige, 2015). The criteria serve as a tool to strengthen organizational performance as a result of customer-focused, data-driven approaches to organizational learning. The criteria offer a guide for aligning individual department goals with the strategic direction of the organization, to provide a road map, and offer role models of best practice to support achieving performance excellence (Baldrige, 2015).

For organizations that have earned Baldrige recognition, creating a culture of learning, embracing change, and learning how to learn as individuals and as organizations are cornerstones to achievement. Grounded in Senge's systems thinking (1990), core values of the Baldrige Award are organizational learning and systems thinking through personal mastery and collaboration. Predicated on EBPs, improvement cycles, participatory decision-making, and learning, it is expected that Baldrige organizations demonstrate learning that is part of daily work practiced at the personal, unit, and organizational levels; the result is demonstrated improvement using a systematic quality improvement structure that leads to effective, significant, and meaningful change (Burke & Hellwig, 2011; Duarte, Goodson, & Arnold, 2013; Shields & Jennings, 2013; Welborn & Bullington, 2013).

Like Magnet designation, Baldrige is focused on leadership, organizational learning, staff participation in successes, continuous improvement, and demonstrated outcomes, but it differs in focus at the organizational level in that it is not centered on a specific discipline. The major focal points are information management, planning, workforce engagement and development, and customer results that are then examined within the sector of industry in which the organization resides (The Foundation for the National Baldrige Quality Award, 2011). The Baldrige Award process starts with a comprehensive inquiry into the operations of an organization to define accountability for patient-centered excellence and executed best practices customized to achieve outcomes and sustain improvements.

Themes found in the profiles of healthcare organizations that have earned the Baldrige Award emphasize their focus on disciplined continuous improvement throughout the organization, attention to quality, innovation, staff development and organizational learning, and measuring successes; these elements have brought these organizations' health systems into sustained success, with exceptional patient satisfaction and strong financial performance in demanding and changing times (see Baldrige Award Testimonials, 2014, for testimonials from Baldrige Award winners in the healthcare industry).

■ Just Culture

In the last decade, the concept of a *just culture* has entered the healthcare arena, via concepts borrowed from the aviation industry, where safety has been studied extensively (ANA, 2010; Boyson, 2013). Interest in just cultures has grown out of changing interpretations of accidents, starting in the 1970s with the Three Mile Island nuclear accident and expanding to include aviation and petrochemical accidents; this interest has led to greater awareness of the need to understand safety and the role that organizations play in promoting it. In health care, culture considered as "the way we do things here" is perceived as an individual value shared by all, suggesting that an individual is responsible for creating and maintaining safety. A culture of safety can be achieved only through organizational commitment by leaders who nurture and perpetuate cultures that value learning, reporting, and fairness (Boysen, 2013; Leonard & Frankel, 2010). When considering the number of preventable deaths (between 44,000 and 98,000) in the United States annually, the response by the healthcare industry has not been as urgent or indignant as that from the airline industry regarding deaths attributed to airline accidents (Griffith, 2010; IOM, 2001).

The principles of a just culture initially seemed out of place when viewed through the lens of the traditional socialization that professionals experience as they enter the health discipline workforce. Today, most corporate disciplinary systems literally prohibit human error. A human error that brings harm to a patient gives rise to social condemnation and disciplinary action, residing in a severity bias in which harm elevates our disdain for an error rather than bringing attention to the underlying system issues that may have been the antecedents to the occurrence (Boysen, 2013; Griffith, 2009). With advances in patient safety, the ability to collectively learn from our errors—whether near-misses or mistakes that bring harm—requires a reevaluation of how discipline fits into the equation (Marx, 2001). A just culture is meant to balance learning from incidents with accountability for their consequences, thus creating a clear line between acceptable and unacceptable behavior (Boysen, 2013; Dekker, 2009).

One defining characteristic of a just culture is the commitment to values—to be a learning culture that resides in fairness, within a system with safe design, high reliability, and effective management of behavioral choices. Although patient safety is a laudable and consistent value that dominates the values of healthcare organizations, alone it is not sufficient to explain why an organization exists or the imperatives that drive performance expectations. Access to care, privacy, compassion, and quality must also be supported. Management dilemmas addressed by a just culture bring questions to the leaders that include how to account for the systems built around caregivers, how caregivers account for their errors and choices within the systems, and how the workplace supports patient safety (Griffith, 2009; Marx, 2001). A just culture establishes a hunger for knowledge and the desire to understand risk at both the individual and organizational levels (Bashaw & Lounsbury, 2012; Griffith, 2009).

Lucian Leape, MD (2000), a member of the Quality of Health Care in America Committee at the Institute of Medicine, provided testimony to the U.S. Congress, noting:

> Approaches that focus on punishing individuals instead of changing systems provide strong incentives for people to report only those errors they cannot hide. Thus, a punitive approach shuts off the information that is needed to identify faulty systems and create safer ones. In a punitive stem, no one learns from their mistakes. (ANA, 2010, p. 2; Leape, 2000)

After this testimony, recognition of and appreciation for the need to shift the view of errors in healthcare delivery away from punishment, litigation, and blame to a space of learning about and acknowledging the influences of processes within a system became more acceptable (ANA, 2010). Greater awareness of systems factors—the interdependent aspects of a healthcare environment comprising direct and indirect relationships among people, equipment, technology, and monitoring relationships—became part of the landscape for clinicians and administrators to examine in complex adaptive systems. Analyzing elements of the system within an organization extended beyond individual culpability to include equipment design, policy, at-risk behavior, and systems factors that contribute to human error (Dolansky & Moore, 2013; North, 2012, Weberg, 2012).

Just culture organizations recognize human error, at-risk behavior, and reckless behavior as each having appropriate (and inappropriate) responses. Human error involves inadvertently doing other than what should have been done, often described as a slip or mistake. Responses to human error often include consoling the person who made the mistake and assisting him or her in making better choices to avoid the error in the future (Griffith, 2010).

At-risk behavior is a choice that increases risk where the risk is not recognized or is mistakenly believed to be justified. Responses to at-risk behavior are similar to human error and often include coaching the individual around his or her risk awareness and removing the barriers or disincentives that lead to noncompliance with rules and procedures. Individual and group norms are often examined for what they may have contributed. Punishment of these errors serves to drive admission or reporting of these choices below the surface. In many organizations, these situations are reported only when they cannot be hidden (Griffith, 2010).

Reckless behavior is a choice to consciously disregard a substantial and unjustifiable risk. Responses to reckless behavior are punishment or discipline. In this, we must recognize the severity bias where the outcome influences how we think about the person involved or how we respond to him or her if we have managerial authority (Griffith, 2010).

Accountability for a just culture resides in the visible priorities of leadership in establishing a reporting culture so that learning and continuous improvement articulate a commitment to learning from and preventing errors (ANA, 2010; Boysen, 2013; Wachter, 2013). Disciplining employees who make honest mistakes does little to improve overall system safety and may drive the errors underground. Mishaps accompanied by intoxication or malicious behaviors present an obvious and valid objection to today's call for blame-free error reporting systems. To gather and utilize productive investigative data, organizational cultures need to make it safe to report errors in the interest of a safe system. Although no one can condone a "blame-free" system in which any conduct is accepted, society rightly requires that some action warrants discipline or enforcement action. It is the balancing of the need to learn from our mistakes and our need for disciplinary action that forms the basis to establish a just culture (Griffith, 2010; Marx, 2001).

A just culture does not equate to a blame-free environment, but rather an environment that engages people in identifying problems and gives them the responsibility of addressing them. Accountability is often defined through a process of retrospective review of a concern or error. In a just culture, our view is shifted to a forward-thinking perspective to create a space to prevent the error from being repeated (Boysen, 2013; Dekker, 2009). A just culture is defined as a culture that is open, fair, and just—a learning culture based on designing safe systems and managing behavioral choices. Individuals are encouraged to report mistakes so that the precursors to the errors can be better understood in order to fix the system issues (ANA, 2010; Marx, 2001). Events are seen as opportunities to improve, with an eye toward both behavioral and system risks (ANA, 2010; Boysen, 2013; Dekker, 2008). Marrying the managerial function of discipline to the human resource function of learning and justice brings the partnership between accountability and learning into focus.

A just culture balances learning from incidents with accountability for their consequences (Dekker, 2008; Griffith, 2010). Traditionally, the healthcare culture has held individuals responsible for error, failing to consider the impact of system failings on individual accountability (Boysen, 2013; Dolansky & Moore, 2013; Dekker, 2009; Marx, 2001). Today's society predominantly recognizes free will as the operant in individual action. Children are taught by parents and teachers to take individual responsibility for their actions. As adults, individual accountability is reinforced through the legal system. In addition, we are cognitively predisposed to view the world in this way. Retrospective analysis of adverse events can be shaped by these biases and precipitate attribution of error to individuals when the actions of others and the system also influence one's actions (Dolansky & Moore, 2013; Yip & Farmer, 2015).

Reason (1997) wrote that a just culture creates trust that encourages and rewards people for providing safety-related information. Additionally, a just culture defines acceptable and unacceptable behaviors; the result is a middle ground between patient safety and a safety culture. Implicitly, learning is fostered through trusting relationships, openness, and a belief that people will be treated fairly when an error occurs. Explicitly, a learning culture exists when active improvement efforts are directed toward redesign, and reporting fuels this learning because staff feel safe from retribution (ANA, 2010; Reason, 1997). In a just culture, human actions are judged fairly and viewed within the complexity of the systems factors (Reason, 1997), and human error is recognized as unintentional and thus not warranting disciplinary action. Effort is placed on balancing error, blame, and discipline with communication and deterrence (Marx, 2001; Dauterive & Schubert, 2013).

A central message of just culture is that expecting perfection has a price. The true path to success starts with understanding what we value, setting our expectations to align with those values, and designing systems to make safe choices meet our expectations. Errors and adverse events will happen, but rather than overreacting to their immediacy, we should focus on managing the risks around us and pursuing high reliability in our process to prevent the events (Griffith, 2010).

As a vivid point of application of, and appreciation for, how a just culture is different from the culture many operate in, an interview with Julie George, the associate executive director of programs for the North Carolina Board of Nursing, summarized how the use of the definitions in a just culture and the application of the decision algorithm offer a consistent and thoughtful approach to errors in healthcare delivery (Comden, 2007).

George recalled an experience early in her career with the state board of nursing. A nurse with 20 years of impeccable practice experience made an error when administering blood. The nurse recognized her error, but there was lingering impact to the patient. She committed a human error. There was no pattern of substandard care, and her behavior was not intentional or reckless. The systems issues were identified, but because the focus was on outcomes and there was harm, it was a sentinel event, and the nurse was reported to the state board. The sanction for this type of incident was a letter of reprimand, the result of which was a disciplinary report held in the national practitioner data bank. The hospital terminated this 20-year nurse with an otherwise outstanding employment record. Everyone lost in this case: the nurse, the community, and the hospital. The nurse never returned to nursing, and her career and self-confidence were destroyed. Had the hospital been using a just culture decision-making model, the nurse would have been consoled for the human error, not terminated (Comden, 2007).

■ Culture of Safety

A review of the patient safety literature often begins with the seminal Institute of Medicine report *To Err Is Human: Building a Safer Health System*. This report found that medical errors kill between 44,000 and 98,000 people in U.S. hospitals each year (IOM, 2004). Even with the lower death estimate, more people die from medical errors than from car accidents, breast cancer, or AIDS. Based on this, the IOM recommended that healthcare organizations create a culture of safety as an organizational imperative driven by leaders (IOM, 1999; Sammer, Lyken, Singh, Mains, & Lackan, 2010). This led to process improvements and acknowledgment of the widespread safety concerns (Leape, Berwick, & Bates, 2002) and questions about how leaders would know that the culture was safe (Pronovost et al., 2003).

Early attention was focused on defining a culture of safety; this definition was in large part framed by the work of the Agency for Healthcare Research and Quality (AHRQ) and the Health and Safety Commission of Great Britain: "The safety culture of an organization is the product of individual and group values, attitudes, perceptions, competencies, and patterns of behavior that determine the commitment to, and the style and proficiency of, an organization's health and safety management" (Health and Safety Commission, 1993, p. 23; see also Sammer et al., 2010). According to the literature, the major predictors of a positive patient safety culture in healthcare organizations are built on mutual trust, good information flow, shared perceptions about the importance of safety, organizational learning, commitment from management and leadership, and presence of a nonpunitive approach to incident and error reporting (DiCuccio, 2014; Sorra, Khanna, Dyer, Mardon, & Famolaro, 2012). Patient safety culture outcomes include the staff members' perception of safety, the willingness of staff members to report events, the number of events reported, and an overall patient safety grade given by staff members to their units (Ammouri et al., 2015; DiCuccio, 2014). It is generally agreed that a safety culture includes a just culture, a reporting culture, and a learning culture. Event reporting, an essential component for achieving a learning culture, can happen only in a nonpunitive environment in which events can be reported without blame (Ammouri et al., 2015; DiCuccio, 2014; El-Jardali, Dimassi, Jamal, Jaafar, & Hemadeh, 2011).

Assessing an organization's existing safety culture is the first step in developing a new safety culture, and these assessments are a requirement of international accreditation organizations (AHRQ, 2015; El-Jardali et al., 2011). These assessments draw attention to practices that require urgent attention, identify strengths and weaknesses of the safety culture, and help individual units identify safety problems by benchmarking scores with other organizations (AHRQ, 2015; Blegen, Gearhart, O'Brien, Seghal, and Alldredge, 2009; Leonard & Frankel, 2010).

As different organizations have put words in place to define a safety culture, what has become apparent in recent years are the different characteristics, knowledge, and implications attributed to the words by different disciplines in health care as well as by the stakeholders and regulators who may have different assumptions, values, and language to describe their expectations. Sammer et al. (2010) critically reviewed the safety literature to identify studies that addressed the beliefs, attitudes, and behaviors central to a culture of safety in hospitals. This led to their belief that a more comprehensive framework to organize the properties of a culture of safety model were needed by leaders to establish or improve a safety culture in organizations. The seven key properties follow:

- Leaders must acknowledge the healthcare environment as a high-risk environment and align the mission, vision, staff competence, and fiscal and human resources, from the frontline to the boardroom, to address safety.
- Teamwork demonstrated by collegiality, collaboration, and cooperation must exist among executives, staff, and independent practitioners. Relationships are open, safe, respectful, and flexible.
- Patient care practices are evidence based and standardized to achieve high reliability.
- Each staff member, no matter what his or her job, has the right and responsibility to speak up on behalf of a patient.
- The hospital learns from its mistakes and seeks opportunities for performance improvement. All members of the organization value learning.
- The culture is just and recognizes errors as system failures but also recognizes the need to hold individuals accountable for their actions.
- Patient-centered care is delivered around the patient and family through active participation. Patients and families act as a liaison between the hospital and the community.

Naevestad (2009) extended the conceptualization of a safety culture and suggested that a major challenge in safety culture research is neglect of the mesosystem—consequentially, an incomplete conceptualization of the relationships among culture, technology, and structure in high-risk organizations. He postulated that the opposition found in the functional and integrative definitions of safety cultures ignores the relationship between high-reliability organizations (HROs) and standardization and compliance, and it negates the importance of professional meaning and values, thereby limiting sustainable change. This parallels the paradigm of understanding why health care should be underscored as a high-risk endeavor similar to high-risk industries such as aviation, nuclear power, and petrochemical; relative to these industries, healthcare and other industries are viewed through the lens of "lower risk" (Boysen, 2013; Ross, 2011; Wachter, 2013; Yip & Farmer, 2015).

Reason (1997) offered that although the concept of safety culture is popular, it is poorly understood. Safety scholars agree that the research on safety culture and its relationship with safety is fragmented and unsystematic (Dauterive & Schubert, 2013; DiCuccio, 2014). Moreover, research is conducted as a stand-alone function rather than integrated into general models of organizational culture. The compartmentalization of problems as patient or nonpatient and harm versus no harm suggests that culture drives structure. Within the Joint Commission standards for the environment of care, safety committees typically composed of service and support managers address the clinical issues and further subdivide the culture (Joint Commission, 2011). Sammer et al. (2010) offered that despite the efforts of the National Patient Safety Foundation, the AHRQ, the Joint Commission, and others, few hospital executives have invested resources in the measurement of patient safety status or the culture of safety (Pronovost et al., 2003). Although true within the past decade, the interest in culture, safety, and outcomes has grown and is now being coupled with construct development and disciplined study to understand the nuances in health care (AHRQ, 2015; Chassin & Loeb, 2011; DiCuccio, 2014; Griffith & Pope, 2015; Pumar-Méndez, Attree, & Wakefield, 2014).

Functionalist scholars understand culture as shared patterns of behavior embraced to be the preferred approach by practitioners and managers (Boysen, 2013; DiCuccio, 2014; Reason, 1997; Yang et al., 2009). That being the case, a limitation of these studies is the superficial conceptualization of culture and the lack of deeper understanding of shared patterns of meaning that motivate, legitimize, and establish identity with an organization; these are important factors in completely understanding safety cultures (Sitterding, 2011). Further, Perrow (1999) and Turner (1978) demonstrated the impact of technology and ignorance on hazards and signals of danger and failures. HRO researchers have argued that the lack of awareness of threats or hazards can be reduced by means of collective mindfulness (Busby & Iszatt-White, 2014; Vogus, Sutcliffe, & Weick, 2010;) but acknowledged the difficulties in translating mindfulness into individual and collective action.

Recent attention to HROs offers a framework to explain and understand how high-risk industries or organizations are able to achieve consistent quality outcomes through meticulous attention to danger signals and embedded strong responses to maintain or restore system function. Hallmarks of an HRO are capable and reliable achievement of quality outcomes and the capability to identify weak danger signals and execute strong responses to maintain or restore system function. In this regard, healthcare reliability is viewed as the ability of a process, procedure, or service to perform the intended function despite varying circumstances (Busby & Iszatt-White, 2014; Despins, 2014; Weick & Sutcliffe, 2001; Yip & Farmer, 2015).

Interest in HROs arose from the gaps identified in understanding of patient safety; identification of these gaps exposed system failures and reliance on compliance with policies or rules as an incomplete approach to facing technologically infused complex organizations. A team or organization's ability to sustain a balance of information flow, diversity and difference, internal and external connections, power, and anxiety brings creative potential to addressing near-misses or errors. The distinctive qualities of HROs are preoccupation with failure; reluctance to accept simplifications; sensitivity to operations; resilience to error; and deference to experience (Blouin, 2013; Despins, 2014; Yip & Farmer, 2015). These principles parallel and support the learning organization, systems thinking, and unrelenting attention to quality improvement processes within just cultures. Kaissi (2012) examined learning and the healthcare industry's ability sustain change and incorporate high reliability behaviors into the culture. Recognizing traditional healthcare training is ineffective in developing HROs because professional role socialization and organizational behaviors are tradition-laden in the clinical environment, experts agree that the development of HROs will require more than decentralizing role structures; behavioral changes as well as knowledge, culture, and perceptions about repercussions will also be necessary (Blouin, 2015; Castel, Ginsburg, Zaheer, & Tamim, 2015; Kaissi, 2012; Sherwood & Zomorodi, 2014; Wood, 2015).

Drawing from best practices in other high-risk, complex organizations such as the military, law enforcement, and aviation, it appears that research, training, simulation, and decision support methods offer the most promise in teaching clinicians how to meet the situational demands of their work environments. Blouin (2013), Wood (2015), and Yip & Farmer, (2015) highlighted that unless providers are clear about what needs to be communicated, exactly who should be communicating what, and how individuals should be communicating, the potential for error in healthcare delivery will always be high. Clarity in high reliability principles borrowed from other industries provides a framework to address concerns in health care.

■ Conclusion

In review of the evidence for organizational systems and change, several themes emerge that have taken shape during the last 30 years. Organizations must be considered within a social context made up of leaders, followers, participants, and patients, with the beliefs, values, and perceptions held by each. Learning, collaboration, communication, interrelationships between process and departments, and information sharing are central to the effectiveness of an organization. Perceptions shape our thinking and actions and are influenced by the norms, expectations, and experiences we hold; the interdependence of these elements creates the space to define and achieve sustainable success. Concepts of systems and system thinking, shared decision-making, autonomy, and striving for excellence underpin the attainment of effective work environments, patient safety, and a just culture in which learning and accountability rest on a platform of continuous and inclusive improvement grounded in EBPs and empirical outcomes.

Central to any discussion about organizations are the mission, vision, and values that guide their existence. Successful organizations have leaders who inspire curiosity, innovation, and demonstrations of excellence irrespective of their title or position in an organization. One of the many challenges that face healthcare organizations in the near term is creating stability in tumultuous environments in which disciplined and systematic approaches to improvement are essential. A backdrop of openness, flexibility, and commitment to finding creative solutions that address the regulatory, financial, and social mandates for improved care delivery outcomes frames the thinking, but none of this can be attained without awareness of what drives our automatic and habitual responses. Acknowledgment of the interdependence of our systems' elements and an unrelenting commitment to change will shift organizational paradigms started by revisions in individual assumptions and then inspired by collective action.

REFLECTIVE ACTIVITIES

1. Consider your unit, service line, or nursing department. Using an organizational lens, what strengths and areas for improvement are you able to identify using concepts from shared leadership, just culture, and organizational learning?

2. You have been hired into a senior leadership position that you consider ideal. How would you design an organizational assessment to establish the current state assessment of shared governance, just culture, and safety? Whom would you include as key stakeholders? What evidence would you request to inform your assessment?

3. You have joined an organization that is struggling with clinical care outcomes and stands to lose significant money in the coming months if the metrics do not improve. What recommendations would you make to the senior leadership team to improve these metrics?

4. You are the senior nursing leader who has been asked to evaluate the value of implementing just culture. What elements of the organization would you examine to inform a report to the board about the time and resources necessary for implementation? How would you describe a return on investment or cost-benefit if just culture became part of the fabric of the organization?

5. Your organization is concerned about values-based purchasing and recognizes the strategic linkages between a culture of safety, patient satisfaction, and Magnet designation. Considering each of these levers, what initiative and framework would you select to achieve outcomes that would benefit values-based purchasing metrics? Why would you select that lever as opposed to others?

REFERENCES

Abdelhandi, N., & Drach-Zahavy, A. (2012). Promoting patient care: work engagement as a mediator between ward service climate and patient-centred care, *Journal of Advanced Nursing, 68*(6), 1276–1287.

Agency for Healthcare Research and Quality. (2015). Surveys on Patient Safety Culture. Retrieved from http://www.ahrq.gov/professionals/quality-patient-safety/patientsafetyculture/index.html

American Nurses Association. (2010). *Just culture position statement*. Retrieved from http://www.nursingworld.org/psjustculture

American Nurses Credentialing Center. (2013). *2014 Magnet Application Manual*. Retrieved from http://www.nursecredentialing.org/MagnetApplicationManual

American Nurses Credentialing Center. (2015a). *Pathway program overview*. Retrieved from http://nursecredentialing.org/Pathway/AboutPathway

American Nurses Credentialing Center. (2015b). *History of the Magnet program.* Retrieved from http://nursecredentialing.org/Magnet/ProgramOverview/HistoryoftheMagnetProgram

American Nurses Credentialing Center. (2015b). *Announcing the model for ANCC's Magnet Recognition Program.* Retrieved from http://nursecredentialing.org/MagnetModel

American Nurses Credentialing Center. (2015d). *Credentialing International.* Retrieved from http://nursecredentialing.org/Magnet/International

Ammouri, A., Tailakh, A., Muliira, J., Geethakrishnan, R., & Al Kindi, S. (2015). Patient safety culture among nurses. *International Nursing Review, 62*(1), 102–110.

Arnold, E. (2013). Improving organizational climate for excellence in patient care. *The Health Care Manager, 32*(3), 280–286.

Arnold, E., Goodson, J., & Duarte, N., (2015). Workforce and leader development: Learning from the Baldrige Winners in health care. *The Health Care Manager (Frederick), 34*(3), 177–186.

Ashanasy, N., Wilderom, C., & Peterson M. (2011). *The handbook of organizational culture and climate* (2nd ed.). Thousand Oaks, CA: Sage Publications.

Baldrige Award Healthcare Criteria. (1995). Retrieved from http://www.nist.gov/baldrige/publications/hc_criteria.cfm

Baldrige Award Testimonials. (2015). *Testimonials from health care.* Retrieved from http://www.nist.gov/baldrige/about/history.cfm

Baldrige Performance Excellence Program. (2015). *History.* Retrieved from http://www.nist.gov/baldrige/about/history.cfm

Bamford-Wade, A., & Moss, C. (2010). Transformational leadership and shared governance: An action study. *Journal of Nursing Management, 18*(7) 815–821.

Barden, A., Griffin, M., Donahue, M., & Fitzpatrick, J. (2011). Shared governance and empowerment in registered nurses working in a hospital setting. *Nursing Administration Quarterly, 35*(3), 212–218.

Bashaw, E., & Lounsbury, K. (2012). Forging a new culture: Blending Magnet® Principles with Just Culture, *Nursing Management, 43*(10), 49–53.

Beglinger, J. (2015). Designing tomorrow transitioning from participation to governance, *Journal of Nursing Administration, 45*(3), 128–129.

Bellot, J. (2011). Defining and assessing organizational culture, *Nursing Forum 46*(1), 29–37.

Blegen, M., Gearhart, S., O'Brien, R., Seghal, N., & Alldredge, B. (2009). AHRQ's hospital survey on patient safety culture: Psychometric analyses. *Journal of Patient Safety, 5,* 139–144.

Blouin, A. (2013). High reliability: Truly achieving healthcare quality and safety. *Frontiers of Health Services Management, 29*(3), 35–40.

Boysen, P. (2013). Just culture: A foundation for balanced accountability and patient safety. *The Ochsner Journal, 13,* 400–406.

Buckman, K., Sellers, D., & Batchellar, J. (2012). An integrated system's nursing shared governance model a system chief nursing officer's synergistic vehicle for leading a complex health care system. *Nursing Administration Quarterly, 36*(4), 353–361.

Burke, K., & Hellwig, S. (2011). Education in high-performing hospitals: Using the Baldrige framework to demonstrate positive outcomes. *Journal of Continuing Education in Nursing, 42*(7), 299–305.

Busby, J., & Iszatt-White, M. (2014). The relational aspect to high reliability organization. *Journal of Contingencies and Crisis Management, 22*(2), 69–80.

Castel, E., Ginsburg, L., Zaheer, S., & Tamim, H. (2015). Understanding nurses' and physicians' fear of repercussions for reporting errors: Clinician characteristics, organization demographics, or leadership factors? *BMC Health Services Research, 15,* 326. doi:10.1186/s12913-015-0987-9

Chassin, M., & Loeb J. (2011). The ongoing quality improvement journey: next stop, high reliability. *Health Affairs, 30,* 559–568.

Christian, M., Bradley, J., Wallace, J., & Burke, M. (2009). Workplace safety: A meta-analysis of the roles of person and situation factors. *Journal of Applied Psychology, 94*(3), 1103–1127.

Christman, L. (1976). The autonomous nursing staff in the hospital. *Nursing Administration Quarterly, 1,* 37–44.

Clavelle, J., Porter-O'Grady, T., Drenkard, K. (2013). Structural empowerment and the nursing practice environment in Magnet organizations. *Journal of Nursing Administration, 43*(11), 566–573.

Cleland, V. (1978). Shared governance is a professional model of collective bargaining. *Journal of Nursing Administration, 8*(5), 39–43.

Comden, S. (2007). *Interview with Julie George, RN, MSN, associate executive director–programs, North Carolina Board of Nursing.* Retrieved from http://www.justculture.org/newsletters.aspx

Crow, G., Nguyen, T., DeBourgh, G. (2014). Virtual nursing grand rounds and shared governance: How innovation and empowerment are transforming nursing practice at Thanh Nhan Hospital, Hanoi, Vietnam. *Nursing Administration Quarterly, 38*(1), 55–61.

Dahinten, V. S., MacPhee, M., Hejazi, S., Laschinger, H., Kazanjian, M., McCutcheon, A., . . . & O'Brien-Pallas, L. (2014). Testing the effects of an empowerment-based leadership development programme. II. Staff outcomes. *Journal of Nursing Management, 22*(1), 16–28.

Dauterive, F., & Schubert, A. (2013). Ethics, quality, safety, and a just culture: The link is evident. *The Ochsner Journal, 13*, 293–294.

Dearmon, V., Riley, B., Mestas, L., Buckner, E. (2015). Bridge to shared government: Developing leadership of frontline nurses. *Nursing Administration Quarterly, 39*(1), 69–77.

Dekker, S. (2008). *Just culture: Balancing safety and accountability.* United Kingdom: Ashgate.

Dekker, S. (2009). Just culture: Who gets to draw the line? *Cognition, Technology & Work, 11*, 177–185.

Despins, L. (2014). Organizational and individual attributes influencing patient risk detection. *Clinical Nursing Research, 23*(5) 471–489.

DiCuccio, M. (2014).The relationship between patient safety culture and patient outcomes: A systematic review. *Journal of Patient Safety, 11*(3), 135–142.

Dolansky, M., & Moore, S. (2013) Quality and safety education for nurses (QSEN): The key is systems thinking. *OJIN: The Online Journal of Issues in Nursing, 18*(3), 71–80.

Drenkard, K. (2010). The business case for Magnet. *Journal of Nursing Administration, 40*(6), 263–271.

Duarte, N., Goodson, J., & Arnold, E. (2013). Performance management excellence among the Malcolm Baldrige National Quality Award Winners in Health. *The Health Care Manager, 32*(4), 346–358.

El-Jardali, F., Dimassi, H., Jamal, D., Jaafar, M., & Hemadeh, N. (2011). Predictors and outcomes of patient safety culture in hospitals. *BMC Health Services Research, 11*(45). Retrieved from http://www.biomedcentral.com/1472-6963/11/45

Foundation for the National Baldridge Quality Award. (2011). Retrieved from http://www.nist.gov/baldrige/

Fray, B. (2011). Evaluating shared governance: Measuring functionality of unit practice. *Creative Nursing, 17*(2):87–95.

George, V., & Sovering, S. (2013). Transforming the context of care through shared leadership and partnership an international CNO perspective. *Nursing Administration Quarterly, 37*(1), 52–59.

Gonzalez, J., Zedreck, J., Wolf, G., Ddujak, L., & Jordan, B. (2015). Impact of Magnet culture in maintaining quality outcomes during periods of organizational transition. *Journal of Nursing Care Quality, 30*(4), 323–330.

Grant, B., Colello, S., Riehle, M., & Dende, D. (2010). An evaluation of the nursing practice environment and successful change management using the new generation Magnet model. *Journal of Nursing Management, 18*(3), 326–331.

Greenslade, J., & Jimmieson, N. (2011). Organizational factors impacting on patient satisfaction: A cross sectional examination of service climate and linkages to nurses' effort and performance. *International Journal of Nursing Studies 48*, 1188–1198.

Griffith, K. (2009). The growth of a just culture. *The Joint Commission Perspectives on Patient Safety, 9*(12), 8–9.

Griffith, K. (2010). Error prevention in a just culture: System design or human behavior. *The Joint Commission Perspectives on Patient Safety, 10*(6), 10–11.

Griffith, J., & Pope, J. (2015). Understanding high-reliability organizations: Are Baldrige recipients models? *Journal of Healthcare Management, 60*(1), 44–62.

Health and Safety Commission. (1993). *Third report: Organizing for safety.* ACSNI Study Group on Human Factors. London, England: HMSO.

Hess, R. (2011). Slicing and dicing shared governance: In and around the numbers. *Nursing Administration Quarterly, 35*(3), 235–241.

Hess, R., DesRoches, C., Donelan, K., Norman, L., & Buerhaus, P. (2011). Perceptions of nurses in Magnet hospitals, non-Magnet hospitals, and hospitals pursuing Magnet status. *Journal of Nursing Administration, 41*(7/8), 315–323.

Higdon, K., Clickner, D., Gray, F., Woody, G., & Shirey, M. (2013). Business case for Magnet® in a small hospital. *Journal of Nursing Administration, 43*(2), 113–118.

Hoying, C., & Allen, S. (2011). Enhancing shared governance for interdisciplinary practice. *Nursing Administration Quarterly, 35*(3), 252–259.

Institute of Medicine. (1999). *To err is human: Building a safer health system.* Washington, DC: National Academy Press.

Institute of Medicine. (2001). *Crossing the chasm: A new health system for the 21st century.* Washington, DC: National Academies Press.

Institute of Medicine. (2004). *Keeping patients safe: Transforming the work environment of nurses.* Washington, DC: National Academies Press.

Jacques, R. (1996). *Manufacturing the employee: Management knowledge from the 19th to 21st centuries.* London, England: Sage Publications.

Jayawardhana, J., Welton, J., & Lindrooth, R. (2014). Is there a business case for Magnet hospitals? Estimates of the cost and revenue implications of becoming Magnet. *Medical Care, 52*(2), 400–406.

Joanna Briggs Institute. (2010). Evidence on determining the impact of Magnet designation on nursing and patient outcomes best practice: evidence-based information sheets for health professionals. *Best Practice, 14*(11):1–4. Retrieved from http://connect.jbiconnectplus.org/ViewSourceFile.aspx?0=5383

Joint Commission. (2011). *Accreditation manual for hospitals.* Chicago, IL: Joint Commission.

Kanter, R. (1977). *Men and women of the corporation.* New York, NY: Basic Books.

Kanter, R. M. (1997). *Rosabeth Moss Kanter on the frontiers of management.* Boston, MA: Harvard Business Review Press.

Kaissi, A. (2012). "Learning" from other industries: lessons and challenges for health care organizations. *The Health Care Manager, 31*(1), 65–74.

Kelly, L., McHugh, M., Aiken, L. (2011). Nurse outcomes in Magnet® and non-Magnet hospitals, *Journal of Nursing Administration, 41*(10), 428–433.

Krive, J. (2013). Building effective workforce management practices through shared governance and technology systems integration, *Nursing Economics, 31*(5), 231–236, 249.

Laschinger, H., & Fida, R. (2015). Linking nurses' perceptions of patient care quality to job satisfaction: The role of authentic leadership and empowering professional practice environments. *Journal of Nursing Administration, 45*(5), 276–283.

Laschinger, H., Nosko, A., Wilk, P., & Finegan, J. (2014). Effects of unit empowerment and perceived support for professional nursing practice on unit effectiveness and individual nurse well-being: A time-lagged study. *International Journal of Nursing Studies, 51*(12), 1615–1623.

Laschinger, H., Read, E., Wilk, P., & Fiegan, J. (2014).The influence of nursing unit empowerment and social capital on unit effectiveness and nurse perceptions of patient care quality. *Journal of Nursing Administration, 44*(6), 347–352.

Leape, L. (January 25, 2000). Testimony, United States Congress, United States Senate Subcommittee on Labor, Health and Human Services, and Education.

Leape, L. L., Berwick, M. D., & Bates, D. W. (2002). What practices will most improve safety? Evidence-based medicine meets patient safety. *Journal of the American Medical Association, 288,* 501–507.

Leonard, M., & Frankel, A. (2010). The path to safe and reliable healthcare. *Patient Education and Counseling, 80*(3), 288–292.

Linnen, D., & Rowley, A. (2014). Encouraging clinical nurse empowerment. *Nursing Management, 45*(2), 44–47.

MacPhee, M., Dahinten, V. S., Hejazi, S., Laschinger, H., Kazanjian, A., McCutcheon, A., & O'Brien-Pallas, L. (2014). Testing the effects of an empowerment-based leadership development programme. I. Leader outcomes. *Journal of Nursing Management, 22*(1), 4–15.

Marx, D. (2001). *Patient safety and the "just culture": A primer for healthcare executives.* Retrieved from http://psnet.ahrq.gov/resource.aspx?resourceID=1582

McHugh, M., Lesley, K., Smith, H., Wu, E., Vanak, J., & Aiken, L. (2013). Lower mortality in Magnet hospitals. *Medical Care, 51*(5), 382–388.

Messmer, P. R., & Turkel, M. C. (2010). Magnetism and the nursing workforce. *Annual Review of Nursing Research, 28,* 233–252.

Naevestad, T. (2009). Mapping research on culture and safety in high-risk organizations: Arguments for a sociotechnical understanding of safety culture. *Journal of Contingencies and Crisis Management, 7*(2), 126–136.

North, N. (2012). A systems perspective on nursing productivity. *Journal of Health Organization and Management, 26*(2), 192–214.

Perrow, C. (1999). *Normal accidents: Living with high risk technologies* (2nd ed.). Princeton, NJ: Princeton University Press.

Porter-O'Grady, T. (2012). Reframing knowledge work: Shared governance in the postdigital age. *Creative Nursing, 18*(4), 152–159.

Porter-O'Grady, T. (2015). Confluence and convergence: Team effectiveness in complex systems. *Nursing Administration Quarterly, 39*(1), 78–83.

Porter-O'Grady, T., & Finnigan, S. (1984). *Shared governance for nursing.* Rockville, MD: Aspen Systems Corporation.

Pronovost, P., Weast, B., Holzmueller, C., Rosenstein, B., Kidwell, R., & Haller, K., Rubin, H. (2003). Evaluation of the culture of safety: Survey of clinicians and managers in an academic medical center. *Quality and Safety in Health Care, 12,* 205–410.

Pumar-Méndez, M., Attree, M., & Wakefield, A. (2014). Methodological aspects in the assessment of safety culture in the hospital setting: A review of the literature. *Nurse Education Today 34,* 162–170.

Reason, J. (1997). *Managing the risks of organizational accidents.* London, England: Ashgate.

Ross, J. (2011) Patient safety outcomes: The importance of understanding the organizational culture and safety climate. *Journal of PeriAnesthesia Nursing, 26*(5), 347–348.

Rundquist, J., & Givens, P. (2013). *Quantifying the benefits of staff participation in shared governance,* 8(3), 38–42.

Sammer, C., Lykens, K., Singh, K., Mains, D., & Lackan, N. (2010). What is patient safety culture? A review of the literature. *Journal of Nursing Scholarship, 42*(2), 156–165.

Schein, E. (Ed.). (1997). *Organizational culture and leadership* (2nd ed.). San Francisco, CA: Jossey-Bass.

Senge, P. (1990). *The fifth discipline: The art and practice of the learning organization.* New York, NY: Doubleday Currency.

Senge, P., Kleiner, A., Roberts, C., Ross, R., & Smith, B. (1994). *The fifth discipline fieldbook: Strategies and tools for building a learning organization.* New York, NY: Doubleday Currency.

Shepard, M. L., Harris, M., Chung, H., & Himes, E. (2014). Using the Awareness, Desire, Knowledge, Ability, Reinforcement Model to build a shared governance culture. *Journal of Nursing Education and Practice, 4*(6), 90–104.

Sherwood, G., & Zomorodi, M. (2014). A new mindset for quality and safety: The QSEN competencies redefine nurses' roles in practice. *Nephrology Nursing Journal, 41*(1), 15–22, 72.

Shields, J., & Jennings, J. (2013). Using the Malcolm Baldrige "Are We Making Progress" survey for organizational self-assessment and performance improvement. *Journal for Healthcare Quality, 35*(4), 5–15.

Sitterding, M., (2011). Overview and summary: creating a culture of safety: The next steps. *OJIN: The Online Journal of Issues in Nursing, 16*(3).

Sorra, J., Khanna, K., Dyer, N., Mardon, R., & Famolaro, T. (2012). Exploring relationships between patient safety culture and patients' assessments of hospital care. *Journal of Patient Safety, 8*(3), 131–139.

Squires, M., Tourangeau, A., Laschinger, H. K. S., & Doran, D. (2010). The link between leadership and safety outcomes in hospitals. *Journal of Nursing Management, 18*(8), 914–925.

Stringer, H. (2010). Workplace transformation: Pathway to Excellence Program aims to improve conditions for RNs. *Nursing Spectrum, 20*(17). Retrieved from https://news.nurse.com/2010/10/18/workplace-transformation-pathway-to-excellence-program-aims-to-improve-conditions-for-rns/

Swartwout, E. (2012). *How implementing the practice standards can improve nursing care, satisfaction, and retention.* Retrieved from http://www.nursecredentialing.org/Pathway/PathwayResources/PathwayBenefitsPDF.pdf

Turner, B. (1978). *Man-made disasters.* London, England: Wykeham Publications.

Vogus, T., Sutcliffe, K., & Weick, K. (2010). Do no harm: Enabling, enacting and elaborating a culture of safety in health care. *Academy of Management Perspectives, 24*(4), 60–77.

von Bertalanffy, L. (1969). *General system theory: Foundations, development, application.* New York, NY: George Braziller.

Wachter, R. (2013). Personal accountability in healthcare: Searching for the right balance. *Quality and Safety in Health Care, 22,* 176–182.

Weberg, D. (2012). Complexity leadership: A healthcare imperative. *Nursing Forum, 47*(4), 268–277.

Weick, K., & Sutcliffe, K. (2001). *Managing the unexpected: Assuring high performance in an age of complexity.* San Francisco, CA: Jossey-Bass.

Weick, K., Sutcliffe, K., & Obstfeld, D. (1999). Organizing for high reliability: Processes of collective mindfulness. In B. M. Staw & L. L. Cummings (Eds.), *Research in organizational behavior* (Vol. 21, pp. 81–123). Grenwich, CT: JAI Press.

Welborn, C., & Bullington, K. (2013). Benchmarking award winning health care organizations in the USA. *Benchmarking: An International Journal, 20*(6), 765–776.

Williams, J. (2015). A systems thinking approach to analysis of the Patient Protection and Affordable Care Act. *Journal of Public Health Management Practice, 21*(1), 6–11.

Wolf, F., Triolo, P., & Ponte, P. (2008). Magnet recognition program: The next generation. *Journal of Nursing Administration, 38*(4), 200–204.

Wood, D. (2009). *ANCC's Pathway to Excellence: Commitment to good nursing environments.* Retrieved from http://www.nursezone.com

Wood, E. (2015). Communication, collaboration, commitment are cornerstones of high reliability healthcare. *OR Manager 31*(3), 18–21.

Yang, C., Wang, Y., Chang, S., Guo, S., & Huang, M. (2009). A study on leadership behavior, safety culture, and safety performance of the healthcare industry. *Proceedings of World Academy of Science, Engineering and Technology, 41,* 1148–1155.

Yip, L., & Farmer, B. (2015). High reliability organizations: Medication safety. *Journal of Medical Toxicology, 11,* 257–261.

CHAPTER 9

The Nature of the Evidence: Microsystems, Macrosystems, and Mesosystems

■ Linda A. Roussel ■

■ Objectives:

- Discuss complexity science and complex adaptive systems (CASs) as a conceptual perspective for understanding microsystems, macrosystems, and mesosystems.
- Describe clinical microsystems as small organized groups of providers and staff caring for a defined population of patients.
- Identify common principles for systems thinking that have implications for microsystems, macrosystems, and mesosystems.
- Describe leadership, change management, and engagement as important to system innovation.

■ Introduction

Complexity science theory provides the concepts and principles for understanding CASs. Microsystems, macrosystems, and mesosystems are CASs. "A complex adaptive system is a collection of individual agents with freedom to act in ways that are not always totally predictable, and whose actions are interconnected so that one agent's actions changes the context for other agents" (Plsek & Greenhalgh, 2001, p. 627). Patterns of relationships in the systems, how these relationships sustain, self-regulate, and self-organize, and outcomes that emerge are inherent in CASs. CASs require that we become adaptable to the chaotic changes all around us.

Health care has become increasingly complex, requiring a greater understanding of systems at all levels: microsystems, macrosystems, and mesosystems. Evidence-based organizational systems provide a framework for understanding complexity and serve providers well in facilitating innovation and improvement science. Other research has described leadership, organizational systems, culture, and work environments, and tools, methods, and strategies have been advanced for translating theory and research-based evidence into excellence in administrative practice. This chapter provides a "deeper dive" into systems-level understanding and gives examples of the utility of viewing systems from a multidimensional perspective.

Complex Adaptive Systems

CASs readily describe our current healthcare system. Properties of CASs, such as diversity, embeddedness, distributed control, nonlinear dynamics, adaptable elements, and emergence, coexist as the paradox of order and disorder. The dynamics of CASs provide a lens for understanding a new and perhaps different way of being in the world, be they microsystems, macrosystems, or mesosystems. From complexity and CASs, we appreciate the concept of relatedness and that connections occur at all levels. Systems thrive on relationships, and it is at the intersections that providers and patients and providers and providers meet. Control is an illusion. Attempts to control the process are often fraught with frustration and aggression, resulting in a sense of powerlessness to influence outcomes.

Using the machine metaphor (a reductionist model), we have been socialized to find the right fix—that is, to break down processes (reducing ambiguity), to come to grips with any paradox by resolving uncertainty and to simplify our situation. Complexity science professes that it is often more effective to work through a variety of methods, allowing for flow and, evolving and shifting over time to options that are working best. Plsek and Greenhalgh (2001) gave examples of Schön's reflective practitioner, Kolb's experiential learning model, and the Plan-Do-Study-Act cycle of quality improvement as means of exploring new ways through trial and error, taking risk, and trying unique methods that may not at first blush be the "right solution" (p. 628). "Believing implicitly in a system as machine, nurses would see the policy making framework as separate from their daily work, and that it should involve rational planning, forecasting, and predictions" (Lindberg, Nash, & Lindberg, 2008, p. 131).

Clinical Microsystems and High-Performing Work Teams

Researchers at Dartmouth University led by Nelson, Batalden, Godfrey, and others studied clinical microsystems in health care, with the aim of identifying characteristics that lead to high-level performance. The authors published their work in the *Joint Commission Journal on Quality and Patient Safety* and also in *Quality by Design: A Clinical Microsystem Approach* (Nelson, Batalden, & Godfrey, 2007). Qualities include:

- High-performing teams that foster a positive culture and advocate for microsystems. This requires leadership and organizational support aiming toward purpose and greater clarity of goals and expectations. This is a primary role of leadership.
- High-performing teams demonstrate authentic relationships that highlight and underscore trust, collaboration, helpful attitudes, appreciation of

complementary roles of staff, and recognition of the contributions of everyone. Cultures should be created to support education, intensive training, and interdependence of the care team. This is aligned when staff are hired with the aims in mind and integrated into the work and culture of the system.

- High-performing teams are patient-centric, with attention to continuity of care and flow, including caring behaviors such as listening, being sensitive to special needs, and engaging patients through relationships with family and community.
- High-performing teams are relentless in their pursuit of results focused on process improvement, creating an environment of learning and redesign. This is facilitated by ongoing monitoring of care, using standards of care to benchmark, and engaging in frequent tests of change. Staff are empowered to have stretch goals and be innovative. Patient outcomes, efficiency in service delivery, and being good stewards of resources are paramount to high-performing work teams. Data are collected to measure outcomes and to further inform positive outcomes.
- High-performing teams seek connections and link information to technology in the quest to provide patient care that is evidence based. Facilitating effective and efficient communication is of the utmost importance in flow and continuity of care. High-performing teams make this job one when providing quality patient services. Being integrated ensures that connections are maintained and that gaps and missteps are avoided.

The authors maintain that quality and value are not created by accident and that frontline care framed through a microsystems lens can begin this process. The lens provides a focus that helps providers see things differently, thus asking different questions and seeking new, innovative answers, and solutions to real concerns. We do not measure what we miss. We miss things when our eyes are not reflecting on new and different ways of viewing the world.

System Qualities Defined

According to Batalden, Nelson, Edwards, Godfrey, and Mohr (2003), a system is perfectly designed to get the results it gets. The overall system can be considered in light of the micro, meso, macro, network, and the geopolitical marketplace. The *microsystem* is the point of care. The *mesosystem* supports the microsystem, occurring within the larger agency, allowing the multidisciplinary team to work, linking the *macrosystem*. The infrastructure of the larger organization is the macrosystem, which allows the other systems and its structures to define the overall care system. For the operations to run smoothly at the point of care (microsystem), policies, resources, and supportive structures are created at the macrosystem level. The regional level or *network* is the integration of health systems across agencies, organizations, and care settings. The network takes into account the entirety of the patient's lived experience in the health and illness continuum. The holistic impact of this experience further informs the other systems created within the network. At the national policy and program level, the *geopolitical marketplace* is represented. The external forces and drivers of the geopolitical marketplace have direct and indirect influences on resource allocation, research, new product development, and healthcare reform initiatives. The clinical microsystem has to contend with such influences as the healthcare experience changing on a sometimes daily basis (Batalden, Davidoff, Marshall, & Pink, 2011).

Nelson et al. (2008) described the microsystems as places where healthcare professionals and leaders develop tailored pathways to health care considering where patients, families, and care teams meet. "The micro system is the place where the combined and unceasing efforts of everyone—health professionals, patients and their families, researchers, payers, planners, administrators, educators—make changes that will lead to better patient outcomes, better system performance, and better professional development" (p. 367). Multiple knowledge systems are necessary to transform health care, and the clinical microsystems focus plays a vital role.

Microsystems Growth and Development

Five stages of microsystem growth and development are described by Batalden et al. (2003), as discussed in the following section.

Stage 1: Awareness

Being mindful of the work on the clinical unit increases awareness of the day-to-day operations as they relate to accomplishing goals, meeting patient demands, and functioning as a high-performing team. It is only with this awareness that staff can "see" what is in front of them, thus pointing out ineffective work practices and patterns. Change is possible only if there is first authentic communication and openness to discussing observations of the care processes, the merit of the flow (or lack of), and the overall team functioning. Heightening awareness of the microsystem as an interdependent group of individuals with the capability to be innovative underscores the power of the group to understand what works and what does not work regarding the care process and how the team functions. "Sleepwalking"—that is, going through the motions, staying under the radar, and not drawing attention to oneself—serves only to bury ineffective processes. This not only thwarts progress, but also can be fatal to care. Empowering the clinical unit to "dig deep" for change opportunities can make all the difference in creating a healthy work environment.

Stage 2: Purpose

Taking the blinders off through increased awareness of the processes allows for the development of aim statements. Defining the purpose of the work—that is, why it exists—promotes shared values and beliefs and a common focus on patients and families. With a clear, focused purpose, meaningfulness in the work to be done grounds everyone in the reason for being together. Our individual and collective work draws the team together to connect our purpose, aim, and shared values and beliefs. Being able to articulate this message keeps the team focused particularly when there is greater complexity in care delivery.

Stage 3: Small Tests of Change

Moving from mindfulness to a compelling shared vision and purpose, the microsystem is then able to effectively take on small changes and is prepared to create improved systems. This can be particularly challenging in light of increasing workloads, increased patient acuity, doing more with less, and taking on new technology and ever-changing "rules" of healthcare business. With this overarching purpose, there is often a lack of drive to respond to strategic challenges, leading to a return to the "path of least resistance." This does not stretch our capacity, nor create a culture of inquiry. Well-defined clinical microsystems are often freer to take on greater opportunity and challenges.

Stage 4: Measurement and Value

Following awareness, a sense of purpose and identity, and making innovation commonplace, the microsystem is poised to measure its value. Tracking and trending are important to demonstrating the value-added changes made to improve safe, quality care. Using a variety of tools such as visual reminders can be useful to the transparency of change initiatives. When progress is visual and clearly tracked, measurement can become rewarding and a true reflection of effort expended to improve processes. Indicators of successful work in the assessment, diagnosis, and treatment of the unit concerns become natural extensions of changes taken on as a microsystem. Problem solving, tracking, and trending can give staff greater insight into the processes of the work, engaging staff in the innovative process. What we do not observe or what we are unaware of we cannot measure; thus, we may miss an improvement opportunity.

Stage 5: Improvement Is the Fabric of the Work

When improvement becomes embedded in the daily work of staff in the microsystem, the culture becomes reflective of the "way we do things around here." Self-awareness is being able to initiate and sustain change through tracking and trending on performance. The microsystem is poised to analyze, change, and customize its own procedures, engaging microsystem members in the daily operation of the unit while being focused on improvement and staff vitality in meeting the needs of patients. The staff are able to be involved in multiple tests of improvement changes while integrating strategies for a healthy work environment that rewards positive, productive work.

Using the 5 Ps—purpose, patient, professional, process, and patterns—microsystems can be assessed, affording greater understanding of the inner workings of the unit. The discussion that follows defines the 5 Ps and offers a useful description of carrying out the assessment. This allows for an integrated approach to making improvements. Assessing the 5 Ps by identifying sources of information and engaging the entire multidisciplinary team in the microsystem in the process provide baseline information for gaining greater knowledge and insight into the current state, leading to improvement opportunities. Becoming familiar with the 5 Ps and its tools begins the identification of the gaps, begins the healthcare provider's development of the needs, and leads to identification of improvement themes and aims.

Health professionals are familiar with assessing, diagnosing, and treating patients; this is basic to our educational processes and socialization of care delivery. Clinical microsystems also can use this framework employing the 5 Ps.

■ The 5 Ps

The 5 Ps assessment allows a unique view of the microsystem anatomy: seeing things differently; asking new, possibly different questions that we have not previously considered; and coming up with new options for future improvements (Nelson et al., 2007).

Purpose

The purpose of the microsystem goes beyond the mission statement. The purpose is reflected in the culture of microsystems—its shared values, beliefs, and attitudes. Understanding the microsystem's culture and climate requires talking to key stakeholders, observing interactions, and how work gets done. This affords the opportunity to reflect on how policies and protocols align with "how we do things around here," giving insights to the inner dynamics of the microsystem. The purpose also considers the aspirations of the people who make up the microsystem, their vitality, and their commitment to the microsystem. Considering the purpose allows for a deeper reflection of what may go unnoticed or untapped with regard to staff commitments. This affords greater clarity and purposeful priority setting and engagement in purposeful decision-making.

Patients

When considering patients, the clinical microsystem focuses on the types of patients and their particular diagnoses, comorbidities, needs, services provided, and the overall routines carried out. A deep dive into understanding the patient population and subpopulation provides essential insight into improving redesign of the care and system in which this happens. Populations encompass a larger view of patients and can include the population specific to the microsystem assessed. For example, if I am a nurse manager or executive, my population would be staff and providers directly caring for patients. Understanding how care is delivered—that is, resources required, barriers to overcome, and capacities to build, would be my focus from a larger systems' perspective.

Professionals

Individuals who contribute to the delivery of health care make up the microsystem's professionals. Roles are respected for every member of the professional team and are important to the overall engagement of the team. Individuals are encouraged to engage in the care process, with each person's unique perspective brought to the microsystem. When assessing for the P that stands for *professional*, it is essential to have an understanding of what the individual does, the hours that he or she works, and his or her perspective of the environment of care and work. It is also important to know how the individual thinks and process information and what is needed regarding his or her learning. Competencies and standards of care of professionals would also be essential to know from the individual and system's perspective specifics to educational needs. This would guide how care is delivered and improved as new practices were required to improve performance. Understanding what each professional aspires to contribute by identifying opportunities for change and improvement is also critical to the team's working together.

Processes

Process includes the steps, tasks, and day-to-day procedures required for patient care in the microsystem. It is important to know how tasks are interrelated and perhaps the overlapping or sequential nature of their various work activities. Achieving a high level of flow requires that professionals "unearth" processes, considering differing views, assumptions, perceptions, and sometimes hidden meanings behind the work. High-level flow, through process mapping, alerts the team of the overall patient experience from admission to discharge. This makes the process transparent, because often a lack of shared knowledge about the process may increase risk and waste as well as reduce the reliability of the microsystem. Process mapping assists in uncovering details of the current state of the microsystem, forming the basis for work redesigns that are more efficient and effective. Failure Mode and Effects Analysis (FMEA) and Root Cause Analysis (RCA) are strategies that are helpful in further drilling down of potential and real failure points (CNA, 2010). These strategies provide opportunities for providers and staff to get a better understanding of their microsystem. Examples of how a deeper understanding can be reached include strategies such as role playing and walking through the process while noting positive and negative experiences. These insights provide greater ways to improve work care processes, thereby fostering healthy work environments.

Patterns

Seeing patterns in the microsystem is critical to understanding how processes come together. In discussing patterns, the team meets regularly to talk about how quality, efficiency (costs), performance, safety, and satisfaction come together. How do team members define quality? How does the microsystem stack up to standards and benchmarks? What measurements and metrics are in place? What purposes do they serve? How are they used to improve the processes? What are the staffing patterns and patient demand patterns? Perspectives from the direct care providers, and those administering and executing policies for daily practices are important to understand the full scope of work processes. Patterns illustrate what happens in the day-to-day work-world processes. Understanding pattern recognition provides baseline information (quantitative and qualitative data) that will be important to improvement work. For example, if my microsystem serves outpatients with depression, am I seeing improvements in mood states using specific assessment tools and evidence-based protocols? How am I measuring success in caring for this population? How do my purpose, processes, and patterns align? Do I have the right number and appropriate providers in caring for this population? Understanding and addressing patterns provide priority areas for improvement, a starting point for the team's work in delivering safe, quality care.

■ Clinical Microsystem and Areas of Practice

The clinical microsystem presents a focus of the clinical setting (patient-centric); it also has utility as an assessment tool for administrative, public health, and informatics practice. As the practitioner in these areas of study, the Patient or Population (P) would also encompass those delivering care to patients and clients as compared to the actual patient. The patient remains at the center of care and service delivery; however, the practitioner assessing their unit of work would focus on those at the sharp end of the microsystem. This would have an impact on processes as well as patterns of care within the microsystem and their impact on staff and patient outcomes. To be clear, the patient remains at the center; however, who delivers the care to the patient and how that care is delivered may be my focus if I serve in an administrative role assuring patients' safe passage during their care experience. The microsystem model can provide a meaningful framework for considering all aspects of the unit of work.

■ Systems, Networks, and Marketplaces

Systems, networks, and marketplaces evolve over time and are often embedded in larger systems and organizations. The clinical microsystem is charged with care delivery for patients, providing a safe, healthy work environment for staff and maintenance of a clinical unit (Capra, 2002; Lindberg, Zimmerman, & Plsek, 2001). "With self-organization and emergence in mind, healthcare professionals appreciate that while results of their actions can never be predicted, they always hold the potential for triggering significant change" (Lindberg et al., 2008, p. 43). Being nimble regarding the ever-changing internal and external demands of our systems is a good way to start our own evolution of innovation and change agency.

In the provision of health care to patients in complex organizational arrangements, the work at the "sharp end" occurs at the clinical microsystems level. It is at this frontline of healthcare delivery that the engagement of patient and provider begins the relationship, making the first connection to mesosystems and macrosystems and possibly to the network. The network may be considered the "soft end." Clinical microsystems are a basic unit of an organizational system, with a purpose, aims, linked processes, and a shared information exchange environment. Microsystems produce performance outcomes as a result of their daily work. The patient care experience occurs at the microsystems level (Batalden et al., 2003). Clinical microsystems are shorthand for a comprehensive approach to providing value for individual and families by analyzing, managing, improving, and innovating in healthcare systems. These systems offer senior leadership strategies and frameworks for competing in an increasingly competitive, data-driven, and value-added medical environment (Nelson et al., 2008, p. 367).

Microsystems occur in every healthcare setting and include primary care clinics, neonatal intensive care units, renal dialysis units, diabetes care clinics, and other systems akin to care at the frontline. Microsystems may or may not be recognized as a functioning unit by the macrosystems or mesosystems or as providing the organizational context for the system's work. This is one perspective; however, leaders in microsystem research take the position that if microsystems are improved, everything about the larger system moves forward (Batalden & Davidoff, 2007; Mohr & Batalden, 2002; Nelson et al., 2007).

■ Characteristics of Microsystems

Mohr and Batalden (2002, p. 47) described characteristics of effective microsystems. In their qualitative analysis of interviews with representatives from 43 microsystems across North America, eight characteristics of clinical microsystems emerged. Using these characteristics, they developed a tool for assessing the function of microsystems. The authors reported that more research is needed to assess microsystem performance, outcomes, and safety. Additionally, replicating their work may further inform best practices in other settings. The eight characteristics identified were:

1. Integration of information
2. Measurement
3. Interdependence of care teams
4. Supportiveness of the larger system
5. Constancy of purpose
6. Connection to the community
7. Investment in improvement
8. Alignment of role and training

Integration of information is essential to high-performing microsystems. With information integration, the microsystem allows for knowledge creation. Microsystems appreciate *measurement,* tracking, and trending outcomes. Macrosystem indicators and measurement may not always be helpful at the microsystem level. *Interdependence of care teams* involves reflection of the importance of the multidisciplinary team approach to care. Systems in silos with low levels of interdependence may have limited means of sharing information and/or communication. *Supportiveness of the larger system* is a hallmark of a well-functioning microsystem. Macrosystems and mesosystems in turn may be helpful or toxic to the microsystem. *Constancy of purpose* is consistent with the aim of the larger systems, guiding the work of the microsystem. When the aim is high and apparent to the microsystem, communication across boundaries facilitates seamless transitions. Larger systems that lack a clearly defined and communicated aim may be destructive to the microsystem and may negatively affect patient care. *Connection to the community* goes beyond clinical care of a defined set of patients on the frontline, extending beyond the microsystem. This interaction considers a symbiotic relationship between the microsystem and community. *Investment in improvement* considers resources such as time, money, and training and involves creating a theoretical perspective of improvement. The support of the larger systems may overlap depending on availability of resources. *Alignment of role and training* considers matching team members' education, training, and licensure with their role. Most team members communicated that alignment leads to higher satisfaction and lower turnover. Some, however, were not comfortable working in expanded roles.

Engaging frontline workers at the microsystems level is an excellent example of sound administrative practice. Tucker and Spear (2006) observed the work environment of hospital nurses that focused on performance of work systems. Their study considered the patient care perspective, particularly information, materials, and equipment required to do nursing's work. The researcher collected minute-by-minute data through primary observations of 11 hospital nurses at the frontline. Semi-structured interviews and surveys were also completed by the nurses. Per 8-hour shift, nurses were observed to experience an average of 8.4 work system failures. Medications, orders, supplies, staffing, and equipment were the five most frequent types of failures and accounted for 6.4 of the failures. The average task time was only 3.1 minutes; however, nurses were interrupted mid-task on an average of eight times per shift. The researchers concluded that nurse effectiveness could be improved by reducing the occurrence of work system failures and eliminating future occurrences. Creating system redesign that reduced fragmentation of work processes also could improve work flow. This study has implications for changes at the microsystem level.

■ Transforming Care at the Bedside

The Institute of Health Care Improvement and the Robert Wood Johnson Foundation in 2003 created the Transforming Care at the Bedside (TCAB) initiative as a nationwide strategy to improve healthcare delivery (Institute for Healthcare Improvement, 2004). TCAB provides an example of improvement science at the microsystem level. Lorenz, Greenhouse, Miller, Wisniewski, and Frank (2008) from the University of Pittsburgh Medical Center Hillman Cancer Center adapted principles of TCAB to their outpatient setting. The TCAB team began their work engaging frontline workers (led by a team) with a series of meetings that included brainstorming and setting priorities guided by facilitators educated in TCAB methods. Issues were identified through deep dives with rapid cycle change strategies implemented for care delivery improvements. The authors noted key improvement within the first 6 months of TCAB, which included reduction in patient wait times, increase in patient and staff satisfaction by 30 percentiles, shortened turnaround for laboratory results, and improvement of visitors' first impressions through new signage and a concierge program. The authors found improved staff involvement, ownership, and accountability as key factors in the TCAB success initiative. Task forces were created to move care delivery improvements forward. Additionally, TCAB was scheduled to be implemented in other University of Pittsburgh Medical Center cancer facilities.

■ Small Troubles, Adaptive Responses (STAR-2): Frontline Nurse Engagement in Quality Improvement

Stevens and Ovretveit (2013) through the Improvement Science Research Network conducted a multisite study considering operational failures at the microsystem's level, which keep frontline staff from providing safe, effective nursing care. Their study, STAR-2, focused on frontline nurse engagement in quality improvement by identifying failure points in care delivery (Stevens & Engh, 2012). For example, if I need to give a medication and it is not available in my medication system, this is an operational failure. Specifically, I will be required to take additional steps to determine why the medication was not there, what happened from the time the medication was prescribed to actual administration. These extra steps take time away from patient care and are not value-added to the patients' experience. Frontline nurses often "workaround" operational failures, often feeling pride in overcoming the problems from their unique care perspective. Frontline staff may not consider workarounds as problematic and possibly leading to fatalities when variations are "handled" individually and not from a system perspective. This leads to not having an appreciation of the variation thus limiting opportunities to reduce potential errors. The authors reported that the broad impact on health come from the premise that most adverse events in health care originate from frontline operational failures that are sufficiently "invisible" to be considered common practice. Although process failures include both errors and "problems" (task interruptions resulting from something or someone not being available when needed), the latter are far more common, yet have drawn far less attention (Tucker, Singer, Hayes, & Falwell, 2008). According to Stevens and her colleagues, these problems happen approximately once per hour per nurse on hospital units and 95% of problems are managed through workarounds (Tucker, et al., 2008). Practice implications are that detecting small problems provides practice-based data about operations that could then drive transformation. Considering operational failures and practice implication, an organizational learning environment can be created that is sensitive and responsive to resolve these latent failures as small troubles often reduce the morale and efficiency of an overextended and overloaded nursing workforce (Stevens et al., 2013).

■ Microsystems, Macrosystems, Mesosystems, and Quality

The need for understanding microsystems, macrosystems, and mesosystems is reinforced by the urgent need to improve quality. The most recent National Healthcare Quality and Disparities Reports, released in April 2010, underscored the need for quality as a continuing issue. Selected concerns include the following (Ulmer, Bruno, & Burke, 2010):

- Necessary care is received by patients only 59% of the time, with an annual improvement rate of a mere 1.4% annually.
- One in seven hospitalized Medicare patients experienced at least one adverse event.
- Four percent of hospitalized patients are harmed by care that is supposed to help.
- Deaths resulting from medical errors are roughly equivalent to the annual death rates for motor vehicle accidents, breast cancer, and AIDS combined.
- More people die annually from medication errors than from workplace injuries.
- Eight percent of hospitalized patients experience preventable negative outcomes.
- More than 32,000 patients experience postoperative infections and other preventable complications.

Healthcare organizations are having to do more with less. Value-based purchasing requires that hospitals in the United States be on guard for rapid cycle changes. Healthcare providers are headed for a transformative reawakening; major shifts in regulation and reimbursement are happening at all levels. Value-based purchasing is the most significant wave of change since the enactment of original Medicare legislation in the mid-1960s. There is and will continue to be an increased demand for service because 30 to 40 million additional individuals will require some level of coverage and will likely increase the demand dramatically in 2020 (Feldman, Dowd, & Coulam, 2015)(Business as usual will be nothing but! Healthcare providers must stretch their capacity, view the way we work through different lenses, and work in creative, innovative ways. There is an urgency that necessitates that we change the way we think about what we do, act accordingly, and transform the healthcare delivery system. Our focus must be on the patient experience, seeking to improve outcomes at every level. We, as healthcare providers, are all about improvement! It is our charge, and it is our moral imperative.

■ Systems Thinking and Organizational Learning

Understanding macrosystems and mesosystems and their interactions and changes allows leaders to establish and maintain a focus on process and to achieve organizational strategy. Senge (1990), as an influential systems thinker, provided us with the learning organization. Based at the Massachusetts Institute of Technology, Senge has authored a variety of books and articles that focus on systems thinking and organizational learning. Senge provided a set of core values of a leadership system framework for change and transformation.

Senge (1990) described 11 laws of systems, supporting an essential understanding of all levels of systems. These laws are (p. 283):

1. **Yesterday's solutions come from today's problems.** This law considers our lack of thinking consequentially, which often leads to the development of new problems.

2. **Pushing harder does not always give you the results you intended.** This refers to our lack of mindfulness about our situation; we often push forward without thinking through strategies. Problems sometimes are solved; however, in our CAS, new challenges are created.

3. **Behavior grows better before it grows worse.** Considering the longer view will, more often than not, provide greater clarity of our situation. When going for a short-term win, we often miss the fundamental issues and problems. The situation often may be worse from the longer view.

4. **The easy way out leads back in.** By going for the "quick fix," the uniqueness of individuals, situations, and context is often not considered. Again, the short-term gain may end up creating greater confusion and chaos.

5. **The cure can be worse than the disease.** Relying on tried and true solutions may lead to dependence on methods that worked in the past but that are not relevant to today's problems. Senge considers this to be possibly addictive and dangerous, noting that it may lead to dependency.

6. **Faster is slower.** Slow growth, particularly when considered in a systematic, reflective way, trumps aggressive, and fast-track methods. Rapid solutions may not lead to sustainable progress and hardwired long-term improvement.

7. **Cause and effect are not always closely related in time and space.** Because we cannot always "see" the consequences of our actions, we cannot anticipate the longer term.

8. **Grand schemes and plans may backfire.** Incremental changes that are consistent and repetitive can make big, important differences.

9. **You can have your cake and eat it too—but not all at once.** Learning organizations profess that decisions do not have to be either-or. Being flexible and fluid in our ways at looking at the world can provide different rules of the system.

10. **Dividing an elephant in half does not produce two small elephants.** Seeing the system as a whole, more than just the sum of parts, provides more ways to see options, thus possibly improving decision-making. This is particularly important when keeping the "big picture" perspective.

11. **There is no blame.** Situations may not always turn out the way we anticipate, and pointing fingers or raising suspicions does not improve matters. The causes of events, situations, problems, and mistakes are often part of the system.

■ Properties

There are properties that inform systems at all levels. Properties can be assessed within the microsystem and larger system perspectives. Properties include flow and variation (Senge, 1990).

Flow

Flow involves engagement of providers, patients, and stakeholders at every level. The patient's progress through an episode of care defines flow. As the patient moves through the system, it is generally not a seamless process, if ever. Providing the right care at the right time for the right patient is an opportunity, yet also a significant challenge in CASs. The ability to flow smoothly with these processes involves deliberate thinking and acting. An example is length of stay: patient discharge is often contingent on provider convenience or delayed for any number of reasons, including waiting for test results, medication, and transportation. Inefficiency within the system should not prolong length of stay; the uniqueness and challenges of each patient are true causes for such inconveniences for patients.

Variation

Variations in standards of care can be costly, ineffective, and redundant. Considering system and process design, any divergence in standards of care can lead to unpredictable results. When variation and unpredictability are the order of the day, it is difficult to understand the system. Working around ineffective processes can create variations that may go unnoticed because of ongoing work to "make it work." Tucker et al. (2008) studied operational failures that resulted from frontline staff perspectives. Observations and focused interviews noted that the two most common types of operational failure—equipment/supplies and facility issues—reduced staff efficiency and created safety risks. Such failures are not priorities in national healthcare initiatives. The researchers concluded that an underused strategy for improving patient safety and staff efficiency was leveraging frontline staff experiences with work systems, particularly those focused on identifying operational failures. "Thus, prioritizing improvement of work systems in general, rather than focusing more narrowly on specific clinical conditions, can increase safety and efficiency of hospitals" (Tucker et al., 2008, p. 1807). Variation and variability are risky. Process variability can be random or have a special cause. For example, random variability related to unknown causes is a "voice of the process," signaling potential issues for attention. Special variation is of known or identifiable cause, is infrequent, and demands immediate analysis. Variation can occur from natural causes (emergency department arrivals, walk-ins, and no shows) or be self-imposed (scheduling anomalies, intentional overbooking, emergencies).

■ Leadership and System Change

Porter-O'Grady and Malloch (2011) described leadership in systems change, seeing everything within the context of "systemness." Understanding the connectedness,

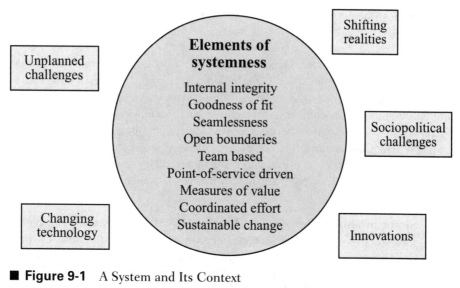

■ **Figure 9-1** A System and Its Context

Reproduced from Porter-O'Grady, T., & Malloch, K. (2011). *Quantum leadership: Advancing innovation, transforming health care* (2nd ed.). Sudbury, MA: Jones & Bartlett Learning.

dynamic relationships, and interactions allows for the creation of strategies for adaptation, thriving through chaos, and sustained improvement. The authors presented a model for a system and its context. Elements of systemness may include internal integrity, goodness of fit, seamlessness, open boundaries, measure of value, sustainable change, and other elements. See **Figure 9-1** for illustration of elements of systemness (Porter-O'Grady & Malloch, 2011, p. 74). The nature of evidence through microsystem, macrosystems, and mesosystems provides a lens through which to consider our work environments, our relationships with each other, and the outcomes we hope to attain. Considering the theoretical underpinnings provides frameworks to advance healthcare priorities in order to sustain improvement efforts.

■ Leadership, Change Management, and Engagement

Leading change is the work of those that provide care and manage systems. Understanding the microsystem with the patient at the center of care provides the infrastructure to begin making changes to meet the Institute of Medicine's Aims for Quality: Safe, Effective, Efficient, Equitable, Patient-Centered, and Timely (IOM, 2001). Transformational leadership theory is not new to business and healthcare. Early work in transformational leader comes from Burns (1978) in the late 20th century. Burns purported that transformational leadership happens when one or more individuals engage with others in a way that leaders and followers move to a higher level of motivation and morality (p. 20). Bass (1985) expanded Burns' leadership theory stating that a transformational leader moves us to do more than what is expected (p. 20). Motivation can be improved by increasing awareness about the essential outcomes and ways to reach them going beyond our own self-interest to the larger good of the team and organization. According to Hickman (1997, p. 2) transformational leaders "create and sustain a context for building human capacity developing leadership and effective followership, utilizing interaction-focused organizational design, and building interconnectedness." Transformational leaders do more than transact business through resource exchange. Considering systems' properties, the transformational leader understands change and is able to manage the many nuances of improvement work. Jones, Aquirre, and Calderone (2004) provide 10 principles for change management. They consider these principles as a set of practices, tools, and techniques:

1. **Systematically addressing the human side of organizations.** People issues are always front and center in improvement work and making change. Collecting and analyzing data on systems flow and "people" interactions will guide a better understanding of the system and how change can be embedded in an infrastructure that facilitates best practices and builds capacity.

2. **Begin at the top.** The leaders' role in setting the tone and modeling the way cannot be overemphasized. Without good examples of how to embrace change, learn new strategies that may be "foreign" to customary practices must be experienced by those who lead the way. Severing as an example for best ways to take on new practices and policies can be taught, although not truly accepted, with observing the "lived experience" of those leading improvement.

3. **All hands on deck.** Involving all layers in the organization is essential to changes that will be embedded, sustained, and spread overtime. There are several ways to involve members of the organization, including chartering teams for improvement, facilitating small tests of change (rapid cycle change), and supporting and mentoring new and senior members through creativity and innovative thinking and action.

4. **Making the case.** Leaders are able to make the formal case for change by confronting reality and assuring organizational members that the improvement work is doable. Leaders model confidence in the process of identifying the realities of the organization that have an impact on progress, as well as maintaining hope and confidence that the organizational capacity exists to follow this through. The transformational leader translates the complexities and helps to make sense of the nuances and ambiguities innate in high-reliability organizations. This requires a deep understanding and reflection of the system and the ability to "make it real" for those at the sharp end of implementation.

5. **Owning the change.** Responsibility and accountability must be built into the change strategy. This requires more than a passive agreement to accept the change. Owning the change requires a deep level of commitment that takes

leaders and followers through the often rough ups and downs of improvement work. Involvement in all aspects of the change through team science and accountability are ways to facility ownership. Influence and incentives are also key considerations in creating ownership.

6. **Messaging for meaning and commitment.** Communicating messages up and down the organizational channels is fundamental to making the case and translating how the change will affect the various layers of the organization. We often believe that our message is clear if we and those closest to us understand the underlying meaning. This is not often the case. Engaging all layers of the organization and how this will likely affect daily workflow is critical to embedding new ways of operating within the system. Aligning messages to the mission and core values of the organization further supports how the change is important to the work of the organization and not a trend or fad that the system takes on.

7. **Culture trumps knowledge.** Organizations often assess the culture too late in the process of making changes. There are any number of tools to assess the organizational readiness for change, key stakeholders to include, and how change happens in the system. Knowing the barriers to overcome and how best to build capacity within the existing organization's culture enhances the change process and positions better outcomes.

8. **Using cultural knowledge to address change.** Knowing through extensive analysis of the organizational culture and climate is not enough. Knowing how to use the information to facilitate change and overcome barriers acknowledges the "what and how" to make the changes. For example, informal leadership, change champions, and opinion leaders often model the way in endorsing changes and speed up the change process.

9. **Consider what could go wrong and worst case scenarios.** It is important to think through possible worst case scenarios that may have an impact on understanding, acceptance, endorsement, and finally enactment of change. Quality improvement strategies such as the 5 Whys and Failure Mode and Effects Analysis can be useful tools in considering failure points (CNA, 2010).

10. **Make it personal.** Understanding the organization's culture and climate and how change happens at a system's level are important. Translating at the individual level recognizes that individuals make up teams, and that the change is more than the "sum of parts" of the system. Change is personal, affecting individuals' workflow, ability to self-manage new ways in which I may be expected to operate in the system, and possibly my sense of self within the system. Addressing the individual as well as the team and larger system only improves successful outcomes.

Engaging individuals and teams can be accomplished through use of change management strategies, as well as mindfulness, intentional communication, and action.

It is important to assess the level of engagement of organizational members. This can be done through quantitative and qualitative methods. For example, staff engagement surveys through rating scales of minimal to total participation and engagement can give organizational leaders a range of scores and a perspective of levels of commitment. Interviews, focus groups, and observation of daily work activities can provide robust descriptions of how individuals are engaged and what patterns may emerge from individual and team involvement in the organization. Using a mixed methods approach (quantitative and qualitative data) can give greater depth to our understanding of the culture and readiness for change.

■ Exemplar One: Implementing the Clinical Nurse Leader Role in an Ambulatory Heart Failure Clinic for the Underserved

Erica Arnold

Background

The current state of the nation's healthcare delivery system requires urgent attention focusing on quality, safety, and cost of delivering effective and equitable care. Thus, the purpose of this paper is to describe how the University of Alabama at Birmingham (UAB) hospital (UABH) and the UAB School of Nursing partnered to implement a grant-funded interprofessional collaborative practice (IPCP) model to address the healthcare needs of an underserved heart failure (HF) patient population with goals to reduce 30-day hospital readmissions and improve patient outcomes. Utilizing a nurse-led clinic with the Triple Aim as a framework, the clinic's goals were to (a) improve the patient experience, (b) improve the health of populations, and (c) reduce the cost of health care in an underserved HF population. As a key team member, the clinical nurse leader (CNL) acts as a lateral integrator of care and patient advocate along the care continuum, serving as an information manager to the multiple disciplines on the IPCP team.

Methods

Within the IPCP model, the CNL contributed care coordination expertise across the healthcare continuum making daily rounds on all HF panel patients hospitalized at UABH. The CNL executed the role coordinating a postdischarge follow-up visit within 7 days prior to patient hospital discharge, making follow-up phone calls on all patients, confirming clinic visits, arranging home visits for new patients, and leading IPCP team morning huddles and postclinic conference meetings on clinic days. Huddles and conferences focused on improving communication among professionals and ensuring customized and coordinated care based on individual patient needs.

Outcomes

Patient care delivery in the grant-funded HF clinic began in late December 2014. Considering objectives of the Triple Aim and using data from the first 8 months of clinic operations, desirable outcomes were achieved: (a) The clinic has exhibited impressive patient satisfaction scores, reflecting optimal patient experiences. Of 124 patient responses, 95% rate responsiveness of staff as very good/excellent, 92% think providers always listen, and 96% think providers always treat them with respect. (b) About 39% of established patients (n = 29) had a clinical improvement in their HF classification. (c) In a short time, there has been a trend toward lower 30-day readmission rates compared to a national average readmission rate of 22.7%, which highlights the clinic's effectiveness in improving patient outcomes and decreasing healthcare costs.

Conclusion and Recommendations

Delivering care that is safe, timely, effective, equitable, efficient, and patient-centered is the primary focus of the CNL. Utilizing the CNL role in an ambulatory HF clinic and implementing an IPCP model around transitional care coordination has demonstrated outstanding achievement in all three dimensions of the Triple Aim. Our findings affirm the value of the CNL's contribution and suggest the CNL skill set has applicability beyond the acute care environment. Therefore, it is recommended that the CNL role be integrated into care environments beyond the in-hospital setting to better address the continuum of care.

■ Exemplar Two: Utilizing an Interprofessional Collaborative Nurse-Led Clinic to Improve the Patient Experience and Decrease 30-day Readmissions in Underserved Heart Failure Patients

Dana Mitchell, Shannon DeLuca, Maria Shirey, and Connie White-Williams

Background

Socioeconomically disadvantaged patients with chronic HF have an increased risk for hospital readmissions. Yet, little evidence exists focusing on this patient population. Multiple barriers including self-care management, educational resources, and access to care have an impact on the patient experience and long-term survival. Therefore, the purpose of this presentation is to describe how the UAB School of Nursing and UABH partnered to establish an IPCP team to implement a transitional care clinic for underserved HF patients.

(continues)

Methods

This nurse-led clinic manages patients along the hospital-home-clinic care continuum. Nurse practitioners, CNLs, social workers, and the collaborating physician comprise the clinic team. This project was funded by the Health Resources and Services Administration (HRSA) and the Nurse Education, Practice, Quality, and Retention (NEPQR) program and guided by the Triple Aim Framework of improving the patient experience, improving the health of populations, and decreasing costs. The IPCP team provides guideline-directed medical management of the patients' HF and also utilizes a patient-centered approach to find resources to address specific barriers to self-care. The project also has access to palliative care resources, a transitional care coach, an informatics expert, and the leadership partners from the UAB School of Nursing and UABH. Patient outcome data, including morbidity, symptom burden, patient satisfaction, self-reported depression, readmission rates, and cost-benefit analyses, are collected. In addition, data regarding the interprofessional collaborative team is collected every 3 months.

Results

Since December 2014, the clinic has established care with more than 60 patients. The clinic has excellent patient satisfaction scores, reflecting optimal patient experiences. Of 124 patient responses, 95% rate think providers always treat them with respect. Twenty-nine established patients (39%) have had a clinical improvement in their HF classification. Early results show a trend toward lower 30-day readmission rates compared to a national average readmission rate.

Conclusion

As the project progresses, the team has encountered both expected and unexpected challenges in regard to the coordination of HF care in this complex patient population. Financial barriers to medications are prevalent as expected, but additional hurdles of high medical acuity, inadequate social support and caregiver buy-in, and very limited health literacy are daunting variables as well. The innovative approaches taken by this team further outline the importance of an interprofessional approach and are facilitated greatly by the direct affiliation with a large academic medical center.

REFLECTIVE ACTIVITIES

1. With interdisciplinary colleagues, select a gap in healthcare quality within the system of care. Using the 5 Ps of the clinical microsystem, outline first steps and next steps to bridge the gap.
2. Consider the gap from Question 1, using the framework for mesosystems and macrosystems, as well as the network perspective.

3. Discuss safety and quality improvement relative to microsystems, macrosystms, and mesosystems, identifying specific strategies from each system's view.
4. Select research articles that describe microsystems, macrosystems, and mesosystems as a conceptual framework for quality improvement.

REFERENCES

Bass, B. M. (1985). Leadership and performance beyond expectations. New York, NY: The Free Press.

Batalden, P., & Davidoff, F. (2007). What is "quality improvement" and how can it transform healthcare? *Quality and Safety in Healthcare, 16,* 2–3.

Batalden, P., Davidoff, F., Marshal, M., & Pink, C. (2011). So what? Now what? Exploring, understanding and using the epistemologies that inform the improvement of healthcare. *British Medical Journal Quality and Safety, 1,* i99–i105.

Batalden, P. B., Nelson, E. C., Edwards, W. H., Godfrey, M., & Mohr, J. J. (2003). Microsystems in health care: Part 9. Developing small clinical units to attain peak performance. *Joint Commission Journal on Quality and Patient Safety, 11,* 575–585.

Burns, J. M. (1978). *Leadership.* New York, NY: Harper & Row.

Capra, F. (2002). *The hidden connections.* New York, NY: Doubleday.

CNA. (2010). Analyzing errors: Improving quality, reducing risks by understanding underlying causes. *In-Brief, 2.* Retrieved from https://www.cna.com/vcm_content/CNA/internet/Static%20File%20for%20Download/Risk%20Control/Medical%20Services/AnalyzingErrors-ImproveQuality,ReduceRiskbyIdentifyingUnderlyingCauses.pdf

Feldman, R., Dowd, B., & Coulam, R.(2015, October). *Medicare's role in determining prices throughout the health care system* (Mercatus Working Paper). Arlington, VA: George Mason University.

Hickman, G. R. (1997). *Transforming organizations to transform society* (Transformational Leadership Working Papers). College Park, MD: Kellogg Leadership Studies Project, The James MacGregor Burns Academy of Leadership.

Institute of Medicine. (2001). *Crossing the quality chasm: A new health systems for the 21st century.* Retrieved from https://iom.nationalacademies.org/~/media/Files/Report%20Files/2001/Crossing-the-Quality-Chasm/Quality%20Chasm%202001%20%20report%20brief.pdf

Institute for Healthcare Improvement. (2004). *Transforming care at the bedside.* Retrieved from http://www.hsi.gatech.edu/erfuture/images/9/99/Bedside.pdf

Jones, J., Aquirre, D., & Calderone, M. (2004). Ten principles of change management, Tools and techniques to help companies transform quickly. Strategy-Business. http://www.strategy-business.com/article/rr00006?gko=643d0

Lindberg, C., Nash, S., & Lindberg, L. (2008). *On the edge: Nursing in the age of complexity.* Bordentown, NJ: Plexus Institute.

Lindberg, C., Zimmerman, B., & Plsek, P. (2001). *Edgeware: Complexity resources for health care leaders.* Bordentown, NJ: Plexus Institute.

Lorenz, H. L., Greenhouse, P. K., Miller, R., Wisniewski, M. K., & Frank, S. L. (2008). Transforming care at the bedside: An ambulatory model for improving the patient experience. *Journal of Nursing Administration, 38*(4), 194–199. doi:10.1097/01.NNA.0000312757.06913

Mohr, J. J., & Batalden, P. B. (2002). Improving safety on the front line: The role of clinical microsystems. *Quality and Safety in Healthcare, 11,* 45–50.

Nelson, E. C., Batalden, P. B., & Godfrey, M. M. (2007). *Quality by design: A clinical microsystems approach.* San Francisco, CA: Jossey-Bass.

Nelson, E. C., Godfrey, M. M., Batalden, P. B., Berry, S. A., Bothe, A. E., McKinley, K. E., . . . Nolan, T. W. (2008). Clinical microsystems. I. The building blocks of health system. *Joint Commission Journal on Quality and Patient Safety, 37*(7), 367–378.

Plsek, P., & Greenhalgh, T. (2001). The challenge of complexity in health care. *British Medical Journal Quality and Safety, 323*(7313), 625–628.

Porter-O'Grady, T., & Malloch, K. (2011). *Quantum leadership: Advancing innovation, transforming health care* (2nd ed.). Sudbury, MA: Jones & Bartlett Learning.

Senge, P. (1990). *The fifth discipline.* New York, NY: Currency Doubleday.

Stevens, K. R., & Engh, E. P. (2011). *Small troubles, adaptive responses (STAR-2): Frontline nurse engagement in quality improvement.* Improvement Science Research Network. Retrieved from http://isrn.net/improvement/index.asp

Stevens, K. R., & Ovretveit, J. (2013). Improvement research priorities: USA survey and expert consensus. *Nursing Research and Practice,* 2013, Article ID 695729. doi:10.1155/2013/695729

Tucker, A. L., & Spear, S. J. (2006). Operational failures and interruptions in hospital nursing. *Health Research and Educational Trust, 41*(3, Pt. 1), 643–662. doi:10.1111/j.1475-6773.2006.00502.x

Tucker, A. L., Singer, S. J., Hayes, J. E., & Falwell, A. (2008). Front-line staff perspectives on opportunities for improving the safety and efficiency of hospital work systems. *Health Research and Educational Trust, 43*(5), 1807–1829. doi:10.111/j.1475-6773.2008.00868.x

Ulmer, C., Bruno, M., & Burke, S. (2010). Future directions for the National Healthcare Quality and Disparities Reports. Committee on Future Directions of the National Healthcare Quality and Disparities Reports, Institute of Medicine. Washington, DC: National Academies Press.

CHAPTER 10

Quality Improvement and Safety Science: Historical and Future Perspectives

■ SHEA POLANCICH, LINDA A. ROUSSEL, AND ANNE MILLER ■

■ Objectives:

- Explore the foundations of QI and safety science.
- Understand the use of QI in the practice of health care.
- Identify contributions of QI science to evidence-based practice (EBP) and research.
- Identify quantitative and qualitative methods for process improvement
- Examine QI methods using a clinical example.

■ Introduction

Understanding the influence of quality imporovement (QI), its vital role in EBP, and its integration into research begins with understanding QI, including patient safety within the healthcare environment. What is QI, and what is its role in health care? This chapter explores principles of QI and change while providing the mental model that we, the authors of this chapter, hold.

Research, EBP, and QI are often blurred (Newhouse & Unruh, 2009; Newhouse, Dearholt, Poe, Pugh, & White, 2007; Newhouse, Perrit, Rocco, & Poe, 2006). The randomized controlled trial has long been deemed the gold standard for changing what care is delivered (Polit & Beck, 2012). Although there is truth in that statement, there is also truth in understanding how care is delivered (Newhouse & Unruh, 2009); this is the most basic mission of QI (Langley, Nolan, Nolan, Norman, & Provost, 2009). QI science is founded in systematic, standardized, and rigorous methods of study that are separate and distinct from "empirical" research (see http://www.improvementscience research.net/). When they are combined, both approaches make powerful contributions to health care.

The purpose of this chapter is to explore the foundations of QI and safety science and to understand the use of QI in the practice of health care and the contribution of improvement science to evidence-based medicine and research. This chapter is written with an operational lens to provide a practical application to QI.

■ History of Quality Improvement in Health Care

A number of individuals are contributing to the development of QI and safety science, with key individuals laying the framework for QI integration into EBP, outcomes, practice variation, and the exploration of error (Leape & Berwick, 2005; Nelson, Batalden, & Godfrey, 2007; Vincent, 2010; Vincent, Batalden, & Davidoff, 2011).

One of the earliest pioneers of the study of outcomes and the integration of those data into the quality care of the patient was Ernest Codman (Chambler & Emery, 1997; Kaska & Weinstein, 1998; Spiegelhalter, 1999). This Massachusetts-based physician was trained at Harvard, then practiced at, and was later removed from, Massachusetts General Hospital for his revolutionary ideas about measuring a surgeon's competence. Codman was a pioneer in QI and safety science and is known for his study of outcomes of surgical care as well as his study of error. He is credited for initiating the first mortality and morbidity conferences at Massachusetts General. Through his relentless pursuit of quality, Codman helped to establish the American College of Surgeons and the Hospital Standardization Program. The Hospital Standardization Program later became known as the principal accreditation body in health care—the Joint Commission (Chambler & Emery, 1997; Kaska & Weinstein, 1998; Spiegelhalter, 1999).

QI within health care has been influenced by efforts undertaken in diverse industry sectors, especially industrial production processes (Scrivens, 1997). Borrowed from manufacturing and process control, some of the earliest notions of QI in health care were defined by inefficiencies in the provision of health care (Drury, 1997; Eklund, 1995, 1997). What makes a system—in this case, the healthcare system—function efficiently and effectively? In the early 1900s, Frederick Taylor and later, W. Edwards Deming, laid the foundations for studying industrial efficiency and effectiveness (Deming, 1986, 2000; Taylor, 1911). Deming's industrial quality assurance standards have been translated into the healthcare environment. Through the use of statistical process control, healthcare processes can be quantified and outcome variation can be studied. Deming's work has been credited as the foundation of the Total Quality Management (TQM) movement. TQM proposes that managers possess a System of Profound Knowledge (Langley et al., 2009). This system contains four key elements: appreciation of a system, knowledge of variation, theory of knowledge, and knowledge of psychology. In essence, these four components set the infrastructure for understanding a microsystem, understanding variation, and understanding the human factors inherent within processes (Deming, 1986, 2000).

One of the most influential persons in QI within health care is Avedis Donabedian (Donabedian, 2003). Donabedian described three key aspects to health care: structure, process, and outcomes. These three elements are integral to the study of quality health care. Structure is the environment in which the healthcare services are provided. Process contains the steps involved in the provision of services. Outcomes are measured indices of the processes within the structure, based on identified criteria. All three components are integrally related and connected, existing only in interdependence. Donabedian (2003) created the theoretical underpinnings on which to base any methodological approaches to the design and study of QI and outcomes research.

Although many other individuals have contributed to QI and the safe care of the patient, the individuals described in the preceding paragraphs provided the foundations from which to understand the translation of EBP (Leape & Berwick, 2005; Nelson et al., 2007; Vincent, 2010; Vincent et al., 2011).

■ Structure, Process, and Outcomes

Donabedian's concepts constitute the lens through which we view the theoretical underpinnings of QI work. Donabedian's framework and its composite elements of structure, process, and outcomes will be explored in more detail because they are foundational for improvement design. Structure defines the conditions under which care may be provided. Structure includes material resources, human resources, and organizational characteristics. Defining and examining a process's structure is necessary to understand the constraints and opportunities in the system that shapes an individual's behavior and the system's capacity to deliver a high quality of care. In some instances, structure may be the major determinant of the quality of care provided by a system. Detailed variations in many system characteristics may have a weak relationship to the corresponding quality—although as an advantage, some attributes of structure are more readily observable, more easily documented, and tend to be more stable (Donabedian, 2003).

Healthcare processes integrate the separate tasks and activities that constitute health care: diagnosis, treatment, rehabilitation, prevention, and patient education (Nelson et al., 2007). Typically, these activities are performed by the professional care provider but also may include contributions made by patients and their families. Detailed characteristics may provide discriminating judgments that validate the quality of care. However, quality is not inherent in the process in and of itself. Quality is established in advance of evidence-based care practices that are found to produce desirable outcomes. Processes are more directly related to outcomes than they are to structure. Processes show smaller variations in quality and are taking place in the "now," thus offering more immediate indications of quality (Donabedian, 2003).

Outcomes are the desirable and undesirable changes that occur in individuals or populations that are the result of health care. Outcomes include changes in health status, changes in patients' and families' knowledge that may influence care, and changes in behaviors of patients and families that may influence health promotion, patient satisfaction, and family satisfaction (Donabedian, 2003). Quantified patient outcomes provide the greatest support for the effect of practice on patient care. There has been great debate regarding the relationship of processes to patient outcomes. The challenge arises with attribution of the outcome to process and the probability that a particular process or set of processes leads to an outcome or set of outcomes. The advantage of using the outcome as a measure of quality is that the outcome reflects not only what was done for the patient but also how well it was done. However, patient outcomes typically depend on both the therapeutic efficacy of a treatment regimen and the effective delivery of that care regimen (Donabedian, 2003; Langley et al., 2009).

Based on a review of structure, process, and outcome, it should be noted that the three aspects of quality should be examined together as a complete approach. Examining all three aspects together provides more comprehensive insight into the contribution that each aspect makes to the quality of care being studied (Donabedian, 2003).

■ Understanding the Microsystem and the Macrosystem

Although it is outside the scope of this chapter to delve into the depth of these concepts, it will be important for the reader to have a basic knowledge of the scope of each. The microsystem is a smaller system within a larger system called the macrosystem (Nelson et al., 2007).

QI typically initially focuses on the microsystem before improvement processes are expanded to the larger system. The analysis of a small work unit, such as a floor or a ward within a hospital, is an example of a microsystem starting point (Nelson et al., 2007). Understanding the relationship between this small system and the stakeholders surrounding and interacting with this system helps narrow the focus of improvement efforts and provides a fertile ground for exploring and testing interventions on a smaller scale. It is more efficient and effective to pilot or test within a limited environment to determine if interventions work locally before more global actions are instituted. However, it is important to understand that microsystem changes may not be entirely transferable to the macrosystem (Nelson et al., 2007).

An analysis of the microsystem provides the starting point for improvement. Analyzing the microsystem requires exploration of the care provided, the expected outcomes, and the associated cost and resources. In analyzing the microsystem, a value compass is produced. The following sections provide an overview of evidence-based processes used to implement a QI project within or after the completion of a microsystem analysis (Nelson et al., 2007).

■ The Methodological Foundation for Quality Improvement: The Model for Improvement

The Plan Phase

To practice improvement science in an evidence-based, rigorous way, it is important to be grounded in an understanding of central methodological frameworks for healthcare quality. The model for improvement has four key elements: *plan, do, study,* and *act,* most often represented by the acronym PDSA (Langley et al., 2009). PDSA provides a structure for designing, implementing, measuring, and disseminating QI work. The PDSA model is used iteratively in rapid cycles to explore an improvement idea, test the merits of the idea, and then evaluate the results. Each component of the PDSA model will be described in detail (Langley et al., 2009).

To *plan* is to design and formalize the QI project. During this phase of the cycle, key tasks must be performed: the development of a charter and the formation of a team. The charter is the written formalization of the work to be done, which defines and describes the aim of the project, the timeline for the project cycle, the measurable criteria and tactics, the resources needed, and the personnel required to complete the various tasks (Langley et al., 2009).

Plan: Quality Improvement Team Development

QI work is best accomplished within the structure of a team that includes all the key stakeholders and subject matter experts (Langley et al., 2009). It is important that the team share a common vision for the work to be accomplished, and this is most readily accomplished by formalizing and documenting a written charter with defined aims for the improvement work. Within healthcare quality improvement, teams are determined by the improvement project but are often multidisciplinary and represented by physicians, nurses, pharmacists, ancillary services, and information technology, to name a few. The level of the participant can range from frontline staff to executive leadership. It is essential to examine the type of improvement needed and to gauge the need of the participant based on what he or she will be able to provide to the group in support of the QI project's aim or goal (Schwarz, Landis, & Rowe, 1999).

Plan: Developing Aims for Quality Improvement

To develop and implement a QI project requires thoughtful consideration of the outcomes desired. To formalize a project, significant time and attention should be devoted to the development of the aims of the study. Aims are the "what," the "how," and the "how much" of the project (Langley et al., 2009). Without the formalization of what is desired, the project lacks an attainable goal or outcome that is quantifiable and measurable. SMART (Specific, Measureable, Attainable, Realistic, Timely) goals are necessary to tailor metrics and an evaluation plan to determine success of the project.

The first consideration for the aim is that it should be something that is deemed an improvement or a "stretch" to accomplish. However, it should be a goal that is attainable with effort or, in this case, improvement. The key to developing the aim or goal of a QI project is often found in examination of baseline information and/or information obtained from a gap analysis of a current process. Understanding the current state provides direction for improvement. The next step is to set the "targeted" level of improvement (Langley et al., 2009).

For example, in an academic medical center, the QI office found that adherence to the National Patient Safety Goals (NPSGs) for universal protocol and timeout had been determined, through observational methods, to be as low as 20% qualitatively for all the required elements (Joint Commission, 2016). An improvement team was chartered with an overall aim: to improve the adherence of providers to the NPSG requirements for universal protocol and timeout in the medical center clinic. With the overall aim defined, specificity of the aim is further refined. Because adherence to the NPSG is central to safe patient care and avoidance of wrong-site procedures, the aim was further refined to be 100% adherence to the standards set for the universal protocol and timeout. Additionally, the tool used to facilitate the adherence was added to the aim, thus defining the "how" component (Joint Commission, 2016).

Once there is an understanding of the current state and targeted level of improvement, consideration is given to how the aim is measurable (Langley et al., 2009). The ability to measure an aim is imperative in the development of the study. Staying with the example of the universal protocol and timeout electronic checklist, measurement could be accomplished both quantitatively and qualitatively. Quantitative measurement can be accomplished by simply pulling the data electronically from the form; however, would this process meet the intent of the improvement project? Knowing what metrics will be relevant to determining success of the improvement strategies, data (and condition of the data) to be collected, and how to analyze and interpret are essential to quantitative measurement. Qualitatively, the baseline showed that adherence to the components was low; therefore, checking the box electronically did not capture the intent. Daily observations provide a qualitative perspective of how processes were actually being carried out (not just documented). So, the aim was further refined to 100% adherence to the requirements based on observational assessment of the process (Joint Commission, 2016).

In QI studies, an aim may be singular or there may be multiple aims (Langley et al., 2009). The overarching goal or aim of the project may be measured by a variety of outcomes. It is important in the planning phase of the cycle to clarify the aim statement(s). In the preceding example, a specific aim on the utilization of the electronic form by the providers also could have been developed. For example, if there had been four providers in the clinic, an aim statement could have been developed around the integration and use of the electronic checklist by 100% of—or all four—providers. At this point, we would like to note that outcome aims for the patient are typically the central focus in improvement work. This example highlights a point that should be addressed. In the patient safety improvement process, such as with wrong-site surgery, the incidence of this event is rare. Therefore, an aim related to a reduction of wrong-site surgery would not be appropriate. However, an aim could be included that would represent zero defects, or "zero" wrong-site surgeries and wrong-site procedures in the given time frame of the improvement work (Langley et al., 2009).

Although aims must be measurable, it is acceptable to propose an aim that is developmental in nature (Langley et al., 2009). The best example of this type of aim in the operational aspects of improvement is in the development of an evidence-based protocol. Evidence-based protocols are tools that are used in the clinical care of the patient that provide guidance to the practitioner on the most appropriate treatment modalities, based on the literature. The development of an evidence-based protocol is based on extensive review of the literature and the integration of clinical practice expertise by key stakeholders in the specified area of practice. An aim of this nature may be written so as to develop and implement an evidence-based protocol within a specified practice setting. The measurable criteria may be in the completion of the evidence-based protocol and the degree of implementation accomplished within a given practice setting (Langley et al., 2009).

In finalizing the planning phase of the cycle, careful consideration should be given to the cycle time of the project (Langley et al., 2009). PDSA cycles are typically considered to be rapid cycles of improvement, but what does that mean? In most instances, the cycle time of the project will depend on the nature of the improvement. However, the shortest cycle time necessary to reach a steady state of the intervention and then measure the impact is recommended. Improvement science has value in the rapid study or exploration of an intervention into clinical practice. Whereas research studies may take years to provide evidence of results, the improvement process provides a way to test and measure results in weeks to months. Although the improvement project will not be initially used to change practice, as in a randomized controlled trial or an experimental design for a treatment modality, it does become the stimulus for change that may result in the improvement of a clinical process or in the development of a research design (Langley et al., 2009).

Plan: Leadership and Resource Support

Outside the aims of the project, the Plan phase of the improvement model also includes defining the resources required and obtaining leadership support for the project (Langley et al., 2009). A key factor in any improvement study is adequate resources to support the projects that will be developed, designed, and implemented. Leaders within an organization must understand the improvement model and be active participants if these projects are to succeed. This leadership engagement includes, but is not limited to, executive, administration, medical, and nursing, ancillary, and information technology staff. Improvement in healthcare quality requires a multidisciplinary approach and is best when there is inclusion of expertise from all domains within the healthcare system (Langley et al., 2009).

Leaders who are engaged and active participants create opportunity for dissemination and are the driving force needed to overcome barriers (Kotter, 1996). Additionally, as participants in the study, these individuals are an integral part of the team. They experience with other participants the successes and failures of the study, and they influence other leaders with firsthand knowledge of the project. Leadership and resource support in an improvement study is intertwined with the operational work of the facility (Langley et al., 2009). Typically, these types of projects do not require the development of a formal proposal for review as in the research domain. However, improvement studies require extensive analysis of the impact of the project on the operations of an organization, thus a "working plan" is important and can serve as a structuring framework (Langley et al., 2009). Thinking through a plan is a key step in the planning phase of the PDSA model. The outcomes of the Plan phase include a written charter, a formed project team with defined aims, a leadership structure, organizing framework, and resource support (Langley et al., 2009).

The Do Phase

The next step in the improvement model is the Do phase (Langley et al., 2009). The planning phase defined what is to be accomplished; the Do phase executes the plan. To carry out the project, the team must assign appropriate tasks. The project plan requires some definition and structure; however, this process does not require sophisticated or expensive tools. Paper-based tools often provide a low-cost approach for a rapid cycle improvement project and the evidence for proof of concept. Tools such as Microsoft Excel and Access are readily available and provide a simple method of storing and analyzing data (Mears, 1995).

Tool development for quality improvement is important to mention because this process is differentiated from research-based instrument development. In the research domain, tools are instruments and are developed and evaluated for validity and reliability through rigorous techniques. In quality improvement, tools are primarily developed for the PDSA cycle to collect information or data about the intervention or the improvement process that is being designed and implemented (Langley et al., 2009). For the purpose of improvement, tools do not require reliability and validity testing because they serve and reflect local needs; thus, they are not expected to generalize beyond the immediate environment. For purposes of improvement, tools are developed within a microsystem and are used for rapid cycle improvement (Nelson et al., 2007). Once the desired outcome is obtained, the tool may be applied to other microsystems and disseminated more broadly within an environment for a defined purpose, most often for data collection. However, if there is an existing valid and reliable instrument that measures the outcome desired, it is appropriate to use the tool for improvement work as well (Mears, 1995).

The Do phase also may incorporate processes such as Lean and Six Sigma methods (Simmons, 2002). Lean was developed out of the automotive manufacturing industry as a method for organizing and reducing waste in a system. This process, as in all improvement work, requires extensive analysis of the processes of the system being studied (including process mapping and spaghetti diagramming) and often takes a SWAT team can be defined as any group of specialists brought in to solve a difficult or urgent problem. Six Sigma is another tool born within industry and focuses on the reduction of defects. Six Sigma techniques are geared toward a reliable system design in which errors result at a rate of 1:1,000,000. Both tools may be useful in improvement studies but may not always be applicable, and they are not required elements of the model (Simmons, 2002). Lean Six Sigma (LSS) includes the following steps: define, measure, analyze, improve, and control. When defining the problem it is important to use internal data to have baseline information to launch improvement efforts. LSS is based on facts, not assumptions, so using measurement to determine improvement is essential in the analyzing phase. Improvement can be determined from baseline data after analyzing measures are instituted to solve the problem. Controlling for variance is important to ongoing sustainability of successful strategies and solutions (Nave, 2002).

To operationalize the Do phase of the improvement model, we will again discuss an example. In the example provided earlier in the chapter regarding the adherence to the NPSG for universal protocol and timeout, the checklist tool would be developed as the intervention and integrated into the work flow of a small microsystem. So, for example, a single clinic would be identified. Baseline information would be collected on the current status of the process by trained observers, and data would be collected. Then, the checklist intervention would be implemented into the work flow. The observers would then collect data regarding the quality of the process after the intervention. All data would be collected and, if possible, stored electronically in some fashion. For performance improvement purposes and a small test of change, this can be as simple as creating an Excel spreadsheet. Using Excel has advantages in that the product was developed for calculation (Mears, 1995). Given this functionality, data may be entered and calculated in one tool.

Qualitative data also can be important to understanding process improvement. Narrative inquiry and rich data that generate themes often give depth to statistics and numbers, which may not tell the "whole story." Sorensen and Bernard (2012) used a case study approach to study practices in their natural environments when considering a change package for the Health Resources and Services Administration's (HRSA) Patient Safety and Clinical Pharmacy Collaborative. The researchers used grounded theory and inductive data analysis techniques to identify strategies, change concepts, and actionable methods that may have been missed using quantitative methods alone.

The Do phase also typically includes an educational component (Langley et al., 2009). To implement a process, educational content specific to the intervention will need to be developed and conveyed to the targeted audience. This education will not only be specific to the intervention but also will incorporate any education that may be needed for any tools that are developed and used during the intervention. The most common mistake found in improvement implementations is failure to provide the needed education in some phase of the project. Poor education may lead to variation of process, which may ultimately lead to failure of the entire project. For example, following the universal protocol example, the quality professional provided education to the clinic staff on the basic requirement of universal protocol and timeout and the need for compliance based on the NPSG (Joint Commission, 2016). The tool was provided to the staff, and observations were completed. The observer found that inconsistent interpretations of the tool's elements and the variation in the process could again lead to a safety failure. Without educating the clinic staff on the appropriate use of the tool and defining the operational definitions for each element, variation entered into the process, and the consultant had to stop the implementation and rework the process.

The Do phase of the improvement model is probably the most extensive work section (Langley et al., 2009). However, the type of "work" or the type of improvement will vary. Tools may be designed and implemented, or the project may be the development of an evidence-based protocol. For this type of project, the Do work is more individual and involves in-depth analysis of the current state of the evidence (Langley et al., 2009). Program evaluation also may be the focus of an improvement project. The improvement work may be based on outcomes examined while exploring the microsystem, and the choice may be made to improve the entire program or certain key areas of the program (Mark & Pines, 1995).

The Study Phase

The Study phase is the analytical phase of the cycle (Langley et al., 2009). Analytics refers to the analysis of the improvement study through an examination of the qualitative and quantitative information collected for the intervention or the process improvement changes. In quality improvement, an analysis may range from being as simple as creating rates and reviewing percent changes in a process to as complex as a statistical process control method with control charts. In this section, we provide a few examples to highlight the Study phase (Langley et al., 2009).

The first example is related to the NPSG for universal protocol and timeout, and developing a checklist tool as the intervention and integrated into the work flow of a small microsystem. The checklist tool that was developed in the Do phase would be used to measure the adherence of providers to the specific components of the universal protocol and timeout quantitatively. Therefore, a report could be designed to provide data regarding the percentage of appropriate utilization of the checklist. The operational metrics of the numerator and the denominator would have been defined in the Plan phase, and now, in the Study phase, the reports are developed based on those definitions. Once the data are converted to a "quantitative" value, an aim can be assessed based on the results of the intervention or the new process that has been implemented within that individual microsystem and structure (Langley et al., 2009; Nelson et al., 2007).

The clinic example also had a qualitative component. It is not enough to measure adherence to the checklist without assessing the quality of the performance of the process. With this in mind, the observational method that was employed in the baseline data collection would have again been used to observe the process after the intervention. Using a tool developed for the observational process, the observer would capture the qualitative assessment of the process. The qualitative assessment would then be converted to a quantitative number for analysis and study. The change in the adherence at this point relates to the qualitative component of the process change, again within the specific structure of the defined microsystem (Langley et al., 2009; Nelson et al., 2007).

"Study" may also be defined as analyzing the gaps in the literature or evidence. For improvement work that is focused on assessing a current state of a process or program, or for developing evidence-based guidelines, the Study component may be quantifying existing literature or identifying gaps in evidence or practice (Langley et al., 2009). Both a quantification of the evidence and a summation of the current state are appropriate analyses used to assess an outcome of an improvement project. However, there is also a higher level of analysis that may be incorporated into improvement work. Similar in nature to research, there are tiers of analyses based on the type of data. Therefore, similar to the parametric statistic for ratio level data, in improvement work, statistical process control methods for analyzing variation in a process may be incorporated. Statistical process control includes run and control chart methods. In-depth discussion of these methods is outside the scope of this chapter; however, we discuss briefly the use of graphical display of data in improvement work (Langley et al., 2009).

As mentioned, Deming popularized the use of control charts on an international level (Deming, 1986, 2000). Control charting is the process of graphically displaying whatever you are measuring over a period that allows for the identification of variation, or a change, in a process. Control charts are used for the purposes of examining special cause and common cause variation. Special cause variation occurs in a process when a change that is made to the system results in the variation of the process. This statement simply means that something that you did resulted in a change. Common cause variation occurs when a change in a process occurs naturally, with no changes to the processes (Deming, 1986).

Control chart methodology includes examining data points based on a mean or median, as well as using an upper and lower control limit (Deming, 1986). One of the most basic ways to examine data is to graph the data points over time and then look for points for runs and trends in the data. A run occurs when there are seven or more consecutive points on either side of the center line. Depending on the measurement, if the consecutive data points are steadily moving upward or downward, this represents a trend in either the positive or negative direction, respectively (Langley et al., 2009). The universal protocol example described earlier was graphed monthly and after 7 months revealed a positive trend noted above the median.

For greater assurance of process changes that can be asserted as special cause or the result of an improvement project, the control chart should be used (Deming, 1986). The control chart uses the mean as the center mark and establishes upper and lower control limits that represent boundaries similar to the standard deviation. Although not the exact same calculation as the standard deviation, the upper and lower control limits are calculated in a similar fashion (Deming, 1986).

In conclusion, during the study phase, the assessment of the improvement work occurs in some fashion using a method discussed in the preceding paragraphs. However, this is the point at which the outcome of the process change would be compared with the aims set for the project. Comparing the outcome with the aim will inform and provide direction for the final phase of the PDSA, the Act phase (Langley et al., 2009).

The Act Phase

The final phase of the PDSA cycle is to "act" (Langley et al., 2009). This is the decision point for the dissemination and spread of the small test of change that has been tested. During this phase, the review of the entire PDSA will yield information on the next step for broader distribution from a microsystem to the macrosystem, or it will require that changes be made to the process and another PDSA piloted in the original microsystem (Langley et al., 2009; Nelson et al., 2007). It is important at this phase to look at failures and successes because they both provide valuable information regarding the ability to spread outside the initial pilot site. Although success of process change in one area may have great applicability to another area, do not be surprised if there is not a one-to-one translation. Different microsystems have different stakeholders, and thus the processes will vary by situation. However, in general, there are typically transferable elements of process changes that will be applicable to broader distribution (Langley et al., 2009; Nelson et al., 2007).

Dissemination and spread of an improvement process change require effective change management skills and knowledge. A brief discussion of change management theory is provided next.

■ Change Management

QI and change management are complementary approaches that are both essential to effectively and efficiently implement change. QI implies the need for change from a current state to some better state of affairs. "Change management" implies a managed process for moving from one state to another (Langley et al., 2009).

John P. Kotter (1995, 1996) described two orientations that are needed for sustained change implementation. The think-analyze-change orientation that is the hallmark of QI provides the evidence and rational basis for change. Think-analyze-change processes define the problem solved by change while identifying the processes and roles that must be changed, including risks and costs-benefits.

Change is hard. Rational approaches specify directions but rarely provide the motivation or the psychological impetus for change (Bradford & Cohen, 1984, 1998; Heath & Heath, 2010; Kotter 1996). Using a see-feel-change orientation change management approach creates the environment for change. Effective change management approaches allow managers and frontline staff to appreciate their clients' and customers' experiences as the reason for change while strengthening organizational commitment through effective leadership, teamwork, and communication at all levels (Bradford & Cohen, 1998; Kotter, 1995, 1996). Spreadsheets do not impel action in the same way that a client's story does, but a story does not prioritize actions like a spreadsheet. Similarly, process diagrams do not reflect the interactions among people that make processes work, but team building does not show the value of the team or its contribution to the organization's outcomes.

QI and change management are two faces of the same coin (Kotter, 1995; Langley et al., 2009). The success of one depends on the inclusion of the other. Healthcare organizations and providers must combine QI and change management approaches to be able to meet the challenges wrought by demands for often radical and rapid change (Varkey & Antonio, 2010).

Given the theoretical underpinnings of change management, how does one translate the knowledge into an operational perspective? How does one implement and achieve sustainable improvement in an efficient and timely fashion? Although there is no one solution that will be the answer for all, some tactics may facilitate this process (Bradford & Cohen, 1998; Kotter, 1996; Kotter & Cohen, 2002). Effective project management is a key component of improvement work. For improvement projects, this includes the development of a timeline with demarcated milestones and an approved budget based on the resources needed to implement the change. These functions are also integral to the research process, but again, the differences, timelines, and budgets for improvement work are integrated into the operational aspects of an organization and will exist within the work flow (Langley et al., 2009).

The greatest challenge that we have found in the Act phase of the PDSA cycle is staying on task and meeting deadlines. A variety of factors contribute to delays, but greater success is achieved when key leaders are in place to prioritize the work and remove barriers. Removing barriers will allow the greatest opportunity for success, which sets the stage for other improvement efforts and iterative PDSA cycles.

■ Quality and Safety Improvement

At the close of this chapter, we would like to distinguish quality and process improvement to incorporate the broader domain of quality, which is inclusive of safety improvement efforts (Langley et al., 2009). Whereas there are distinct sciences that address variation and reliability applicable most specifically to patient safety, improvement science is applicable to processes in quality and safety. The PDSA model can be applied globally to improvement work across all aspects of quality, which, by our definition, includes safety improvements as well (Langley et al., 2009). Additionally, the lines of what distinguishes "quality" and "safety" projects often tend to merge, and throughout this chapter, the universal protocol adherence project highlighted is an example of an improvement project that crosses both domains.

Quality and Safety Improvement as an Impetus for Research

Finally, it is hoped that throughout the pages of this chapter, it is clear to the reader that QI may become the impetus for research. Whereas the rigor with which an improvement project is performed will differ from that of a research design, improvement work clearly incorporates evidence and research into the design of the processes (Langley et al., 2009). Additionally, improvement work nationally has become the testing bed for the integration of evidence-based standards into the healthcare process. The first national pay-for-performance project was a combination of evidence-based research tied to process measures for delivering care (O'Hare, 2005; Williams, 2006). This project formed the basis for examining processes over time from an improvement design to change care. At this point in the evolution of the project, there is a focus on the impact of the processes on outcomes (Donabedian, 2003). This has become an opportune time to translate improvement evidence into translational research design.

■ **Exemplar One: Implementation of Cardiac Assessment Team and Cardiac-Specific Pediatric Early Warning Score Reduces Emergency Events on Inpatient Pediatric Cardiology Unit**

Clare Krantz

Background

A large tertiary pediatric hospital in Dallas, TX implemented a policy to assist bedside nurses on inpatient units to predict patient acuity of illness help prevent emergency events from occurring. The policy incorporated a pediatric early warning score (PEWS) along with a rapid response team (RRT) to assist in care of deteriorating patients. This policy was implemented hospital-wide, with one exception, the heart center. This was due to concerns that the PEWS tool would not appropriately identify deteriorating cardiac patients. Over the subsequent 4 years, the inpatient cardiology unit was found to have the highest number of emergency events outside of an intensive care unit (ICU); emergencies included acute respiratory compromise (ARC) and cardiopulmonary arrest (CPA).

Method

Under the leadership of a nurse practitioner, a multidisciplinary group within the heart center was formed with one driving objective: To prevent emergency events on the inpatient cardiology unit by developing a cardiac-specific RRT. An exhaustive literature search revealed an abundance of evidence in support of PEWS and RRTs in pediatrics, but there was little evidence to support its use in patients with congenital and acquired heart disease. Emergency events that occurred on this unit over the 4-year period described previously were reviewed in detail, along with those events that ensued within 24 hours of transfer to the cardiac ICU (CICU). The group also met with those who created the hospital PEWS and policy adopted 4 years prior.

With this data, the hospital-adopted PEWS was modified to include more variables specific to the pediatric cardiac patient population. An escalation algorithm was developed outlining assessment frequency, notification, and documentation. A cardiac assessment team (CAT) was created to respond to CPEWS-identified deteriorating patients prior to the hospital-wide RRT deployment. The CAT included nurses and providers from both the inpatient cardiology unit and CICU. The primary goals of the CAT were to improve communication and eliminate silos, establish a working care plan, and determine a time frame for reevaluation. A trial of this procedure was conducted and modified prior to implementation along with exhaustive staff education.

Results

One year after implementation of this system, the rate of emergency events was dramatically reduced. Specifically, CPAs fell from a rate of 0.79 (events per 1000 patient days) to a rate of zero, 3 years after implementation.

Conclusion

The CPEWS tool appropriately identifies the deteriorating cardiac patient. The cardiac-specific RRT allows for improved communication and timely interventions, which reduces out-of-ICU emergency events on pediatric inpatient cardiology units.

▪ Exemplar Two: Evaluation of Nursing Practices Within a Heart Failure Protocol

Quinton P. Ming

Purpose

The doctoral project Evaluation of Nursing Practices within a Heart Failure Protocol provides an illustration of how using best practice guidelines can have an impact on readmission rates, patients' length of stay, and cost. The doctoral project consisted of identifying, tracking, and examining communication and documentation practices of nurses who cared for heart failure (HF) patients before and after implementation of an HF protocol. More specifically, practices within the protocol examined if nurses (a) weighed patients daily, (b) notified medical providers when HF medications were held, and (c) educated patients about HF management.

Conceptual Framework

Donabedian's framework is an interdependent model consisting of three domains: structure, process, and outcomes, which allows information to be categorized so

(continues)

that inferences about the quality of care can be evaluated and improvements can made (Donabedian, 1980). Through the use of the Donabedian's framework, variables were categorized into the appropriate domains to examine the communication, documentation, and patient education practices of nurses to improve the delivery of care to HF patients as a result of using an HF protocol.

Methods

A retrospective chart review was conducted to examine the period between June 1, 2014 and November 30, 2014. There were 121 participants included in the study. Males accounted for 49.6%, and females accounted for 50.4% of the sample. Inclusion criteria are as follows: Hospitalist patients admitted through the emergency department with a diagnosis of HF, 19 years of age or older, no mental/psychiatric history, and not requiring continuous intravenous diuretics or cardiac medications. Nursing variables examined were (a) documentation of patients' daily weights, (b) documentation of medical provider(s) being notified when HF medications were held, and (c) documentation of HF patient education provided. Outcome variables examined were patients' length of stay, readmission rates, and costs.

Results

Findings indicated that of the variables examined, nurses educating patients about HF management and obtaining patients' daily weights were significant predictors of hospitalization costs. An independent sample t-test was performed to evaluate whether HF education differentiated participants based on the cost pertaining to their hospital visit. Findings indicated that there was a significant difference, $t(119) = -2.754$, $p = 0.007$. More specifically, those who received HF education ($M = 30,155.00$, $SD = 35,652.21$) had significantly lower hospitalization cost compared to those who did not receive HF education ($M = 45,544.81$, $SD = 38,425.69$). A multivariate linear regression was conducted to determine what independent variables significantly predicted variability in cost. HF education and daily weights were significant predictors of cost in the regression model, $F (2, 118) = 12.956$, $p < 0.001$. The predictors accounted for 12.5% of the variability in cost based on the model ($R^2 = 0.180$, $R = 0.424$). HF education ($r = 0.183$, $p = 0.022$) and daily weight ($r = 0.322$, $p = 0.000$) were both positively correlated to cost. However, follow-up t-tests revealed that obtaining daily weights was the most significant predictor, $t(118) = 4.158$, $p < 0.001$. HF education was also significant, $t(118) = 2.420$, $p = 0.017$.

Conclusion

The project identified that the use of an HF protocol based on best practice guidelines has helped nurses to more consistently educate patients about HF management and has helped medical providers to better monitor and manage some HF symptoms, such as weight gain–related fluid retention. The use of an evidence-based protocol for HF management is fairly new at the academic medical center, and evidence from the study suggests that as more medical providers and nurses consistently use the protocol, medical teams will be able to better manage the care of HF patients.

References

Donabedian, A. (1980). *The definition of quality and approaches to its assessment.* Ann Arbor, MI: Health Administration Press.

National Center for Biotechnology Information (2015). *Conceptual frameworks and their application to evaluating care coordination interventions.* Retrieved from http://www.ncbi.nlm.nih.gov/books/NBK44008/

REFLECTIVE ACTIVITIES

1. Identify a gap in your current practice. Using the PDSA framework, describe how each step contributes to developing an action plan for improvement.
2. Consider qualitative methods in the Do phase of the PDSA cycle. How might your qualitative data add richness to your process, particularly in describing outcomes?
3. Using your answer to question 1, describe effective change management and leadership approaches used in improving the process.

REFERENCES

Bradford, D. L., & Cohen, A. R. (1984). *Managing for excellence: The leadership guide to developing high performance in contemporary organizations.* Hoboken, NJ: Wiley.

Bradford, D. L., & Cohen, A. R. (1998). *Power: Transforming organizations through shared leadership.* Hoboken, NJ: Wiley.

Chambler, A. F., & Emery, R. J. (1997). Lord Moynihan cuts Codman into audit. *Annals of the Royal College of Surgeons of England, 79*(Suppl. 4), 174–176.

Deming, W. E. (1986). *Out of crisis.* Cambridge, MA: MIT Press.

Deming, W. E. (2000). *The new economics for industry, government, and education* (2nd ed.). Cambridge, MA: MIT Press.

Donabedian, A. (2003). *An introduction to quality assurance in healthcare.* New York, NY: Oxford University Press.

Drury, C. G. (1997). Ergonomics and quality movement. *Ergonomics, 40*(3), 249–264.

Eklund, J. (1995). Relationship between ergonomics and quality in assembly work. *Applied Ergonomics, 26*(1), 15–20.

Eklund, J. (1997). Ergonomics, quality and continuous improvement ± conceptual and empirical relationships in an industrial context. *Ergonomics, 40*(10), 982–1001.

Heath, C., & Heath, D. (2010). *Switch: How to change things when change is hard.* New York, NY: Random House.

Joint Commission. (2016). *Facts about patient safety.* Retrieved from http://www.jointcommission.org/facts_about_patient_safety/

Kaska, S. C., & Weinstein, J. N. (1998). Historical perspective. Ernest Amory Codman, 1869–1940. A pioneer of evidence-based medicine: The end result idea. *Spine, 23,* 629–633.

Kotter, J. P. (1995, March–April). Leading change: Why transformation efforts fail. *Harvard Business Review, 73*(2), 59–67.

Kotter, J. P. (1996). *Leading change.* Boston, MA: Harvard Business School Press.

Kotter, J. P., & Cohen, D. S. (2002). *The heart of change: Real-life stories of how people change their organizations.* Boston, MA: Harvard Business School Press.

Langley, G. L., Nolan, K. M., Nolan, T. W., Norman C. L., & Provost, L. P. (2009). *The improvement guide: A practical approach to enhancing organizational performance* (2nd ed.). San Francisco, CA: Jossey-Bass.

Leape, L. L., & Berwick, D. M. (2005). Five years after To Err Is Human: What have we learned? *Journal of the American Medical Association, 293,* 2384–2390.

Mark, M. M., & Pines, E. (1995). Implications of continuous improvement for program evaluation and evaluators. *Evaluation Practice, 16*(2), 131–139.

Mears, P. (1995). *Quality improvement tools and techniques.* New York, NY: McGraw-Hill.

Nave, D. (2002). How to compare Six Sigma, Lean and the theory of constraints: A framework for choosing what's best for your organization. *Quality Progress, 35*(3), 73–78. http://www.lean.org/Search/Documents/242.pdf

Nelson, E. C., Batalden, P., & Godfrey, M. (2007). *Quality by design: A clinical microsystems approach.* San Francisco, CA: Jossey-Bass.

Newhouse, R. P., Dearholt, S., Poe, S., Pugh, L. C., & White, K. (2007). *Johns Hopkins nursing evidence-based practice model & guidelines.* Indianapolis, IN: Sigma Theta Tau International.

Newhouse, R. P., Perrit, J. C., Rocco, L., & Poe, S. (2006). The slippery slope: Differentiating between quality improvement and research. *Journal of Nursing Administration, 36,* 211–219.

Newhouse, R. P., & Unruh, L. (2009, October). *Empirical outcomes: What's the difference between research and quality improvement?* Paper presented at ANCC National Magnet Conference, Louisville, KY.

O'Hare, P. K. (2005). Pay for performance: Will your hospital be ready? *Healthcare Financial Management, 59*(5), 46–48.

Polit, D. F., & Beck, C. T. (2012). *Nursing research: Generating and assessing evidence for nursing practice* (9th ed.). Philadelphia, PA: Lippincott Williams & Wilkins.

Schwarz, M., Landis, S. E., & Rowe, J. E. (1999). A team approach to quality improvement. *Family Practice Management, 6*(4), 25–30.

Scrivens, E. (1997). Putting continuous quality improvement into accreditation: Improving approaches to quality assessment. *Quality in Health Care, 6,* 212–218.

Simmons, J. C. (2002). Using Six Sigma to make a difference in health care quality. *The Quality Letter for Healthcare Leaders, 14*(4), 2–10, 1.

Sorensen, A. V., & Bernard, S. L. (2012). Accelerating what works: Using qualitative research methods in developing a change package for a learning collaborative. *The Joint Commission Journal on Quality and Patient Safety, 38*(2), 89–95

Spiegelhalter, D. (1999). Surgical audit: Statistical lessons from Nightingale and Codman. *Journal of the Royal Statistical Society: Series A, 162*(Part 1), 45–58.

Taylor, F. W. (1911). *The principles of scientific management.* New York, NY: Harper & Row.

Varkey, P., & Antonio, K. (2010). Change management for effective quality improvement: A primer. *American Journal of Medical Quality, 25,* 268–274.

Vincent, C. (2010). *Patient safety* (2nd ed.). Oxford, England: Wiley Blackwell.

Vincent, C., Batalden, P., & Davidoff, F. (2011). Multidisciplinary centers for safety and quality improvement: Learning from climate change science. *BMJ Quality & Safety, 20,* i73–i78. Doi:10.1136/bmjqs.2010

Williams, T. R. (2006). Practical design and implementation considerations in pay-for-performance programs. *American Journal of Managed Care, 12*(2), 77–80.

CHAPTER 11

Improvement Science: Impact on Quality and Patient Safety

■ Mary E. Geary and Linda Roussel ■

■ Objectives:

- Describe the evidence base for quality and patient safety.
- Define the human factor theory and its relationship to the patient safety movement.
- Relate high-reliability organizations (HROs) to achieving a culture of quality and patient safety.
- Describe the Plan-Brief-Execute-Debrief (PBED) model, incorporating specific safe practices that promote teamwork, collaboration, and communication.
- Identify crew resource management as a set of communication skills that promote safe practices, utilizing the communication and team training program TeamSTEPPS.

■ Introduction

Quality programs have existed in hospitals and other healthcare organizations for decades. Their emphases have evolved from quality control and quality assurance to quality and performance improvement and now include patient safety. A major shift in hospital quality activities is measuring practices and outcomes that are supported by research evidence. Quality management professionals in healthcare organizations recognize that scientific principles are used to systematically measure performance and improve processes. Regardless of whether an initiative is unit specific or an organization-wide improvement effort, quality projects need to be a planned effort. This chapter will discuss the focus of quality programs today in health care and give some examples of improvements for both quality and patient safety.

▪ Basic Concepts of Quality and Patient Safety

The basic concepts for quality control and statistical analysis used by healthcare quality professionals today come from two American industrial theorists, Walter Shewhart and W. Edwards Deming. Shewhart's early work with Bell laboratories in the 1920s was the foundation of his quality theory, which combines statistics, engineering, and economics. He advocated measuring processes and using the data to statistically evaluate performance and outcomes. The ideas that every process will have either common cause or special cause variation and that it is important for managers to recognize the difference to determine when actions are needed come from his work. Shewhart believed that reducing the amount of variation in a system would improve the consistency and quality of a product. His research provided statistical process control tools for plotting data that are used today by healthcare quality professionals. Control charts and run charts show data trends over time and process variation, which helps ensure that improvement actions are guided by the data. Shewhart is also the author of the commonly used quality model Plan-Do-Check-Act (PDCA) cycle as an improvement model. The PDCA model is often referred to as the Plan-Do-Study-Act quality model. Both provide quality teams with a systematic problem-solving approach to guide improvement initiatives (Best & Neuhauser, 2006).

W. Edwards Deming is known for his theory of profound knowledge, which consists of four elements: systems thinking, process variation, theory of knowledge, and psychology (Lighter, 2011). He encouraged managers to use data to evaluate the effectiveness of the processes and systems when outcomes were not those desired. Deming recognized that process measurement is as important as measuring outcomes in accurately determining what specifically needs improvement. He believed that organizational management needed to shift away from blaming individuals when outcomes were not as expected and to review the involved processes instead (Williams & Geary, 1999). Deming encouraged organizational leaders to invest in training all employees in quality improvement (QI) principles. This shared knowledge would build teamwork among the workforce and foster a sense of ownership in the organization. Creating such a work environment would encourage employees to voice their opinions and not fear reprisal from mistakes or poor outcomes. Deming's philosophy was adopted by Japanese engineers and executives, which contributed to that country's overall improvement in the quality of its products. Healthcare quality programs used his process variation principles and statistical process tools in the 1990s in their performance improvement programs. However, Deming's ideas of systems thinking and creating a work culture of process review and moving away from casting individual blame was not adopted by the majority of hospitals until later (Deming, 2000).

It took the publication of the Institute of Medicine (IOM) report *To Err Is Human: Building a Safer Health System* in 2000 to capture the attention of the American public and begin the shift away from individual blame to examining systems and processes (Kohn, Corrigan, & Donaldson, 2000). The report's finding that 44,000 to 98,000 deaths per year in this country were attributed to medical errors was the catalyst for the current patient safety movement. This enormous number of patient deaths could not be attributed to individual mistakes or poor performance by healthcare providers. Other explanations had to be sought, and solutions other than individual discipline and blame needed to be identified. Because healthcare organizations traditionally viewed errors from the "person" approach as opposed to the "system" approach, a paradigm shift in quality programs was needed. After the IOM report, the Joint Commission soon began requiring hospitals to have a patient safety program, implement policies to adhere to National Patient Safety Goals (NPSGs), and begin analyzing sentinel events related to medical errors. Hospital quality departments expanded their role to become patient safety leaders and establish patient safety programs. Quality specialists began reviewing adverse patient events in relation to hospital systems and processes of care. Instead of automatically becoming risk management's possible litigation concern shrouded in secrecy, unexpected patient deaths or unforeseen complications became a trigger to review hospital processes and were viewed as an opportunity to improve the overall performance quality. Patient safety partnered with quality, changing the evolution in healthcare quality once again (see **Figure 11-1**).

The IOM report recommended that hospitals adopt a systems approach to error prevention and recommended using the human factors theory (Kohn et al., 2000). Human factors theory assumes that all human beings will make mistakes because of inherent limitations associated with human cognitive abilities. Leape (1997) stated that human errors are commonly suggested from human factors research. Loss of attention because of distractions, lapses in memory, poor concentration from fatigue,

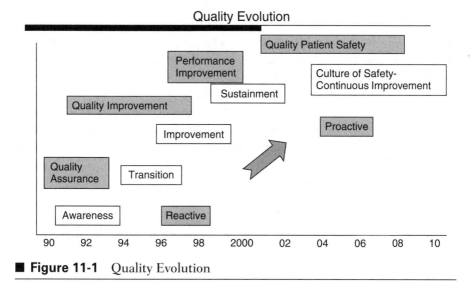

■ **Figure 11-1** Quality Evolution

and multiple stimuli may all contribute to human error. A systems approach to errors uses human factor theory principles of identifying the human elements, environmental effects, and system design issues that may contribute to an error occurring. James Reason's (1990) work regarding human factors theory has been applied to many healthcare quality and patient safety programs. According to Reason, an error occurs when a planned sequence of mental or physical activities fails to achieve the intended outcome. Performance is affected by multiple work environment characteristics, including how people interact, the ability to use equipment, and effects of other physical environmental factors on work outcomes. Too many demands placed on human performance can exceed an individual's capability and have an impact on outcomes. Human performance is enhanced when work environments are created that help decrease demands. Just as Shewhart's work recommended decreasing process variation, human factors theory suggests having standardized processes and types of equipment so that people have fewer rules to follow and steps to remember (Best & Neuhauser, 2006).

Incorporating patient safety into hospital quality programs has brought back Deming's philosophy of creating an organization culture in which everyone is part of the overall team and outcomes are viewed in relation to the involved systems (Deming, 2000). To prevent medical errors, nurses must be able to report unsafe situations and error occurrences to identify potential risks and systems that need safety changes. A positive culture of safety encourages errors to be reported and examined without the fear of ridicule, punishment, or shame (Morath & Leary, 2004). Research has shown that the frequency of hospital staff reporting active errors and near-misses depends on the type of culture the organization has regarding patient safety (Berwick, 2003; Leape, 1997). Implementing a safety culture that promotes a nonpunitive process of error review requires continual education of staff and commitment by hospital leaders. Deming recommended both of these approaches, which include adopting a new philosophy in which everyone feels responsibility for the quality of service, staff are offered training on systems and processes, and leadership embraces process improvement and drives out individual fear. Hospital quality professionals facilitate multidisciplinary reviews of all sentinel events and identify all processes contributing to the adverse events. This root cause analysis not only leads to identifying actions needed to improve hospital systems but also assists in creating an organization culture of safety by removing individual blame. Thus, the early quality theorists Shewhart and Deming continue to provide a foundation for healthcare quality programs even as the focus has expanded to encompass patient safety (Best & Neuhauser, 2006; Deming, 2000).

■ High-Reliability Organizations

HROs are organizations with systems in place that are exceptionally consistent in accomplishing their goals and avoiding potentially catastrophic errors (Chassin & Loeb, 2011). This is addressed through steady changes that health systems make to progress toward reliability and accountability. Leadership's commitment is first and foremost to achieving zero patient harm. Awareness of and a fully functional culture of safety throughout the organization is essential along with deploying robust improvement tools (Chassin & Loeb, 2013). Five key concepts of HROs include (Chassin & Loeb, 2011):

- **Sensitivity to operations:** Ongoing awareness of risks, to prevent harm and safety breaches.
- **Reluctance to simplify:** Avoids looking for the "obvious" solution to a deep-rooted problem interfering with workflow and patient safety. A good example would be automatically going to an educational intervention, when there is not enough information about the failure to "fix it."
- **Preoccupation with failure:** Always on the lookout for what could go wrong and not viewing near-misses as evidence that the system has effective safeguards "caught the mishap," but instead seeing close calls as symptomatic of areas in need of more attention.
- **Deference to expertise:** A keen sense of awareness of those at the sharp end of care delivery having true insights into the workflow and patients' experiences. It is essential that leaders and supervisors listen and respond to staff who know how processes work and the risks patients really face. Without a culture of inclusiveness, it is unlikely that an organization can achieve high reliability.
- **Resilience:** Admitting failure points and being ready to respond when the system fails.

Healthcare environments have many of the characteristics of industries in which accidents often result in fatalities (nuclear power plants, amusement parks). For example, the characteristic of hypercomplexity describes hospitals with layers, and levels of hierarchies that are complicated and often convoluted. A culture of safety relies on the effective coordination of physicians, nurses, pharmacists, therapists, technicians who maintain equipment, and support staff who provide specialized services and maintain the physical environment. Healthcare leaders recognize that this coordination is critical, yet far from perfect. Other characteristics that make acute healthcare systems ready for HROs are tight coupling (overdependence on multiple tasks carried out by multiple providers), multiple decision-makers, high accountability, and compressed time constraints. Striving to be an HRO facilitates an enhanced culture of safety through leadership and a strong improvement focus.

■ Incorporating Patient Safety in the Quality Model

Improving an organization's culture of safety is a key strategic goal for healthcare organizations today. Reducing medical error and providing high-quality care are strategic goals in many hospitals today and are becoming more important as publicly reported measures continue to be mandated and linked to reimbursement. Quality professionals over the past decade have expanded their responsibilities beyond facilitating QI projects to also promote patient safety practices. However, the current QI models that have been used for the past 20 years, such as PDCA, do not incorporate patient safety. This dichotomy can keep quality and patient safety as parallel processes in the minds of many hospital leaders and staff, when in fact, the two should exist simultaneously. A new improvement model is needed to integrate patient safety with quality while still providing a structured problem-solving approach. Revising the PDCA model to a PBED model incorporates specific safe practices of briefs and debriefs, promoting teamwork, collaboration, and communication (Murphy, 2005; see **Figure 11-2**).

Comparisons have been made between aviation and healthcare work environments since the IOM report *To Err Is Human: Building a Safer Health System* was published in 2000 (Kohn et al., 2000). Both are high-risk industries, but aviation safety practices far exceed those in hospitals. Successful characteristics and factors that exist in high-reliability aviation outcomes have been identified for healthcare organizations to implement in order to achieve safer patient outcomes (Helmreich, 2000; Lyndon, 2006). Three of these characteristics are teamwork, collaboration, and communication. Teamwork is consistently discussed in patient safety literature as being critical to reducing medical error and patient harm (Barach & Small, 2000; Grogan et al., 2004; Sexton, Thomas, & Helmreich, 2000; Vincent et al., 2000). The impact of medical teamwork on clinical outcomes has been studied in intensive care units, labor and delivery (L&D) units, surgical suites, and emergency departments. Teamwork training became one of the safe practices discussed in the National Quality

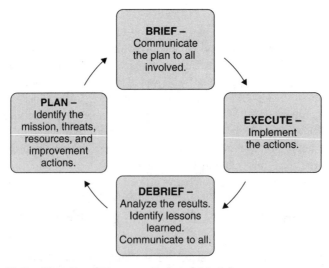

■ **Figure 11-2** Plan-Brief-Execute-Debrief Model

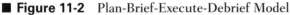

Forum's *Safe Practices for Better Healthcare: A Consensus Report* (Agency for Healthcare Research and Quality [AHRQ], 2016).

Collaboration among team members is recommended in the IOM's report *Crossing the Quality Chasm* to ensure that appropriate patient information is shared that is needed to provide safe care (Briere, 2001). Teams cannot be collaborative or effective without adequate communication. The Joint Commission cites poor communication as the number one contributing factor in reported sentinel events. In addition, the Department of Veterans Affairs National Center for Patient Safety reported that communication breakdown was a primary cause in approximately 75% of 7000 actual and near-miss events (Dunn et al., 2007). Aviation has successfully established practices of effective communication that promote collaborative teamwork.

Crew resource management is a set of communication skills taught in aviation to promote safe practices and was used in the communication and team training program TeamSTEPPS. TeamSTEPPS stands for Team Strategies and Tools to Enhance Performance and Patient Safety and was developed for healthcare professionals by the Agency for Healthcare Research and Quality and the U.S. Department of Defense (King et al., n.d.). This team training curriculum is an evidence-based framework based on safety research from other high-risk industries, such as aviation and nuclear power, and is available for hospitals to use. The training incorporates human factors and focuses on specific skills that support team performance principles such as leadership, mutual support, situation monitoring, and communication. An evaluation study of the TeamSTEPPS training program was conducted within an operating room (OR) service line and found that the trained group had significantly increased team behaviors and perceptions of patient safety compared with a nontrained control group (Weaver, Salas, & King, 2011). Team training and implementation in a surgical and pediatric intensive care unit was also evaluated and found to positively affect patient outcomes and staff perception of safety (Mayer et al., 2011). Many studies have been published regarding the usefulness of implementing specific aviation communication practices such as standardized checklists, closed-loop conversations, and structured communication formats such as SBAR (situation, background, assessment, recommendation) into hospital settings. An evidence-based practice (EBP) study regarding SBAR collaborative communication found that staff transferred evidence, knowledge, and skills into practice to achieve enhanced communication, collaboration, satisfaction, and patient safety outcomes (Beckett & Kipnis, 2009).

Success in team training programs depends on organizational factors such as leadership support, alignment of team training objectives with organizational goals, involvement of frontline care providers, facilitation of the application of trained teamwork skills, and a commitment to data-driven change (Salas et al., 2008). The challenge for hospitals is to sustain the principles taught and ensure that the practices that can prevent errors become daily habits for nurses, physicians, and other healthcare providers. The training and concepts need to be part of what the organization does and consist of policies and procedures that support teamwork (Salas, Gregory, & King, 2011).

Revising the quality model to incorporate aspects of team training is one way to sustain the training and actualize the practices. The PBED model is a more recently developed quality model that incorporates patient safety practices by including steps that require teamwork and communication. The PBED problem-solving model is easily learned by staff because the steps are similar to those in the familiar QI model. Briefings and debriefings are structured communication events that have been shown to improve communication and create teamwork (Leonard, Graham, & Bonacum, 2004; Shannon, 2011). Other communication skills and aspects of a team training program can be incorporated into the various steps of this model, again creating opportunities to implement these safe care practices (see **Figure 11-3**).

The Plan step is similar to the planning phase of the traditional PDCA model in identifying a group with which to address a specific issue. One difference, however, is having a standardized planning tool that ensures consistency of the planning process. Process consistency is a human factors principle, and when applied to a planning initiative, it can keep a group focused on the problem or issue of concern. The six steps of planning are:

1. Determine the objective or goal
2. Identify the threats to accomplishing the objective
3. Identify the resources available and those needed
4. Evaluate lessons learned from related improvement efforts previously tried
5. Develop a course of action to include identifying who will do what by when
6. Proactively identify any needed contingency plans

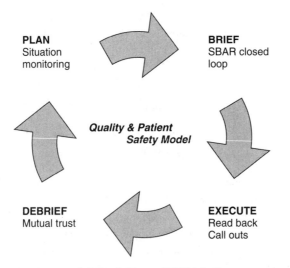

■ **Figure 11-3** PBED Model With TeamSTEPPS Communication Skills

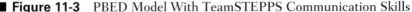

This planning format can be used for large organization-wide initiatives or individual units planning the team's daily plan (Murphy, 2005).

The second step is to *brief,* or communicate the plan to all those who will be involved as well as affected. Briefings are discussed in the patient safety literature and also have been referred to as huddles. One hospital reported its success in implementing frontline staff safety huddles to review patient safety events and proactively identify preventive safety practices. Gerke, Uffelman, and Chandler (2010) found that the implementation of huddles created a blame-free environment for staff to discuss the process improvements needed to promote patient safety and that it contributed to teamwork among the staff. Another hospital reported that implementing briefings and debriefings after team training led to continued teamwork and improved patient outcomes and patient and staff satisfaction (Beckett & Kipnis, 2009). Two major types of briefings are patient care briefings and process improvement briefings. Patient care briefings can be done at the beginning of a shift to focus the team on the daily plan; at the beginning of a procedure or surgery, to update and include a new team member; and whenever there is a change in a situation or the plan needs to be updated. The Brief step in the process improvement model is to inform everyone affected by any process or policy change needed of any pilot project being started or any part of the plan that relates to his or her responsibilities. Keeping everyone informed of change before it occurs helps create cooperation and support for the improvement activity. Characteristics of an effective brief include being organized and to the point and always encouraging questions from participants to ensure understanding (Murphy, 2005).

The Execute step is similar to the Do step in the PDCA quality model. This is the implementation phase of the plan and should start only after it has been fully communicated. A key part of this communication is to identify who will do what, what will be done, and when it will be done. Making the Execute steps this specific ensures that everyone is aware of his or her responsibilities and what is going to occur. Again, this promotes team communication and helps to eliminate assumptions (Murphy, 2005).

The Debrief step brings a team back together and is an opportunity for learning. Debrief discussions should include what went well, what can be learned, and what should be done differently. Debriefing a QI initiative should include evaluation of any data gathered to determine if the executed plan was successful or if any revisions are needed. All this information is then communicated to everyone involved and affected by the project. Debriefs also can be held after patient events such as falls or emergency surgeries. Primary reasons for conducting debriefs are to promote teamwork, accelerate learning, and generate improvement ideas or actions (Murphy, 2005). Team debriefs have been shown to be helpful in L&D following emergency cesarean sections. One study described an L&D team debrief that identified the need for improved communication among all staff; this discussion resulted in the hospital purchasing walkie talkies for staff to have behind closed doors of a labor room as a means to keep other team members informed of the situation (Shea-Lewis, 2009).

Debriefs are best done immediately after an event or a procedure. Some guidelines for debriefing include being crisp and to the point, allowing everyone on the team to contribute to the conversation, and avoiding judgment. Debriefs should be nonpunitive, and individual performance should never be criticized in a debrief setting. Situations and processes involved need to be reviewed without blaming individuals or departments. The facilitator should always end the debriefing on a positive note. Briefs and debriefs should be done concisely and in a format familiar to all team members so that they know what to expect and want to participate (Murphy, 2005). A large prospective study evaluated the implementation of an OR briefing and debriefing tool. Over a 17-month period, 37,133 briefings and debriefings were conducted. The analyses found that the majority of caregivers involved perceived that both communication and teamwork were improved as a result of using this tool, and on average, the briefing prior to the procedure and the debriefing after the procedure took less than 3 minutes each (Berenholtz et al., 2009).

This quality/patient safety model can be used for QI projects and patient safety initiatives and promotes effective communication among healthcare teams. Briefs and debriefs are evidence-based structured communication events. Merging known patient safety practices into a problem-solving approach can assist an organization in creating a culture of safety.

■ Examples of Model Application

Much of what hospitals monitor for quality of care and patient safety has been determined by the Joint Commission, the Centers for Medicare and Medicaid Services (CMS), the American Nurses Association (ANA), and the AHRQ. All these organizations have taken the majority of their quality and patient safety initiatives from the National Quality Forum (NQF) Safe Practices for Better Healthcare. The NQF is a voluntary consensus standard-setting organization whose mission is to improve the quality of American health care by setting national priorities and goals for performance improvement (NQF, 2009). Thirty-four best practices are evidence-based and have been demonstrated to be effective in reducing the occurrence of adverse healthcare events. Included in these NQF practices are preventable adverse events that CMS refers to as hospital-acquired conditions, which will no longer be reimbursed. The AHRQ has identified patient safety indicators that include some of these preventable hospital-acquired conditions. The ANA has NQF-endorsed nursing measures, the Nursing Database of Nursing Quality Indicators (NDNQI), that assist nurse leaders in evaluating the effectiveness of specific nursing care practices. The Joint Commission began including NPSGs in its accreditation requirements in 2004 to ensure that hospitals have processes in place to prevent adverse events. **Table 11-1** shows a crosswalk of the specific NQF best practices that are also CMS, AHRQ, ANA, and/or Joint Commission measures.

Following are three examples of use of the PBED quality/patient safety model to improve processes of care and prevent patient harm and medical errors.

TABLE 11-1 Selected Measures of NQF, CMS, AHRQ, NDNQI, and the Joint Commission

NQF Best Practice	CMS Hospital-Acquired Conditions	AHRQ Patient Safety Indicators	NDNQI Measures	Joint Commission National Patient Safety Goals	CMS and Joint Commission Core Measures
Nursing workforce			✓		
Direct caregivers			✓		
Order readback—Abbreviations				✓	
Medication reconciliation				✓	
Hand hygiene				✓	
Influenza prevention					✓
Central line bloodstream infection prevention	✓				
Surgical site infection prevention	✓	✓		✓	✓
Care of the ventilator patient		✓			
Multidrug-resistant organism prevention		✓		✓	
Urinary catheter-associated UTI prevention	✓	✓		✓	
Wrong-site, procedure, wrong-person surgery prevention				✓	
Pressure ulcer prevention	✓	✓	✓		
Venous thrombus embolism prevention	✓	✓			✓
Glycemic control	✓	✓			✓
Falls prevention	✓		✓		

Venous Thrombus Embolism Prophylaxis in the Surgical Patient

Issue

The goal for the core measure regarding perioperative thromboembolism prophylaxis was set to be in the top 10 percentile nationally (100%). The team consisted of nurses, OR staff, surgeons, and quality specialists.

Plan

Current patient cases that did not meet the core measure requirement were reviewed to identify the most common reasons. Process improvements were needed to assist in standardizing treatment and documentation.

Brief

A new policy was written and approved by the medical staff to allow defined groups of surgical patients to automatically receive sequential compression devices prior to surgery. In addition, the postoperative note was revised to include an area for surgeons to document the reason that thromboembolism prophylaxis may not be appropriate for a specific patient. All surgeons and OR staff were included in these changes prior to implementation.

Execute

The new policy was implemented and the postoperative form revised. The core measure was monitored for improvement.

Debrief

Venous thrombus embolism prophylaxis measures improved from 88% in Q1 2010 to 100% in Q4 2010 based on actions implemented. This success was shared at the medical staff meetings, surgery staff meetings, and organization-wide when celebrating achievement of this core measure goal.

Surgical Site Infection Prevention

Issue

Reducing sternal wound infections. Team members included cardiovascular surgeons, nurses, infection prevention specialists, and quality specialists.

Plan

Current literature was reviewed for EBPs and recommendations regarding prevention of surgical site infections.

Brief

Organization policy and practices were reviewed by the team members and compared with the research. Policies and procedures were revised and sent to the appropriate committees for approval. All those involved received communication regarding the changes.

Execute

Specific practices implemented included preoperative chlorhexidine baths for cardiovascular surgery patients; changing povidone-iodine (Betadine) to chlorhexidine for surgical site preparation; introducing disposable electrocardiogram leads in the intensive care unit (ICU); scheduling sternal dressing changes at 48 hours with chlorhexidine cleaning; replacing current bath basins with patient bath cloths; and revising preprinted postoperative surgical orders to include postoperative glucose control. Monthly infection rates by surgical site were monitored.

Debrief

Sternal wound infection rates were communicated to the medical staff committees, individual surgeons, and nursing staff on an ongoing basis. The sternal site infection rate decreased from 2.7% in Q3 2009 to 0% in Q1 2010 and continues to be 0% since actions were implemented.

Patient Fall Prevention

Issue

Patients in the rehabilitation unit are at higher risk for falls because of their impaired functional and/or cognitive status. The team consisted of all rehabilitation department staff, including nurses, nurse assistants, and therapists.

Plan

The plan was to decrease patient falls by involving all staff in identifying contributing factors to a patient fall and future preventive measures. A fall debrief was developed to use after a patient fall to facilitate this communication and contribute to teamwork among all care providers.

Brief

All staff members were educated on the process of conducting a postfall debrief immediately after any patient fall to identify additional prevention measures and decrease the overall number of patient falls.

Execute

The postfall debrief was implemented using the form, which provided a standardized format. The debrief was facilitated by the unit manager or team leader. It followed nonpunitive guidelines, involved all staff available on the unit for greatest learning benefit, and kept debriefs to the point. Patient falls were monitored monthly for improvement.

Debrief

The average number of patient falls decreased from 5.4 prior to implementation of the postfall debriefs to 3.14 afterward. The success of this activity in patient fall reduction was shared with the nursing division, and the practice was implemented in all patient care units.

■ Quality Improvement Commentary

Selected Websites

http://www.qualityforum.org/Home.aspx

The National Quality Forum provides a medium for the healthcare system to measure, report, monitor, and constantly improve as we strive to continually improve our own systems, policies, and processes. This site continually evaluates and benchmarks the steps taken and the systems established to reach the goal of higher quality health care in America.

http://www.ihi.org/Pages/default.aspx

An independent not-for-profit organization based in Cambridge, Massachusetts, the Institute for Healthcare Improvement focuses on motivating and building the will for change, identifying and testing new models of care in partnership with both patients and healthcare professionals, and ensuring the broadest possible adoption of best practices and effective innovations.

http://www.squire-statement.org/

The SQUIRE Guidelines help authors write excellent, usable articles about QI in health care so that findings may be easily discovered and widely disseminated. The SQUIRE website supports high-quality writing about improvement through listing available resources and discussions about the writing process.

http://www.nhsiq.nhs.uk

NHS Improvement's strength and expertise lie in practical service improvement. It has more than a decade of experience in clinical patient pathway redesign for cancer, diagnostics, heart, lung, and stroke and demonstrates some of the most leading-edge improvement work in England that supports improved patient experience and outcomes.

REFLECTIVE ACTIVITIES

1. Using the PBED model, incorporate specific safe practices of briefs and debriefs promoting teamwork, collaboration, and communication.
2. Working with a team, cross-reference specific NQF best practices that are also CMS, AHRQ, ANA, or Joint Commission measures.
3. Attend a performance improvement team meeting. Observe the roles of the various team members, attention to quality indicators, and recommendations to improve quality based on improvement programs.

REFERENCES

Agency for Healthcare Research and Quality. (2016). *Safe practices for better healthcare: Summary*. A consensus report. Retrieved from https://psnet.ahrq.gov/search?topic=Culture-of-Safety&f_topicIDs=656&pageSize=100&f_resource_typeID=66

Barach, P., & Small, S. D. (2000). Reporting and preventing medical mishaps: Lessons from non-medical near miss reporting systems. *British Medical Journal, 320*(7237), 759–763. doi:10.1136/bmj.320.7237.759

Beckett, C. D., & Kipnis, G. (2009). Collaborative communication: Integrating SBAR to improve quality/patient safety outcomes. *Journal for Healthcare Quality, 31*(5), 19–28. Doi:10.1111/j.1945-1474.2009.00043.x

Berenholtz, S. M., Schumacher, K., Hayanga, A. J., Simon, M., Goeschel, C., Pronovost, P. J., & Welsh, R. J. (2009). Implementing standardized operating room briefings and debriefings at a large regional medical center. *Joint Commission Journal on Quality and Patient Safety, 35*(8), 391–397.

Berwick, D. M. (2003). Disseminating innovations in health care. *Journal of the American Medical Association, 289*(15), 1969–1975. doi:10.1001/jama.289.15.1969

Best, M., & Neuhauser, D. (2006). Walter A. Shewhart, 1924, and the Hawthorne factory. *Quality and Safety in Health Care, 15*(2), 142–143. doi:10.1136/qshc.2006.018093

Briere, R. (Ed.). (2001). *Crossing the quality chasm: A new health system for the 21st century*. Washington, DC: National Academies Press.

Chassin, M.R., and J.M. Loeb. 2011. The Ongoing Quality Improvement Journey: Next Stop, High Reliability. Health Affairs 30(4):559–68.

Chassin, M. R., & Loeb, J. M. (2013). High-reliability health care: getting there from here. *The Milbank Quarterly, 91*(3), 459–490.

Deming, W. E. (2000). *Out of the crisis*. Boston, MA: MIT Press.

Dunn, E. J., Mills, P. D., Neily, J., Crittenden, M. D., Carmack, A. L., & Bagian, J. P. (2007). Medical team training: Applying crew resource management in the Veterans Health Administration. *Joint Commission Journal on Quality and Patient Safety, 33*(6), 317–325.

Gerke, M. L., Uffelman, C., & Chandler, K. W. (2010). *Safety huddles for a culture of safety: Patient safety and quality of care*. Retrieved from http://www.psqh.com/mayjune-2010/516-safety-huddles-for-a-culture-of-safety.html

Grogan, E. L., Stiles, R. A., France, D. J., Speroff, T., Morris, J. A., Nixon, B., & Pinson, C. W. (2004). The impact of aviation-based teamwork training on the attitudes of health-care professionals. *Journal of the American College of Surgeons, 199*(6), 843–848.

Helmreich, R. L. (2000). On error management: Lessons from aviation. *British Medical Journal, 320*, 781–785.

King, H. B., Battles, J., Baker, D. P., Alonso, A., Salas, E., Webster, J., & Salisbury, M. (n.d.). *TeamSTEPPS: Team strategies and tools to enhance performance and patient safety*. Retrieved from http://www.ahrq.gov/downloads/pub/advances2/vol3/Advances-King_1.pdf

Kohn, L. T., Corrigan, J. M., & Donaldson, M. S. (2000). *To err is human: Building a safer health system*. Washington, DC: National Academies Press.

Leape, L. (1997). *The leading cause of death in the United States is the healthcare system*. Retrieved from http://www.angelfire.com/az/sthurston/Leading_Cause_of_Death_in_the_US.html

Leonard, M., Graham, S., & Bonacum, D. (2004). The human factor: The critical importance of effective teamwork and communication in providing safe care. *Quality and Safety in Health Care, 13*(Suppl. 1), 85–90.

Lighter, D. (2011). *Advanced performance in health care: Principles and methods*. Sudbury, MA: Jones & Bartlett Learning.

Lyndon, A. (2006). Communication and teamwork in patient care: How much can we learn from aviation? *Journal of Obstetric, Gynecologic, & Neonatal Nursing, 35*(4), 538–546.

Mayer, C. M., Cluff, L., Lin, W., Willis, T. S., Stafford, R. E., Williams, C., & Amoozegar, J. B. (2011). Evaluating efforts to optimize TeamSTEPPS implementation in surgical and pediatric intensive care units. *Joint Commission Journal on Quality and Patient Safety, 37*(8), 365–374.

Morath, J., & Leary, M. (2004). Creating safe spaces in organizations to talk about safety. *Nursing Economic$, 22*(6), 344–354.

Murphy, J. (2005). *Flawless execution.* New York, NY: HarperCollins.

National Quality Forum. (2010). *Safe practices for better healthcare: 2010 update.* Retrieved from file:///C:/Users/lroussel/Downloads/Safe%20Practices%2010%20Abridged.pdf

Reason, J. (1990). *Human error.* New York, NY: Cambridge University Press.

Salas, E., DiazGranados, D., Klein, C., Burke, C. S., Stagl, K. C., Goodwin, G. F., & Halpin, S. M. (2008). Does team training improve team performance? A meta-analysis. *Human Factors, 50*(6), 903–933.

Salas, E., Gregory, M. E., & King, H. B. (2011). Team training can enhance patient safety: The data, the challenge ahead. *Joint Commission Journal on Quality and Patient Safety, 37*(8), 339–340.

Sexton, J. B., Thomas, E. J., & Helmreich, R. L. (2000). Error, stress, and teamwork in medicine and aviation: Cross sectional surveys. *British Medical Journal, 320,* 745–749.

Shannon, D. W. (2011, April). Team training in obstetrics: Improving care by learning to work together. *Patient Safety & Quality Healthcare.* Retrieved from http://www.psqh.com/marchapril-2011/800-team-training-in-obstetrics-improving-care-by-learning-to-work-together.html

Shea-Lewis, A. (2009). Teamwork: Crew resource management in a community hospital. *Journal for Healthcare Quality, 31*(5), 14–18. doi:10.1111/j.1945-1474.2009.00042.x

Vincent, C., Taylor-Adams, S., Chapman, J. E., Hewett, D., Prior, S., Strange, P., & Tizzard, A. (2000). How to investigate and analyze clinical incidents: Clinical risk unit and association of litigation and risk management protocol. *British Medical Journal, 320*(7237), 777–781. doi:10.1136/bmj.320.7237.777

Weaver, S. J., Salas, E., & King, H. B. (2011). Twelve best practices for team training evaluation in health care. *Joint Committee Journal on Quality and Patient Safety, 37,* 341–349. Retrieved from http://psnet.ahrq.gov/resource.aspx?resourceID=22712

Williams, T. P., & Geary, M. E. (1999). Cascading data sets: Putting the pieces together. *Journal for Healthcare Quality, 21*(3), 35–40.

CHAPTER 12

Health Policy and Evidence-Based Practice: The Quality, Safety, and Financial Incentive Link

■ JAMES L. HARRIS ■

■ Objectives:

- Identify how health policy and evidence are linked to quality, safety, and value-based practice.
- Discuss how health policy is influenced by evidence.
- Identify strategies for translating evidence into practice and achieving financial incentives.
- Recognize how health policies result in unintended consequences.
- Identify evidence-based tools used in eliminating and/or reducing unintended consequences imposed by health policies.
- Discuss global impact(s) of evidence-based health policy on the health of individuals and society.

■ Introduction

The fast-paced healthcare environment and wide-ranging health policy literature provide insights into the inherent relationship and relevance of evidence-based practice (EBP) methodologies. The literature is replete with key health policy issues, drivers, and approaches that support interprofessional development and the use of EBP interventions. As an organizational culture of EBP becomes increasingly commonplace in all care environments, quality, safety, and financial incentives will be realized. An organizational culture of EBP is an indicator of success and becomes pivotal as health policies are developed and implemented. In organizational cultures embracing EBP, the inclusion of theoretical and evidence theories, provider expertise, preferences, and values are fundamental attributes. These attributes culminate in clinical decisions that create quantifiable quality outcomes (Melnyk & Fineout-Overholt, 2005).

Central to further dialogue among providers and developers of health policy is the inherent relationship of health policy and evidence. If the question is whether health policy should inform clinical practice, will it then be answered as health services are improved and funded and evidence-based protocols are adopted and sustained? As future health policies are developed and enacted, the EBP process will be pivotal to informing, creating, and changing how health care is delivered and funded. Parallel to the process is how outcomes are managed and data collection systems inform organizational policies. Health policies promote the well-being of citizens, institutional policies govern the workplace and workforce, and organizational policies are positions of organizations (Mason, Leavitt, & Chaffee, 2007).

Throughout this chapter, influences of health policy and EBP will be central themes. An overview of how care systems are realizing the value of evidence-based health policy through financial incentives will be provided. Outcomes are and will continue to be aligned with reimbursement and regulatory issues to ensure the quality, safety, and cost-effectiveness of care.

■ Health Policy, Evidence, and Evidence-Based Practice Defined

To provide context for this chapter, health policy, evidence, and EBP are defined. Examples supporting these definitions are provided, as applicable. The World Health Organization (WHO) broadly defines health policy as actions initiated local, state, and national governments to advance and achieve healthcare goals of the public (WHO, 2015). It is not a singular process or action, but a series of regulatory and legislative initiatives framed around the healthcare goals of a society. It is the component of health policy that focuses on any organization, the finances, and provision of healthcare services—a proviso grounded in the US Constitution. An example of how health policy guides care is a wellness center funded through an employee-sponsored health insurance, individual policies, or Medicare. Using a systematic process, data are collected to provide evidence that wellness centers offer cost-effective treatment options to advance the health and well-being of individuals. As the findings are disseminated, additional wellness centers will offer evidence-based programs.

Health policy may achieve multiple outcomes. These include a vision for the future that launches new venues for the short-term and long-term priorities and roles of interprofessional teams and groups. Ultimately, consensus occurs, allowing leaders and society to become informed, whether locally, nationally, or globally (WHO, 2015).

"Evidence is defined as facts, whether actual or stated, intended for use in support of a conclusion" (Lomas, Culyer, McCutcheon, McAuley, & Law, 2005, p. 6). Evidence tends to prove or disprove the existence of an idea or finding. Some statements are considered fundamentally true, such as the provision in the Declaration of Independence stating, "We hold these truths to be self evident . . ." (Library of Congress, 2014). Multiple sources of evidence are available; however, not all evidence is of equal use. Consideration must then be given to how a decision to use evidence was derived.

Facts originate from events that are experienced and arise from many different forums and media. Consideration should be given to how facts drive informed decisions (International Council of Nurses, 2012). Ruland (2010) concluded that this increases the decision quality, diminishes errors, and strengthens the adoption of EBPs.

The International Council of Nurses (2012) define EBP as "a problem-solving approach to clinical decision making that incorporates a search for the best and latest evidence, clinical expertise and assessment, and patient preference values within a context of caring" (p. 6). Fielding and Briss (2006) provide support for this definition by identifying that evidence-based approaches are linked to the best available evidence and preferences that include possibilities for informing health policy decisions. Evidence substantiates the kinds of practice, procedures, and protocol implementation, including their relevancy. At the time a practice intervention or protocol is accepted and implemented it becomes the best evidence. As new information is acquired, interventions or protocols may change.

During deliberations for new or improved health policies, individuals review the available evidence, needs and preferences of healthcare consumers, expertise of care providers, and clinical judgment. A common and reliable process includes asking a pertinent clinical question using a format such as population, intervention, comparison, outcome, and time frame (PICOT) (Melynk & Fineout-Overholt, 2015).

The PICOT process is an organized strategy that describes the parts of the vital question occurring during an analysis. The P delineates the population of interest. The I is the intervention that is related to the population. The C is the comparison to the intervention, commonly used in current practice. The O is the outcome of relevant interest that will be examined based on the intervention. The T is the time frame for investigating the influence and impact on the proposed outcomes (Melynk & Fineout-Overholt, 2015).

Understanding each of these descriptions and their link to one another are foundational to team engagement, policy development, and advocacy for evidence-based health policies. These do not occur in isolation and require that evidence be widely disseminated to advance science, meet population needs, and provide cost-effective care.

■ Historical Influences and Drivers of Health Policy and Evidence-Based Practice

History plays an important role in shaping and guiding actions of individuals and groups. This includes the preparation and communication of evidence-based health policies that influence health status, funding for programs, care improvements, and their universal adoption. Health policy and clinical practice are often shaped by history. For example, Wailoo's work on the history of blood diseases was influenced by societal attitudes about sex, race, and social class. Using this knowledge, Wailoo illustrated how modern understanding of disease and genetics influences policy decisions about who should receive specific blood, drug, and genetic testing and the rationale for each (Fairman & D'Antonio, 2013; Wailoo, 1999).

Recognizing and understanding what influences health policy and EBP beyond the role that history plays are invaluable. Both are complex and inclusive of complicated processes. Making sense of each is easier when one considers three domains. The domains include process, content, and outcomes. Process provides the context necessary to understand approaches that enrich health policy adoption. Content includes specific elements of the policy that are most likely to have relevance and be effective. Outcomes provide venues for documenting the efficacy and policy impact(s). Outcomes are further evident as data are prepared and communicated, analytic tools are used effectively, outcomes documented, and new evidence emerges (Brownson, Chriqui, & Stamatakis, 2009). A good example of the importance of these three domains is provided by Tobbell (2011) in an analysis of the pharmaceutical industry. Tobbell's work revealed how evidence is socially embedded. The analysis provided insight into how a prescription can be influenced by human agents (prescribing groups and pharmaceutical industry) rather than evidence of drug efficacy. This underscores the importance of how the domains offer an approach to understanding health policy and the value of evidence when adopting any policy.

Stevens (2006) stated that history provides evidence that guides policy-makers and provide direction when choices are vague or lack evidence. There are multiple examples in the Patient Protection and Affordable Care Act and how to accomplish the Triple Aim (Stiefel & Nolan, 2012). Each of the examples has major financial impacts, incentives, and potential disincentives if unmet. In an era of fragmented health care and limited care access, policy-makers are challenged to explore new ways of examining all options before advocating for enactment of certain policies. Evidence plays a vital role in preventing further care fragmentation. One option is questioning if additional funds should be allocated for advanced nurse practice preparation. Also, removing scope of practice restrictions remains a debatable topic and requires policy-makers to examine all evidence before arriving at decisions or taking action. Thoughtful hesitation from an immediate situation allows reflection versus reaction before decisions or actions. Nurses are key players in giving voice to policy changes and educating policy makers to recognize the value of history and evidence that guide their decision and actions before changes occur.

As discussed in the preceding paragraphs, evidence-based policy historically has and will continue to levy profound impacts on the health and well-being of individuals. Beyond historical influences is recognition and identification of health policy and EBP drivers. The drivers cannot be understated in the constant healthcare changes and demands imposed by consumers. Birkland (2005) stated that health policy is often driven by the values and biases of the policy decision-makers or their constituent's influence. While policy makers have a desire that decisions are based on evidence and creditability, it is a call for action by society to inform and advocate for evidence-based health policies. Policy-makers should not negate public awareness of evidence given the exponential explosion of media and connectivity among individuals. This is and will continue to remain a key driver for health policy and providers.

Cost, quality, and access provide a context for understanding health policy issues and EBP drivers (O'Grady & Johnson, 2009). As healthcare managers and policy-makers continue to respond to cost containment and ensuring quality and access, innovation will be required. Innovation is a critical value of alignment between the multiple forces affecting health care and decisions that follow (Porter-O'Grady & Malloch, 2015). Both mangers and policy-makers must ensure engagement by teams because their actions are directly and indirectly linked to cost, quality, and access. The convergence of team efforts forms a network of evidence-based health knowledge for policy development and advocacy.

During past decades, multiple cost containment approaches were attempted with varied success. Whereas some approaches were based on evidence, others were only a short-term solution that lacked substantiated proof. Policies and strategies to contain cost cannot be created in isolation and must include impacts imposed by cultural influences, demographic changes, and technology. As advances in care delivery continue and technology evolve, consumers will demand more. The health research enterprise and technology advances do not happen without a cost. Policy developers, care providers, and related groups have a social responsibility to develop and promote policies that are based on evidence, reduce cost, and ensure access is available to all.

A broad interest in ensuring quality care is present from governmental agencies to accreditation bodies. The interest has been fueled by the Institute of Medicine (IOM, 2001) publication and the Center for Medicare and Medicaid Services (CMS, 2014a, 2014b) charged to ensure effective and efficient use of public funds for quality care. Foundational to quality care is patient safety and measuring quality based on data. With the publication of *Crossing the Quality Chasm* in 2001, six domains provide a framework for quality and subsequent measurement. The six domains include (IOM, 2001):

- **Patient safety:** Service provision in a safe environment
- **Effectiveness:** Interventions for improving health and function
- **Patient centeredness:** Patient needs at the center of the health system
- **Efficiency:** Care provision in a cost-effective manner
- **Timeliness:** Care and services when needed
- **Equity:** Care and services distribution based on need versus ability to pay

Data generated from healthcare facility accreditations offer consumers options for informed decisions when choosing a facility or provider. Policy-makers must continue to ensure public reporting of quality outcomes and their availability for consumers of care (CMS, 2014a). Standards and outcomes will continuously provide opportunities to plan and evaluate care based on processes, planning, interprofessional activity, statistical reasoning, and analysis.

Translating evidence into health policy is essential for providers and consumers seeking care. Being effective in this translation is a provider requisite skill, often referenced as political competence in the policy arena. Political competence is the ability to assess the impact of public policies on an area of responsibility and influence public policy-making (Longest, 1998). Longest (2006) further contended that organizations form policy communities that influence the political process. Political competence becomes the avenue for providers to assist policy-makers to propose laws that are based on evidence and are able to remove or mitigate barriers to quality care. As providers master political competence, they can anticipate risk that mitigates loss. Opportunities become available to create value-added advice. Possessing political competence and strategic foresight will be beneficial as health care becomes increasingly regulated, unpredictable, and globalized (Habegger, 2009).

As nurses and other interprofessional providers of care are working collaboratively to advance evidence-based healthcare policy, all must understand health care and the political landscape of organizations. Political savvy becomes a tool for this to be accomplished.

DeLuca (1999) defined political savvy as one's ability to cut across organizational, cultural, and global boundaries to establish priorities and actions. DeLuca further identified behaviors of the political savvy leader to include the following:

- Ability to acknowledge differences
- Remove personal or defensive biases
- Aware of unclear scenarios
- Remain approachable
- Be consistent in leader style and behavior
- Remain open to innovation
- Able to compromise
- Thankful and appreciative
- Deliver on agreements

As discussed, providers who are politically competent and savvy create opportunities to describe what is affecting delivery of care and those policies that should be changed (Porter-O'Grady & Malloch, 2015). As graduate doctoral education has embedded health policy and political competence in programs of study, providers are prepared to anticipate need, consider risk, and offer sound advice as evidence is translated for health policy developers and interprofessional clinical teams (American Association of Colleges of Nursing, 2006a).

■ Translating Evidence Into Health Policy for Success

Who would not want health policy to be based on evidence? It seems paradoxical that one would question this notion. However, one must not negate the importance of ensuring that data provide evidence that can be translated for an actual category or type of decision. For example, evidence collected on a benefit to an individual may not be beneficial to health policies aimed at health inequalities (Smith, Ebrahim, & Frankel, 2001). The lag time from discovery of a treatment and practice adoption ranges from 15 to 20 years (Balas & Boren, 2000). Similarly, lags in health policies often limit timeliness in funding, innovation, and further inquiry.

Translating evidence into the development of health policy is rarely a linear process. A need is defined and evidence is readily available to fully support the policy, but additional considerations cannot be dismissed. If one ascribes to a linear model of evidence translation in the policy development process, evidence will be judged primarily in terms of the impact on policy. Few question the need to base health policies on evidence in order to benefit individual health and well-being. However, one cannot forget that when policy is being considered and developed, the impact of evidence must be quantifiable. A substantial return-on-investment is required in the current healthcare arena (Black, 2001; Buxton & Hanney, 1996; Haines & Donald, 1998).

All healthcare systems have a desire for evidence-based health policies that are easily transferrable to practice and create value. It is imperative for providers to assist policy-makers to interpret evidence to avoid misinterpretation of data and lessen variations based on personal values. Otherwise, translation of available evidence in health policy is marginalized.

For continued translation of evidence in health policy, care environments must be changed and aligned toward improvement for change to occur. Four areas of environmental change are proposed: (a) an infrastructure that supports dissemination and application of new knowledge, (b) information technologies, (c) payment policies, and (d) a prepared healthcare workforce (IOM, 2001).

Translating evidence in future health policies will have a profound impact on getting treatments to patients sooner. Obstacles, gaps, and unintended consequences are considerations necessary to drive processes of discovery, natural outgrowths of care, innovation, and incentivized health policies. Without these considerations, tangible progress toward accomplishing evidence-based health policies will be diminished.

■ Health Policy Barriers, Gaps, and Unintended Consequences of Evidence

Numerous barriers, gaps, and unintended consequences of evidence-based policies exist in contemporary health care. This imposes multiple challenges in meeting the IOM's goal that 90% of clinical decisions will be evidence-based by 2020 (McClellan, McGinnis, Nabel, & Olsen, 2007). Meeting the goal and overcoming challenges can be a daunting task for providers and managers of healthcare agencies. Inadequate knowledge about EBPs and their value requires a fast-paced gain. Only in the last 5–10 years has EBP been included in curricula.

The pace required by care providers to deliver efficient care rapidly is a major factor today. When organizational cultures do not support and recognize the importance of evidence, advocacy for its inclusion in health policy is a limitation. Allowing providers time to seek evidence and make application is needed. The role and functions of all providers and managers are vital to positive outcomes (Finkelman and Kenner, 2013; Hinshaw & Grady, 2011). This includes point-of-care providers who seek and apply evidence to the management officials who engender a culture of EBP.

The creators of health policy are also confronted with barriers as their goals go beyond clinical effectiveness, including social, financial, strategic alliances, and electoral (Black, 2001). This may create barriers that subsequently result in unintended consequences. Evidence may be dismissed as irrelevant in certain geographical regions, cultures, and groups. Evidence may be moderated when scientific controversy and differing opinions exist. This results in evidence not being included in health policy legislation and those that never move beyond a motion or committee.

Social environments also may be a barrier because they are not conducive to policy change based on the current evidence. An impression is that using the evidence will result in lower morale and discord. Many of policies result in unintended consequences. Five examples of health policies that may be based on evidence but are influenced by barriers with unintended consequences include:

1. Decisions to aim at drug prevention in affluent localities
2. Introduction of a new procedure to reduce cholesterol levels that only included randomized studies among one population
3. Requirements for immunizations of infants and preschoolers
4. Decisions to implement medical homes throughout a healthcare system
5. Lack of trust when evidence is generated from industry-funded studies

Overcoming the barriers is not an easy task. This requires the actions of all team members as users of evidence, advocates, and interpreters of evidence for policy makers. Using available tools and resources becomes a passage for reducing or eliminating the barriers.

■ Evidence-Based Tools for Overcoming Barriers, Gaps, and Unintended Consequences

Overcoming or diminishing the impact of barriers and consequences requires much thought and purposeful actions using evidence-based tools. Otherwise, a disconnect will prevail between health policy and evidence. Various authors and observers have developed tools and criteria to diminish the disconnect (Hunt, 2003). One such tool is informed decision-making supported by systematic, empirical evidence. Decisions that incorporate evidence during the proposed development of health policy strengthen the likelihood of adoption. Using a systematic review offers a comprehensive approach to locating and synthesizing the evidence on an identified issue or question. Through an organized, transparent, and replicable process, some initial barriers are overcome (Littell, Corcoran, & Pillai, 2008). A scale of proposed health benefit emerges, and the fit with an existing or proposed policy, consideration of potential for harm, ease of application, and enactment is possible.

Identifying barriers and consequences is insufficient if health policy and evidence are linked. Often situations arise and an immediate defense of what may not be immediately measurable occurs. Paralysis and lack of action follow. A health policy may or may not become reality, and in the event it does, there is lack of support for a practice improvement. Therefore, unintended consequences may follow. Lloyd (2004) purported that there is strong support and foundation for the science of improvement in such instances. Deductive (general to specific) and inductive (specific to general) phases of the scientific method are integrated to create opportunities that support evidence-based health policies.

Other tools to overcome barriers and consequences include accreditation standards. One such example is the standards that form the framework for Joint Commission accreditation (2004). The standards encompass three major areas:

1. **Patient-focused functions:** Rights, ethics, and responsibilities; provision of care, treatment, and services; medication management; and surveillance, prevention, and control of infection
2. **Organizational functions:** Improving organizational performance, leadership, management of the environment of care, management of human resources, and management of information
3. **Structures and functions:** Medical staff, nursing

Other organizations also have tools for overcoming barriers. These include the National Quality Forum, Institute for Healthcare Improvement, and Robert Wood Johnson Foundation. A final example used to diminish barriers and unintended consequences is healthcare report cards. The report cards provide specific performance data organizationally at designated intervals focusing on quality and safety (Finkelman & Kenner, 2010).

Continuously acting to eliminate barriers and unintended consequences and link health policy to evidence is required for healthcare agencies to remain solvent. Disincentives can rapidly occur, leading the best organization to engage in rapid cycle improvements and using whatever evidence is able to correct deficits. Many financial incentives have arisen during the past decade based on evidence-based health policy, as discussed in the following section.

■ Financial Incentives of Evidence-Based Health Policy

Incentives that balance innovation with value have sizeable implications for survival in the current healthcare arena. Since the enactment of healthcare reform, value has become a national strategic goal. The shift from volume-based to value-based care has required leaders to shift previous mental models of care to those that ensure advancement of the health of a nation (CMS, 2013; US Department of Health and

Human Services [DHHS], 2011). Balancing innovation with value requires processes in which evidence-based policy-making is supported and adopted. This calls for actions that reflect all the work processes and activities subject to constant inquiry and reassessment (O'Grady & Malloch, 2015).

Under increasing pressure to demonstrate effectiveness with fewer resources, many state governments have expanded the use of evidence-based programs that are grounded in rigorous outcome evaluations. As states commit to evidence-based programs, the efficiency and accountability to achieve improved outcomes for residents emerge. Some 100 state statutes were enacted between 2004 and 2014 to promote evidence-based, data-driven programs (Pew-MacArthur Foundation, 2015). Each of the statutes used the best available evidence and program outcome data to inform the budgetary process, policies, and management decisions. As a result, wasteful spending was reduced, successful programs were expanded, and accountability was strengthened.

Previously, governments lacked data, thus limiting policy-makers' ability to make informed budget decisions. As a result of evidence-based policy-making, some state governments now require agencies to create inventories of funded programs and categorize them based on effectiveness through rigorous research (Pew-MacArthur Foundation, 2015).

Creating robust economic data and evidence of program value produces avenues for an economic model aligning care provided with incentives. Each incentive is inclusive of evidence-based indicators. Active participation by interprofessional teams follows, and the quality of care is improved while reducing costs.

Two things can occur simultaneously when teams are working collaboratively. First, fragmented care decreases. Second, new approaches to greater clinical integration and efficiencies are found. Achieving these results has provided the impetus for greater attention to value-based purchasing through state insurance exchanges included in the Patient Protection and Affordable Care Act (US DHHS, 2011).

As care incentives flourish and economic healthcare models are approved, windows of opportunity have occurred for researchers. Data can change health policy only when it is reliable and valid. This does not occur rapidly, but is an iterative process of inquiry underscoring the value of evidence-based data that creates healthcare incentives. One such example is the enactment of Public Chapter 585 in Tennessee, in which additional funds were allocated for evidence-based programs offering researchers opportunities for program evaluations (National Juvenile Justice Network, 2007).

Changes in evidence-based policy-making have increased state-funded grants when implementing evidence-based programs. In 2014, Massachusetts established a competitive grant program directed at testing and expanding evidence-based research and practice methods to reduce recidivism. Using a cost-benefit model, programs were evaluated based on implementation with their fidelity to the original submitted designs (Massachusetts General Court, 2014). Additionally, California's Community

Corrections Performance Incentives Fund Act evidenced great success as evidence-based programs aimed at risk and needs assessments, offender supervision, and management strategies were initiated (Judicial Council of California, 2014).

Incentives based on evidence-based health policy-making are a powerful mechanism when economic models are included. Effective programs follow, and widespread inequities from cost shifting, practice variation, and ad hoc consensus judgments of appropriateness are mitigated. There is general agreement that evidence-based incentives are fair when based on evidence-based economics. Evidence-based incentives have an intuitive appeal because patient's benefit is the central focus, and the rules for penalty and reward are explicitly defined (Diamond & Kaul, 2009).

Evidence is and will continue as the hallmark heralding the next great revolution in healthcare reimbursement. Present and future evidence-based programs will continue to shape how policy-makers base decisions. This will certainly influence the landscape of global evidence-based health policy-making and reimbursement reforms.

■ Global Impact of Evidence-Based Health Policy and Reform

As one nation initiates evidence-based health policies and reforms, conceivably other nations will observe the outcomes and act accordingly. Health policies and reforms that are supported by evidence have a considerable solidarity on a global level. Nevertheless, sustainability is a key determinant that depends on a complex set of structural variables such as economic growth and a guarantee that the population's health problems are addressed.

Achieving equilibrium between social protection and financial solidarity offers a regimen to ensure that health policy–makers consider all available evidence. Mitigating loss and providing quality, safe, and value-based care is the primary objective. Scientific and economic evidence allows a nation to learn from others and create greater certainty and efficiency for the delivery of care.

■ Conclusion

The idea that evidence transforms into policy is a reality. Linking inquiry and health policy sets an agenda for others to follow in the fast-paced healthcare environment. Adopting a culture of evidence and inclusivity of others offers roadmaps by which leaders, health policy-makers, and interprofessional teams will transform the future landscape of healthcare delivery, reform, and economic stability.

History will continue to play an important role in how health policies are formulated. Learning from our past is leverage for future prosperity of the health and well-being of society. Using past and present knowledge offers opportunities for overcoming obstacles and creating prospective alliances among policy-makers, providers, and stakeholders. Using evidence to base decisions on and ongoing inquiry will ensure a world in which shared enterprises create continuous chances for quality, safe, and efficient care. The immediacy for action is now to inquire, test, prove, and use findings that result in health policies that are limitless.

REFLECTIVE ACTIVITIES

1. Considering the current healthcare environment and constant changes, what individual, team, and organizational actions are required to ensure health policy is evidence-based?
2. Reflect on care that is delivered by you or others and identify what actions contributed to quality, safe, and value-based outcomes.
3. Professional care models have exhibited varied outcomes. Consider how you would develop a care model that includes evidence-based outcomes yielding fiscal incentives. How would you present the model to a health policy-maker?
4. We live in a global society influenced by cultural, economic, historical, and societal influences. What actions can interprofessional teams take that will contribute to the spread of evidence-based, innovative projects globally? Further, how can health professionals be more proactive in health policy-making?

REFERENCES

American Association of Colleges of Nursing (AACN). (2006a). *The essentials of doctoral education for advanced nursing practice*. Washington, DC: AACN.

Balas, E., & Boren, S. A. (2000). Managing clinical knowledge for health care improvement. *Yearbook of Medical Informatics*. Bethesda, MD: National Library of Medicine.

Birkland, T. A. (2005). *An introduction to the policy process: Theories, concepts and models of public policy making* (2nd ed.). Armonk, NY: M. E. Sharpe.

Black, N. (2001). Evidence based policy: proceed with care. *British Medical Journal*, 323, 275–279.

Brownson, R. C., Chriqui, J. F., & Stamatakis, K. A. (2009). Understanding evidence-based public health policy. *American Journal of Public Health*, 99(9), 1576–1583.

Buxton, M., & Hanney, S. (1996). How can payback from health services research be assessed? *Journal of Health Services Research Policy*, 1, 35–45.

Centers for Medicare and Medicaid Services. (2013). Bundled payments for care improvement (BPCI) initiative: General information. Retrieved from http://innovation.cms.gov/initiatives/bundled-payments/

Centers for Medicare and Medicaid Services. (2014a). Cost report by fiscal year. Retrieved from https://www.cms.gov/Research-Statistics-Data-and-Systems/Downloadable-Public-Use-Files/Cost-Reports/

Centers for Medicare and Medicaid Services. (2014b). Hospital outpatient prospective payment: final rule with comment. Retrieved from https://www.cms.gov/Medicare/Medicare-Fee-for-Service-Payment/ASCPayment/ASC-Regulations-and-Notices-Items/CMS-1613-FC.html

DeLuca, J. R. (1999). *Political savvy: Systematic approaches to leadership behind the scenes*. Berwn, PA: EBG.

Diamond, G. A., & Kaul, S. (2009). Evidence-based financial incentives for healthcare reform. *Cardiovascular Quality and Outcomes*, 2, 134–140.

Fairman, J., & D'Antonio, P. (2013) History counts: How history can shape our understanding of health policy. *Nursing Outlook*, 61, 346–352.

Fielding, J. E., & Briss, P. A. (2006). Promoting evidence-based public health policy: Can we have better evidence and more action? *Health Affairs*, 25(4), 969–978.

Finkelman, A., & Kenner, C. (2010). *Professional nursing concepts: Competencies for quality leadership*. Sudbery, MA: Jones & Bartlett Learning.

Finkelman, A., & Kenner, C. (2013). *Professional nursing concepts: Competencies for quality leadership* (2nd ed.). Burlington, MA: Jones & Barlett Learning.

Habegger, B. (2009). Strategic foresight: Anticipation and capacity to act. *CSS Analyses in Security Policy.* Retrieved from http://www.css.ethz.ch/content/dam/ethz/special-interest/gess/cis/center-for-securities-studies/pdfs/CSS-Analyses-52.pdf

Haines, A., & Donald, A. (1998). Making better use of research findings. *British Medical Journal, 317,* 72–75.

Hinshaw, A. S., & Grady, P. A. (2011). *Shaping health policy through nursing research.* New York, NY: Springer.

Hunt, D. J. (2003). Evidence-based policy and practice: riding for a fall? *Journal of the Royal Society of Medicine, 96*(4), 194–196.

Institute of Medicine. (2001). *Crossing the quality chasm: A new health system for the 21st century.* Washington, DC: National Academies Press. https://www.nationalacademies.org/hmd/~/media/Files/Report%20Files/2001/Crossing-the-Quality-Chasm/Quality%20Chasm%202001%20%20report%20brief.pdf

Institute of Medicine. (2011). *The future of nursing: Leading change, advancing health.* Washington, DC: National Academies Press.

International Council of Nurses. (2012). *Closing the gap: From evidence to action.* Geneva, Switzerland: International Council of Nurses.

Joint Commission. (2004). *The Joint Commission press kit.* Retrieved from http://www.jointcommission.org/NewsRoom/PressKits/

Judicial Council of California. (2014). *Report on the California Community Corrections Performance Incentives Act of 2009: Findings from the SB 678 Program.* Retrieved from http://www.courts.ca.gov/documents/jc-20140627-itemC.pdf

Littell, J. H., Corcoran, J., & Pillai, V. (2008). *Systematic reviews and meta-analysis.* New York, NY: Oxford University Press.

Lloyd, R. (2004). *Quality health care: A guide to developing and using indicators.* Sudbury, MA: Jones & Barlett Learning.

Lomas, J., Culyer, T., McCutcheon, C., McAuley, L., & Law, S. (2005). *Conceptualizing and combining evidence for health system guidance.* Ottawa, Canada: Health Services Research Foundation.

Longest, B. (1996). *Health policymaking in the United States* (4th ed.). Chicago, IL: Health Administration Press.

Longest, B. (1998). Managerial competence at senior levels of integrated delivery Systems. *Journal of Healthcare Management, 17,* 299–307.

Mason, D. J., Leavitt, J. K., & Chaffee, M. W. (2007). *Policy & politics in nursing and health care.* St. Louis, MO: Elsevier.

Massachusetts General Court. (2014). House Bill 4242, 188th Legislature. Retrieved from http://www.malegislature.gov/Bills/BillHtml/137923?generalCourtId=11

McClellan. M. B., McGinnis, M., Nabel, E. G., & Olsen, L. M. (2007). *Evidence-based medicine and the changing nature of health care.* Washington, DC: National Academies Press.

Melnyk, B. M., & Fineout-Overholt, E. (2005). *Evidence-based practice in nursing and healthcare: A guide to best practice.* Philadelphia, PA: Wolters Kluwer/Lippincott Williams & Wilkins.

Melnyk, B. M., & Fineout-Overholt, E. (2015). *Evidence-based practice in nursing and healthcare: A guide to best practice* (3rd ed.). Philadelphia, PA: Lippincott Williams & Wilkins.

National Juvenile Justice Network. (2007). Tennessee Public Chapter 585, Senate Bill 1790. Retrieved from http://www.njjn.org/uploads/digital-library/1790.pdf

O'Grady, E. T., & Johnson, J. E. (2009). Health policy issues in changing environments. In A. B. Hamric, J. A. Spross, & C. M. Hanson (Eds.), *Advanced Practice Nursing: An Integrative Approach* (4th ed). St. Louis, MO: Saunders.

Pew-MacArthur Foundation. (2015). Legislating evidence-based policymaking: A look at state laws that support data-driven decision-making. Retrieved from pewtrusts.org/resultsfirst

Porter-O'Grady, T., & Malloch, K. (2015). *Quantum leadership: Building better partnerships for sustainable health.* Burlington, MA: Jones & Barlett Learning.

Ruland, C. (2010). Translating evidence into practice. In W. L. Holzmer (Ed.), *Improving Health Through Nursing Research*. Geneva, Switzerland: International Council of Nurses.

Smith, G. D., Ebrahim, S., & Frankel, S. (2001). How policy informs the evidence: "Evidence based" thinking can lead to debased policy making. *British Medical Journal*, 322, 184–185.

Stevens, R. (2006). Introduction. In R. Stevens, C. Rosenberg, & L. R. Burns (Eds.), *History and health policy in the United States: Putting the past back in*. New Burnswick, NJ: Rutgers University Press.

Stiefel, M., & Nolan, K. (2012). *A guide to measuring the Triple Aim: Population, health, experience of care, and per capita cost*. Cambridge, MA: Institute for Healthcare Improvement.

Stone, D. (2002). *Policy paradox: The art of political decision making (revised)*. New York, NY: W. W. Norton.

Tobbell, D. (2011). *Pills, power, and policy: How drug companies and physicians resisted federal reform in Cold War America*. Berkeley, CA: University of California Press.

US Department of Health and Human Services. (2011). *Hospital value-based Purchasing program*. Retrieved from https://www.cms.gov/Medicare/Medicare-Fee-for-Service-Payment/SNFPPS/Down loads/SNF-VBP-RTC.pdf https://www.cms.gov/Medicare/Medicare-Fee-for-Service-Payment/SNF PPS/Downloads/SNF-VBP-RTC.pdf

Wailoo, K. (1999). *Drawing blood: Technology and disease identity in twentieth century America*. Baltimore, MD: The Johns Hopkins University Press.

World Health Organization. (2015). Health Policy. Retrieved from http://www.who.int/topics/health_policy/en/

■ Notes from the Field: Advanced Practice Nursing Legislation: Engaging Support for HR 1247—Improving Veterans Access to Quality Care Act and S 297: Frontlines to Lifelines Act

---

Background

Motivated by recommendations of the Institute of Medicine report *The Future of Nursing: Leading Change, Advancing Health* that support the policy of advanced practice nurses (APNs) practicing to their full scope and the National Council of State Boards of Nursing Consensus Model, the Department of Veterans Affairs (VA) sought to continue innovating in effective and efficient healthcare delivery. Limiting scope of APNs in the VA impedes access to care, risks limiting delays, increases costs, and restricts promotion of patient safety. Engaging congressional action and stakeholder support for HR 1247 and S 297 is imperative to align the VA with other federal settings (the Army, Air Force, Navy, Indian Health Services, and Combat Support Hospitals). This allows APNs to practice without physician supervision.

Using Evidence to Inform Policy Change and Engender Congressional Support

Removing practice barriers is an expansive proposition that must be based on evidence and engagement of numerous stakeholders, including the US Congress. Twenty-one states and the District of Columbia do not limit the scope of practice for nurse practitioners. With the support of the Congress and stakeholders, it is possible for all four APN roles to practice at their full practice authority.

Gaining support to change practice requires a high level of evidence. Systematic reviews can prove useful, as in the case of the VA, in gathering supportive data on advanced practice outcomes in healthcare delivery, promotion and education, and patient satisfaction. Additional evidence was gathered during systematic reviews on APN and physician practices in terms of cost, access, quality, safety, and patient satisfaction. No appreciable differences were found. This evidence provided support for congressional and stakeholder engagement.

Lessons Learned

Policy change is not limited to one group, but requires the actions by many individuals. Two key lessons learned in the process, including (a) dedicating staff to the policy change who were practicing as APNs and (b) staffers who understood the legislative process and could speak the language understood by Congress. Through a series of evidence seeking, education of staff and stakeholders, open forums for discussion, and publishing frequently asked questions, the policy process culminated in the introduction of HR 1247 and S 297.

As demands for healthcare providers increase in the current decade, allowing full practice authority for APNs is timely. Access to quality, safe, and cost-effective care will continue to require mindful actions of policy-makers, managers, and Congress to meet demands, especially in rural and underserved areas. Care for America's heroes, veterans, cannot be dismissed nor forgotten, and full APN practice authority is a zero-cost, zero-delay, and zero-risk solution.

■ RECOMMENDATION

■ Notes from the Field: Doctor of Nursing Practice (DNP) Student

Debra Berger, RN, MSN, JD, CRNP

Ms. Berger is currently in a doctoral program. She was interviewed about her unique project as it related to a proposed policy change affecting physician–nurse collaborative practice. Ms. Berger addresses her process of integrating research, practice, and proposed policy change.

1. **How did research evidence inform your proposed policy change?**
   I have a very keen interest in healthcare policy and the politics of health care. I noticed a recurring discussion topic in both nurse practitioner (NP) and

(continues)

medical journals over the past couple of years. That topic was the issue of whether NPs should be independent healthcare providers. Related topics that cannot be ignored, because of their impact on the topic that I have already mentioned, include the safety and effectiveness of health care rendered by NPs and the shortage of healthcare providers in the United States, and particularly in Louisiana.

In Louisiana, our healthcare report card is very poor. This includes various health statistics. One included statistic is poor access to primary care. And the state continuously ranks 49th or 50th in health. This of course is directly related to poor access to care. Louisiana has been designated a healthcare physician shortage area (HPSA). Statistics published by our state medical school, Louisiana State University School of Medicine, and also by the Louisiana Office of Primary Care, reflect a steady decline in family physicians, despite efforts to improve the numbers. These primary care providers are essential to primary and preventive services. The number of NPs in the state is significant enough to help mitigate the poor access to primary and preventive care. However, despite their education and clinical training as excellent primary care providers, when NPs must work with the constraints and impending financial and legal problems associated with collaborative practice agreements, they are reluctant to invest in and open offices that could increase access to care throughout the state.

My research revealed that 17 states and the District of Columbia permit full practice rights for NPs. When I say "full practice rights," I mean the ability to practice without a collaborative practice agreement with a physician. Stated differently, I mean the right to practice independently while engaged in all aspects of patient care, including physical examinations, ordering of labs and diagnostic tests, establishing diagnoses, and prescribing treatment regimens, both pharmacological and nonpharmacological. With 17 other states allowing independent practice by NPs, I believed that the time was ripe for Louisiana to embark upon the move to progress Louisiana nurse practitioners into the same practice venue.

Additional evidentiary research revealed support for such a change from major medical and advanced practice nursing advocates. Some examples include: (1) the IOM, (2) the Macy Foundation, (3) the American Academy of Nurse Practitioners (AANP), (4) the National Council of State Boards of Nursing, (5) the AARP, and (6) the Robert Wood Johnson Foundation. Even Dr. Jeffry Susman, physician editor in chief of the *Journal of Family Practice,* commented positively about NPs being permitted to practice without physician oversight.

The topic of safe and effective NP-rendered care was also researched. This was extremely important because it would be against public policy and morally wrong to engage in a legislative effort that had a significant potential to harm the citizens of the state. Thus, I researched and read articles that also addressed this issue. The articles retrieved indicated that NP-rendered healthcare services were equivalent to those of MDs. Adding credibility to this statement, a couple of the articles included an MD author and were published in a major medical journal, the *New England Journal of Medicine*.

With all this positive evidence, I decided to move forward with the project of a legislative repeal of the statutorily required collaborative practice agreement for Louisiana NPs.

2. **Describe the legislative process involved in bringing forth the research evidence (supporting greater access for patients with NPs as primary care providers).**

The legislative process has many prongs to it. As you well know, a single person would not make this legislative change. Thus, a team of bill supporters works on the project together. The Louisiana Association of Nurse Practitioners (LANP) is the organization that supports this bill and is funding related efforts. I work very closely with the president and public policy chairman of LANP to create the change. I presented these two individuals with information and published documentation about the state healthcare provider shortages and resulting decreased access to primary and preventive care services and proposed that this be the platform for promoting the bill. They both agreed.

However, the task does not end with that consensus of agreement. A few of the major steps in the process include (1) writing a bill repealing the old law and including supplemental language to create a viable bill, (2) retaining a representative to author the bill, (3) educating our lobbyists, and (4) educating the general public and members of the legislature. To these ends, it was first necessary to write a viable bill that all the movers and shakers in the project agree upon. This involved writing several versions of the bill, presenting it to the project parties for a consensus of which bill should be proffered, and then presenting it to the author of the bill so that individual can retain an official bill drafter. The public policy chair is actually electing an author for the bill. In drafting the preliminary bill, a purpose of the bill, a bill abstract, and a bill synopsis that details what the proposed law will do was drafted and these three items were incorporated in the preliminary draft. Discussions and explanations were provided to the representative bill author, and he was given an opportunity to ask any questions prefiling, and also an ongoing opportunity. The bill author was also provided a copy of *Compendium for Legislative Support*.

The *Compendium* was considered to be a major aspect of the DNP project. It was drafted to be provided to all parties who required an explanation of the bill and its rationale. I considered this to be critical to bill passage. Even our NPs needed to have the information contained in the *Compendium* at their fingertips. Also it was a valuable tool for any person who would testify at legislative hearings in support of the bill. I know you are wondering what the

(continues)

Compendium included. Well, it included a paper written by me, offering a clear explanation of the bill, its rationale, and its purpose, including citations. A copy of the cited articles and papers was also included. Also incorporated were change needs assessment facts and statistics, articles, and white papers by parties and institutions that support independent NP practice. As you might well imagine, it is like having an answer to almost any question at one's fingertips.

3. **Lessons learned?**
   Just as there is evidence-based medicine, evidence-based nursing, evidence-based business, and so on, there is also evidence-based legislation. As an attorney, this was new to me. I discovered articles surrounding evidence-based legislation to be a strongbox of information. It was a very useful discovery. Evidence-based legislation predicts successful legislative efforts result when a public policy issue is attempted to be resolved through the legislation. The query became, should the tenets of evidence-based legislation be included in the legislative bill, or in the *Compendium*? In this project, I opted for inclusion in the *Compendium* to help preclude repeal of the new law, should the reasons therefore, healthcare physician shortages, ever cease to be the norm in the state.

4. **How did you engage others (from a research evidence perspective) in the process?**
   Involved in this project was actually the bill author, who needed some persuading. This was accomplished in face-to-face discussions explaining the state needs assessment, the safety and effectiveness of NP-rendered health care, and the anticipated improved outcomes statewide. The public would also require some persuasion so as not to telephone their representatives and tell them to vote against the bill. To this end, the project parties developed a communications team that retained an advertising firm to do educational and promotional advertising, promoting NPs as safe and effective independent healthcare providers. To assist with success of this prong of the project, I furnished the advertising firm with two clear and succinct documents: one that explained what LANP is attempting to achieve via the new legislation, and another detailing the rationale for the bill.

PART III

Scholarship of Clinical Practice

CHAPTER 13

Philosophical and Theoretical Perspectives Guiding Inquiry

■ Heather R. Hall and Linda A. Roussel ■

■ Objectives

- Inform the philosophical underpinnings that shape theory development and conceptual frameworks.
- Distinguish between a theory, model, and framework.
- Describe clinical question development through framework utilization.

■ Introduction

Humans have invested great amounts of time and effort in attempting to comprehend the world, specifically its workings. It is in the "making sense" that philosophical and theoretical underpinnings guide the questions and the subsequent work to be done. Science related to these efforts is "characterized by systemic, rigorous, and reproducible modes of inquiry" (Magnan, 2013, p. 102). Organized and supported explanations regarding phenomena (items and actions) in the human experience world are made by scientists in a particular field. The general goal is to further the progress of these explanations to the level of theoretical development. Theory is a respected outcome of the inquiry of science (Magnan, 2013).

Students working toward a research doctorate (i.e., PhD) are enrolled in programs that prepare them to develop theory for practice, whereas students working toward a practice doctorate (i.e., DNP) are being prepared to apply theory in their practice (Magnan, 2013). Theory development and application of theory are both essential to a professional discipline. The purpose of this chapter is to discuss the components of philosophy and theory development in research and the application of theory in practice.

■ Philosophy

Philosophy can be described as the pursuit of wisdom, a search for an understanding of values and reality. Philosophy of science is a branch of philosophy that attempts to describe and understand the nature of scientific inquiry, observational procedures, patterns of argument, methods of representation and calculation, metaphysical presuppositions, and evaluation of the grounds of their validity. This can be pursued from the points of view of a number of perspectives, including empiricism, naturalism, and foundationalism (Okasha, 2002).

Empiricism is a perspective related to the basis of all knowledge and not just knowledge regarding science. Empiricism is defined as a theory of knowledge that purports that knowledge comes to us through our sensory experiences. Emphasis is on the role of experience and evidence, specifically sensory perception in the form of ideas. When comparing and contrasting empiricism to rationalism, innate ideas such as basic logical and mathematical laws are considered formal and of no value as compared with experiential knowledge learned through sensing (Dahnke & Dreher, 2011). The tradition of an empiricist is that there is a tendency to view the differences between science and the thought processes of each day "as the differences of detail and degree" (Godfrey-Smith, 2003, p. 8). Medicine has a history of example events of breakthroughs by people willing to conduct empirical tests. These scientists conducted tests even when faced with doubt, arrogance, and resistance from others (Godfrey-Smith, 2003). In the mid-19th century, physician Ignaz Semmelweis was employed in a Vienna hospital, and by using straightforward empirical tests, he demonstrated that if doctors washed their hands prior to the delivery of a baby, the maternal infection risk would vastly decrease. Semmelweis was ultimately forced out of the Vienna hospital for his controversial claim (Best & Neuhauser, 2004).

Godfrey-Smith (2003) described a more basic empirical example related to the breakthrough regarding drinking water's role in the spread of cholera. In the 18th and 19th centuries, cholera was a crisis in cities, causing death because of severe diarrhea. With inadequate sanitation, cholera remained an issue. This was secondary to the disease's transmission via diarrhea in the water consumed by those living in such deplorable conditions. To better understand what was occurring, a number of theories were posited as to the cause of cholera. The infectious disease role of bacteria and additional microorganisms had not been discovered. Conventional wisdom purported that the disease was caused by miasmas, the foul gases rising from the ground and swampy areas (Godfrey-Smith, 2003). London resident John Snow declared his hypothesis that cholera was being spread through drinking water. He reported one cholera epidemic occurring in London and concluded that it was focused on a specific pump for public drinking water. After much persuasion on his way of thinking and reasoning, he convinced the authorities to remove the pump's handle, and cholera was eradicated. This event marked a milestone in the history of medicine (Vachon, 2005).

Decades after Snow came to his conclusion, Robert Koch and Louis Pasteur developed the *germ theory of disease,* associating microorganisms with the causes of diseases like cholera. Koch isolated the specific bacteria that caused cholera (Ullmann, 2007). Max Josef von Pettenkofer, "a principle founder of public health medicine," which he referred to as "hygiene" (Trout, 1977, p. 1569) did not believe Koch, so he consumed a glass of water that contained the bacterial culprit responsible for cholera. Pettenkofer suffered no consequence from drinking the water. He sent Koch a note reporting disproval of his theory. It was postulated that Pettenkofer could have had an increased acid level in his stomach that protected him from developing the infection. Another theory put forth was that the bacteria had decreased in that specific sample of water. This example is a reminder that direct empirical tests are not guarantees for success (Holdrege, 2001).

According to historians and sociologists, social structure provides a backdrop for a development critical of empiricism. It has been alleged that empiricism expects individuals to distrust authority and trust only their own judgment. This is only partially true. Most steps made by a scientist are dependent on complex collaboration, relationships, and trust networks. Therefore, science would not be able to move beyond simple ideas if each person was adamant about testing each item individually and refused to involve others in the scientific process. Collaboration and history of others who have submitted results are essential to the advancement of science. The example of John Snow is unusual. His reliance on the reports of others during his assessment of the cholera epidemic before and subsequent to the intervention as it related to the pump is testimony to the reflection on discoverers and discoveries that precede us (Godfrey-Smith, 2003).

Godfrey-Smith (2003) maintained that two essential components to science are trust and collaboration. Trust is the cornerstone of collaborative efforts within the context of discovery. Regardless, good science requires the scientist to determine which types of experiences are important to the work. These decisions are critical to decision-making, particularly those related to a scientist's ability to choose relevant data and reliable sources (Godfrey-Smith, 2003).

Naturalism is a philosophy that depends on understanding, explanation, and science to improve and extend perception of truth and civilization's position in truth and authenticity. Human understanding is the essential foundation and validation for all information and awareness. Knowledge has collected in human remembrance and tradition, steadily generating intelligence processes (e.g., logic and science). Logic and science are not totally dissimilar processes because the scientific method is actually an expansion of logic (Shook, 2006).

Naturalism accentuates the progressive and growing understanding that observation and science offer. Science persistently modifies knowledge of physical truth. Philosophical naturalism accepts the duty for developing a complete and logical world perception that is established on understanding, logic, and science. In addition, philosophical naturalism accepts responsibility for shielding science's absolute privilege to investigate and hypothesize about all truth. When intellect disagrees with science, science reaches out to philosophy for rational advice and influence. Naturalistic philosophy clarifies, validates, and enhances scientific method. When science is under political condemnation for the purpose of complicating or hindering scientific research or teaching, science again connects with philosophy for justification and protection of intellectual freedom. Naturalistic philosophy creates and preserves a broad-minded political order to defend science (Shook, 2006).

Foundationalism is the idea that we must attain the philosophy of science from an outside and safe viewpoint (Godfrey-Smith, 2003). The requirement of foundationalism is that we do not make assumptions about the accurateness of scientific thoughts while completing the philosophy of science. This is secondary to the fact that prior to the establishment of a theory of philosophy, the standing of the work of the science is uncertain. A way to explain naturalism is to state that it is against foundationalism within philosophy (Godfrey-Smith, 2003).

Decision-making has been a subject in philosophical deliberations. Decision-making calls into play the way we think about situations, our reasoning abilities, and our rationality (Godfrey-Smith, 2003). A specific action is thought to be instrumentally rational if it is a good method of achieving a specific goal. Instrumental rationality involves practical reasoning and helps a person figure out ways to perform in any given situation, such as completing technical tasks and solving problems (Dahnke & Dreher, 2011). In the assessment of actions related to another's instrumental rationality, the concern is not related to the original thought process behind the goal or whether the goal is appropriate; the question asked is whether it is probable that the action accomplishes the desired outcome (Godfrey-Smith, 2003).

Philosophical underpinnings provide a beginning foundation for understanding how the world in which we, as individuals, live is viewed. As individuals experience the many conundrums in life, questions arise and assumptions are brought to light. Individuals reflect on how the guidance is received in the choices, in the decisions we make, and in actions we take every day. When an individual is grounded in his or her thinking, he or she might be better prepared to make sense of everyday problems and to resolve life's difficulties.

■ Theory, Model, and Framework

A model and theory are applied to explain, clarify, or predict a phenomenon (Peterson & Bredow, 2009). The conceptual underpinnings of research studies are the frameworks (Polit & Beck, 2012). An abstraction that gives an explanation related to the interrelationships among phenomena (concepts) is a theory. Researchers may design a study for the purpose of producing a new theory, or they may test a theory. Significant and interpretable research findings are secondary to theories. Research is stimulated by theories because they provide the direction and drive for inquiry of a concept (Mateo & Benham-Hutchins, 2009).

Quantitative research begins with a theory. Using theory as the foundation, predictions can be made related to the behavior of specific phenomena in a real-world situation "if the theory is true" (Polit & Beck, 2012, p. 50). Predictions based on theory will be tested in the course of a research study. The results of the study may uphold, eliminate, or alter the theory (Polit & Beck, 2012).

Theory assists with guiding inquiry and interpreting data collected using qualitative research methods (Polit & Beck, 2012). In some qualitative research studies, theory is the outcome of the study. In these studies, the researcher has a goal to develop theory and uses participants' experiences to explain phenomena as they are presented, not from a presumption. There is a role for theory in both quantitative and qualitative research methods (Polit & Beck, 2012).

Theory-guided practice is the acknowledgment and use of models, concepts, and theories from all disciplines in a healthcare provider's work with patients. Theories offer a foundation to understand the patient's health issues and plan interventions to assist him or her. A higher quality of care is attained when theory guides practice (Eldridge, 2011).

Trustworthiness of research-based evidence is strengthened by conceptual frameworks (Goetz & LeCompte, 1984). Frameworks are considered to be broad theories. One might compare a conceptual framework with a map from a worldview perspective (Tappen, 2011).

The evaluation of a model related to the philosophic underpinnings includes questions identifying biases and principles. In addition, an explanation is included related to the integration, depiction, and associations of the necessary model concepts in the research and how the connections are applicable in practice (Mateo & Benham-Hutchins, 2009).

No one discovers theories, conceptual frameworks, and models; they are produced, invented, and emerge through the evolution of our work (Polit & Beck, 2012). The process of building a theory depends not only on the facts and evidence that can be observed, but also on the ingenuity of the creator in putting the facts in logical order. Theory construction is an innovative and scholarly endeavor that someone can take on as long as he or she has the following characteristics: (a) is insightful, (b) has a solid case of existing evidence, and (c) has the skill to connect evidence in a pattern that is considered scholarly (Polit & Beck, 2012).

The structural components of a theory are the concepts. A plan that identifies associations among the concepts is included in classic theories. The generality and abstraction levels are different among theories. In nursing, the most common theories include grand theory, middle-range theory, and practice theory (Polit & Beck, 2012).

Grand Theory

Grand theories are considered to be general in scope. The concepts and suggestions are less abstract and broad than those concepts of a conceptual model (Fawcett, 2005). An example of a grand theory is Newman's Theory of Health as Expanding Consciousness (Newman, 1994).

Middle-Range Theory

Middle-range theories are not as general as grand theories. A small number of concepts and proposals are written at a concrete and detailed level. Every middle-range theory includes detailed information regarding the phenomenon, including a description, why it happens, and how it happens (Fawcett, 2005). An example of a middle-range theory is Swanson's Theory of Caring (Swanson, 1991).

Practice Theory

Practice theories are in greater detail than middle-range theories and create specific recommendations for practice. These theories provide an understanding related to nursing practice, how nurses carry out their practice, and the outcomes. Practice theories include limited, simple concepts (Fain, 2009). An example of a practice theory is Theory of End-of-Life Decision-Making.

■ Ladder of Abstraction

A reasoning process with a foundation in philosophy, theory, and empirical summary is used in all disciplines. When the levels meet systematically, this process is logical. The abstraction ladder (see **Figure 13-1**) is a system for establishing and communicating the following three levels: "philosophical, theoretical, and empirical" (Smith & Liehr, 2008, p. 13).

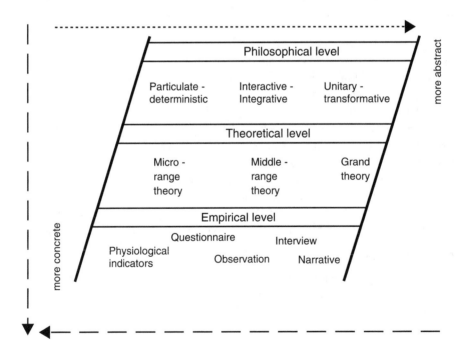

■ **Figure 13-1** Ladder of Abstraction

Source: Smith, M. J., & Liehr, P. R. (2008). *Middle range theory for nursing* (2nd ed.). New York, NY: Springer.

On the ladder of abstraction, Smith and Liehr (2008) described the highest level as philosophical, the middle level as theoretical, and the lowest level as empirical. These levels represent different ways of relating ideas. The philosophical level represents the ideas and assumptions recognized to be true and essential to the next level, which is theory. When coherence of the levels occurs, the theoretical step is led by a clear process that assists with the understanding and application of theory in research and advanced practice. The process of reasoning is the cornerstone to understanding theory at every level. Inductive reasoning is used to make a decision related to the phenomena when moving from the lowest step of the ladder. Deductive reasoning is the progression from the highest philosophical step to the theoretical step and, finally, to the empirical step (Smith & Liehr, 2008).

"Assumptions, beliefs, paradigmatic perspectives, and points of view" are included on the philosophical level of the ladder of abstraction (Smith & Liehr, 2008, p. 16). Assumptions are basic to the process of reasoning in a circumstance related to advanced practice and research in nursing. Assumptions are often beneath the surface and through processing may rise to the level of a belief and value. A worldview that includes specific values and views on a philosophical level is a paradigm (Smith & Liehr, 2008).

"Concepts, frameworks, and theories" are included on the theoretical level of the ladder (Smith & Liehr, 2008, p. 18). A mental representation of a piece of reality that is expressed using words to explain the significance of phenomena important to the discipline is a theoretical concept. An arrangement of interconnecting concepts that clarify the significance of a phenomenon is a theoretical framework. The literature explains a theory at every abstraction level (Smith & Liehr, 2008).

Multiple definitions of theory exist (Magnan, 2013). Polit and Beck (2012) defined a theory as "an abstract generalization that offers a systematic explanation about how phenomena are interrelated" (pp. 126–127). The usefulness of a theory is related to the organization offered for (a) ideas, (b) viewing, and (c) understanding the observation (Fawcett, 2005).

The empirical level signifies a conversation that ultimately puts theory into research and practice. "Physiologic indicators, what can be learned from questionnaires, observation, and interview and narrative," are included in empirics (Smith & Liehr, 2008, p. 20). The organization of abstraction continues even within the lowest level of the ladder of abstraction. The nurse is related to the level of empirics in both research and practice. Theory is applied when empirics are used by the advanced practice nurse when caring for others in the experience of human health. Philosophy and theory guide judgments regarding empirics. It is essential that the advanced practice nurse choose empirics that relate to philosophic and theoretical viewpoints (Smith & Liehr, 2008).

■ The Double ABCX Model of Family Behavior

Theoretical frameworks guide research and practice. To better understand how this works, the Double ABCX model of family behavior will be described. Family dynamic details and the specifics related to a family being able to progress and function from each developmental level and through typical and crisis situations have resulted in the growth and complexity of theories and research related to families. Family stress theory has become a key area in research with families (LoBiondo-Wood, 2008).

The Double ABCX model of family behavior (McCubbin & Patterson, 1983) is a middle-range theory. To completely understand the foundation of the Double ABCX model, one must understand the family stress theory. Reuben Hill was the original developer of the family stress theory after World War II (Hill, 1949). Hill's work focused on a family's reaction to war, separation caused by war, and, ultimately, re-union of family members. Three components that create a crisis were part of the original ABCX family crisis model: the stressor event (a), the family's crisis meeting resources (b), and the definition the family makes of the event (c) produce (x) the crisis (McCubbin & Patterson, 1983, p. 8). The interaction among these factors represented the family's vulnerability to crisis. A vital piece of information regarding the origination of family stress theory is that it was based on a family consisting of a father, mother, and children (Hill, 1949).

McCubbin and Patterson (1983) conceptualized the Double ABCX model as an expansion of Hill's original model (see **Figure 13-2**). Post-crisis concepts predicting adaptation of families over a length of time were added to Hill's model. It is important to note that each concept contributes to family adjustment and adaptation in a negative or positive manner. Family stressors such as long-term illness, cancer, and care of the elderly have been studied using the Double ABCX model (McCubbin & Patterson, 1983).

Theory Concepts of the Hill ABCX Family Crisis Model
Stressor and Hardships (a Factor)

Originally defined by Hill (1949), the stressor represented an event. This definition was subsequently extended by McCubbin and Patterson (1983) as the event in life or the transition that affects the family as a unit and creates change in the social system within the family. With the demands of the stressor, the potential exists to affect all features of life as a family (McCubbin & Patterson, 1983).

Resistance Resources (b Factor)

Every family has some form of resources. The concept of existing resources centers on the family using community and inside-family resources. The stressor is observed as the resources used by family members begin to interact to serve as a safeguard for crisis opposition. A resource can be financial or social and may include toughness and spiritual components (McCubbin & Patterson, 1983).

Focus on Stressor (c Factor)

The perception of the stressor is the importance given to the crisis event by the family and the entire situation that guided the crisis (McCubbin & Patterson, 1983).

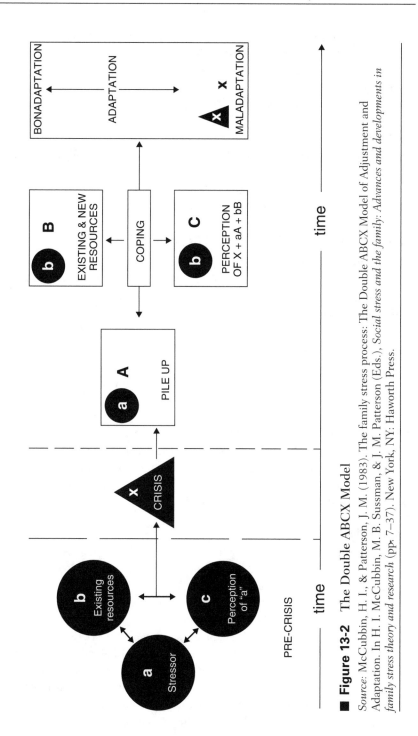

■ **Figure 13-2**   The Double ABCX Model

Source: McCubbin, H. I., & Patterson, J. M. (1983). The family stress process: The Double ABCX Model of Adjustment and Adaptation. In H. I. McCubbin, M. B. Sussman, & J. M. Patterson (Eds.), *Social stress and the family: Advances and developments in family stress theory and research* (pp. 7–37). New York, NY: Haworth Press.

The problem-solving skill of the family contributes to the ability of the family to explain every characteristic of the issue. In addition to the family's cultural points of view, the subjective understanding of the outcome of the stressor event is the key. The concept of perception centers on the view of the family related to whether members can manage the stressor (McCubbin & Patterson, 1983).

Crisis (x Factor)

The crisis in the model is considered to be the inability of the family to sustain stability in a situation in which constant struggle is required. The stressor (a), connecting with the resources (b), and the perception of the family related to the stressor (c), lead to the crisis (x) (McCubbin & Patterson, 1983).

Theory Concepts of the Double ABCX Model

Pile-Up (aA Factor)

The pile-up in the model reflects demands or changes emerging from (a) members of the family, (b) the family as a system, and/or (c) the community, which includes the family and all members (McCubbin & Patterson, 1983).

Adaptive Resources (bB Factor)

When observed over a length of time and in response to a crisis, the adaptive resources of the family seem to be either existing or expanded resources of the family (McCubbin & Patterson, 1983).

Definition and Meaning (cC Factor)

The meaning provided by the family relates to the whole crisis state and includes the stressor thought to have been the cause of the situation. This also includes additional stressors, resources (previous and new), and thoughts related to what it will take to restore balance within the family (McCubbin & Patterson, 1983).

Family Adaptive Coping

As families attempt to attain family functioning balance, coping is the bridging concept that includes cognitive and behavioral elements in which resources, views, and behavioral reactions interrelate (McCubbin & Patterson, 1983).

Family Adaptation Balancing (xX Factor)

Family adaptation is valuable when explaining the family post-crisis adjustment outcome. Three components are stressed as being important in family adaptation: (a) the individual, (b) system of the family, and (c) the community. Family adaptation is attained with relationships that are shared and one's demands are met by the ability of another individual; therefore, a "balance" is attained at the same time at two key levels of communication (McCubbin & Patterson, 1983).

Use in Nursing Practice

Health care for families and each family member has been enhanced by technology; however, the number of people diagnosed with chronic illnesses has increased. The Double ABCX model includes concepts that focus on illness trajectory aspects related to the experience of the family. The theory can be valuable "in assessing, planning, and implementing practice interventions" (LoBiondo-Wood, 2008, p. 237). It is vital to assess the contribution of the family dynamics to stress and adaptation as a plan is being developed (LoBiondo-Wood, 2008).

Example Study Using the Double ABCX Model

A pilot study was conducted to examine the parents' views related to their child's behaviors with autism, resource availability for their child, and parenting stress (Hall & Graff, 2010). Hall and Graff used the Double ABCX model of family behavior (McCubbin & Patterson, 1983) as the theoretical framework to conduct a follow-up study with families of children diagnosed with autism. The purpose of this study was to investigate the relationships among the adaptive behaviors of children with autism, support networks for the family, parenting stress, and coping. The sample for this descriptive correlational study consisted of 75 parents/primary caregivers of children diagnosed with autism. Four concepts of the model were measured: "(a) the adaptive behaviors of the child diagnosed with autism (aA factor); (b) the family support networks (bB factor); (c) parenting stress (cC factor); and (d) parental coping (bridging concept) of the Double ABCX Model" (Hall & Graff, 2011, p. 9). The findings of the study suggest that parents recognize that their child diagnosed with autism has low adaptive behaviors, their parental stress is increased, they have difficulty coping as parents, and more support is needed for the family. The Double ABCX model (McCubbin & Patterson, 1983) guided the understanding of how the findings strengthened the relationships as described in the model and are consistent with the interconnection of the variables measured in families of children with autism (Hall & Graff, 2011).

■ Complexity, Change, and Sense Making: Theoretical Perspectives of Administrative Practice

A theoretical approach to organizational change and improvement can incorporate a number of conceptual perspectives. Reductionism has essentially "ruled" organizational science for a long time. A system of reductionism refers to the breaking down of anything being examined into the parts that make up the whole. It proposes that if we have an understanding of the parts, we will better understand how the whole system works. From this "breakup," we may know more about the individual pieces but do not necessarily come away with a greater comprehension of the subtle nuances and synthesis of the system (Stacey, 2001). Specifically, this method is not always effective as a means of investigating our complex adaptive system (CAS).

When comparing ordered and chaotic systems with CASs, the relationship of the system and agents that act within it must be considered. The level of constraint in an ordered system is noted when all agent behavior is limited to the rules of the system. The agents in a chaotic system are unconstrained, susceptible to statistical and other analysis. The system and the agents coevolve in a CAS. It is noted that there is lightly constrained agent behavior. The agents modify the system by their interaction with it. Approaches to strategy in CAS seek to know the nature of system constraints and agent interaction and take on an evolutionary or naturalistic approach to strategy. The following attributes are noteworthy in CAS (Stacey, 2001):

1. The system does not distinguish between "trivial" and "nontrivial" parts.
2. The system has memory or includes a feedback mechanism.
3. The system can adapt itself according to its history or feedback.
4. The system relationship and its environment are nontrivial or nonlinear.
5. The system can be influenced by, or can adapt itself to, its environment.
6. The system is highly sensitive to initial conditions.

Complexity science advances our need to reflect on the interconnections of the system, relationships, and patterns. Used in the fields of strategic management and organizational studies, complexity theory proposes an understanding of how organizations or businesses adapt to their environments (Plsek & Greenhalgh, 2001). Organizations or firms are treated as a collection of strategies and structures. Survival of these CASs is dependent on the definitive nature of the small number of relatively simple and loosely connected structures. Organizational theorists who have contributed and integrated a greater understanding include Herbert Simon (1991) (decomposable systems and computational complexity), Karl Weick (1995) (loose coupling theory and interest in causal dependencies), Burns and Stalker (1961) (contrast between organic and mechanistic structures), Charles Perrow (1986) (link between complex organization and catastrophic accidents), and James March (1994) (contrast between exploration and exploitation).

Complexity has always been a part of the environment, and many scientific fields deal with complex phenomena and systems (Plsek & Greenhalgh, 2001). This has led some fields to create specific definitions of complexity. A more recent movement involves regrouping observations from a variety of fields to investigate complexity in and of itself; this approach uses examples such as anthills, human brains, and stock markets. An interdisciplinary group of fields considers relational order theories. Health care is an example of such complexity (Plsek & Greenhalgh, 2001).

Displaying variation without necessarily being random is essential given the rewards found in the depth of exploration and reflection (Campbell, Flynn, & Hay, 2003). In a complex system, nonlinear interactions between component parts create effective and evolving states far from equilibrium in a way that is highly dependent on connections within the system and its environment. Because complex systems are highly dimensional, nonlinear, and hard to model, they are often a challenge to apply to "real-world" situations (Campbell et al., 2003).

Complexity science and chaos theory have been informed by systems theory, given the concern for understanding complex systems that are biological, economic, and technological in nature. The development of chaos and complexity theories has gained greater recognition with the advent of computers able to undertake extensive computations necessary to uncover the mysteries of complexity. Hawking and Mlodinow (2010) noted, "The next century will be the century of complexity" (p. 55). Examples of concepts used in complexity are now mainstream, including tipping points, the butterfly effect, and six degrees of separation (Plsek & Greenhalgh, 2001).

Using one theory or integrating several theoretical models provides a framework not only for guiding the improvement process, but also to help in the understanding of relationships and interconnections of the system. Making improvements within CASs using *change theory* further frames best positioning for collaboration for best outcomes. A number of change theorists have provided foundation work in guiding process improvements in organizational systems. For example, Gladwell (2002) provided a framework for change within a framework of complexity. An organic approach to change considers the context of change, those involved in the change making, and the change itself. Kotter (2008) contended that there are eight steps to leading change. This theoretical framework has served as a conceptual model for designing the clinical nurse leader role, guiding development of the assumptions and competencies for curriculum and position development. Another example of application of Kotter's change model is TeamSTEPPS. This system is an evidence-based teamwork system focused on optimizing patient outcomes by improving communication and teamwork skills among healthcare professionals. Kotter's eight steps provide an intensive approach to creating this innovative, interdisciplinary approach to safety (Kotter, 2008).

■ Clinical Question Development Using Frameworks

Developing a clinical question is a multifaceted process (Polit & Beck, 2012). Similar to building a house, any clinical question must have stability to ensure a durable structure. Clinical questions do not appear as a whole; rather, they are the result of the sum total of carefully designed pieces. The underlying thought or idea that inspires the creation of the question is the phenomenon of interest (POI). The POI is the general basis from which the framework for the question is crafted. A conceptual framework may be selected "after the fact"—that is, devising a theoretical context to frame a question. Polit and Beck (2012) cautioned the researcher that such an after-the-fact linkage to theory may not always enhance the study. "Fitting a problem to a theory after the fact should be done with circumspection" (Polit & Beck, 2012, p. 142). Arranging linkages of problems to theoretical frameworks weakens nursing's evidence base. Without strong, sound linkages, decisions about what to measure and how, and interpretation of the findings, flow from the conceptualization of the study may not be supported.

REFLECTIVE ACTIVITIES

1. Read the Mock et al. (2007) article (see the reference that follows). Draw a conceptual map of the study using the integration of the Levine conservation model guiding the investigation of an exercise intervention to mitigate cancer-related fatigue.
2. Mock, V., St. Ours, C., Hall, S., Bositis, A., Tillery, M., Belcher, A., . . . McCorkle, R. (2007). Using a conceptual model in nursing research mitigating fatigue in cancer patients. *Journal of Advanced Nursing, 58*(5), 503–512. doi:10.1111/j.1365-2648.2007.04293.x
3. Reviewing Mock et al. (2007), critique the conceptual framework using the following selected questions:
   a. Is the conceptual framework adequate for understanding the conceptual basis of this study?
   b. Is the model described in such a way that the reader is able to determine the usefulness of the framework for this study population?
   c. Do the research aims (hypotheses) flow from the framework, or does the relationship between the aims (hypotheses) seem forced?
   d. Are the concepts sufficiently defined in a way that is aligned with the theory?
   e. Was the intervention (exercise) aligned with a cogent theoretical basis or rationale for the intervention?
   f. Did the conceptual framework guide the methodology of the study? That is, do the operational definitions correspond to the conceptual definitions (Polit & Beck, 2012, p. 145)?

REFERENCES

Best, M., & Neuhauser, D. (2004). Heroes and martyrs of quality and safety: Ignaz Semmelweis and the birth of infection control. *Quality and Safety in Health Care, 13*, 233–234. doi:10.1136/qshc.2004.010918

Burns, T., & Stalker, G. M. (1961). *The management of innovation.* London, England: Tavistock.

Campbell, J., Flynn, J. D., & Hay, J. (2003). The group development process seen through the lens of complexity theory. *International Scientific Journal of Methods and Models of Complexity, 6*(1), 33. Retrieved from http://www.nosmojournals.nl/ojs/index.php/ISJMMC/article/view/7

Dahnke, M. D., & Dreher, H. M. (2011). *Philosophy of science for nursing practice: Concepts and application.* New York, NY: Springer.

Eldridge, C. R. (2011). Nursing science and theory: Scientific underpinnings for practice. In M. E. Zaccagnini & K. W. White (Eds.), *The doctor of nursing practice essentials: A new model for advanced practice nursing* (pp. 1–36). Sudbury, MA: Jones & Bartlett Learning.

Fain, J. A. (2009). Applying appropriate theories and conceptual models. In J. A. Fain (Ed.), *Reading, understanding, and applying nursing research* (3rd ed., pp. 63–74). Philadelphia, PA: F. A. Davis.

Fawcett, J. (2005). *Contemporary nursing knowledge: Analysis and evaluation of nursing models and theories.* Philadelphia, PA: F. A. Davis.

Gladwell, M. (2002). *The tipping point.* New York, NY: Little, Brown.

Godfrey-Smith, P. (2003). *Theory and reality: An introduction to the philosophy of science.* Chicago, IL: University of Chicago Press.

Goetz, J. P., & LeCompte, M. D. (1984). *Ethnography and qualitative design in educational research.* San Diego, CA: Harcourt Brace Jovanovich.

Hall, H. R., & Graff, J. C. (2010). Parenting challenges in families of children with autism: A pilot study. *Issues in Comprehensive Pediatric Nursing, 33*(4), 187–204. doi:10.3109/01460862.2010.528644

Hall, H. R., & Graff, J. C. (2011). The relationships among adaptive behaviors of children with autism, family support networks, parental stress and coping. *Issues in Comprehensive Pediatric Nursing, 34,* 4–25. doi:10.3109/01460862.2011.555270

Hawking, S. W., & Mlodinow, L. (2010). *The grand theory.* New York, NY: Random House.

Hill, R. (1949). *Families under stress: Adjustment to the crises of war separation and reunion.* New York, NY: Harper & Row.

Holdrege, C. (2001). The art of thinking: Helping students develop their faculties of thinking and observations. *Renewal.* Retrieved from http://www.natureinstitute.org/txt/ch/thinking.htm

Kotter, J. P. (2008). *A sense of urgency.* Boston, MA: Harvard Business School Press.

LoBiondo-Wood, G. (2008). Theory of family stress and adaptation. In M. J. Smith & P. R. Liehr (Eds.), *Middle range theory for nursing* (2nd ed., pp. 225–241). New York, NY: Springer.

Magnan, M. A. (2013). The DNP: Expectations for theory, research, and scholarship. In L. A. Chism (Ed.), *The doctor of nursing practice: A guidebook for role development and professional issues* (2nd ed., pp. 101–129). Burlington, MA: Jones & Bartlett Learning.

March, J. G. (1994). *A primer on decision making: How decisions happen.* New York, NY: Free Press.

Mateo, M. A., & Benham-Hutchins, M. (2009). Theoretical and conceptual frameworks. In M. A. Mateo & K. T. Kirchoff (Eds.), *Research for advanced nurses: From evidence to practice* (pp. 105–114). New York, NY: Springer.

McCubbin, H. I., & Patterson, J. M. (1983). The family stress process: The Double ABCX Model of Adjustment and Adaptation. In H. I. McCubbin, M. B. Sussman, & J. M. Patterson (Eds.), *Social stress and the family: Advances and developments in family stress theory and research* (pp. 7–37). New York, NY: Haworth Press.

Newman, M. A. (1994). *Health as expanding consciousness* (2nd ed.). New York, NY: National League for Nursing.

Okasha, S. (2002). *Philosophy of science: A very short introduction.* New York, NY: Oxford University Press.

Perrow, C. (1986). *Complex organizations: A critical essay.* New York, NY: Random House.

Peterson, S. J., & Bredow, T. S. (2009). *Middle range theories: Application to nursing research* (2nd ed.). Philadelphia, PA: Lippincott Williams & Wilkins.

Plsek, P. E., & Greenhalgh, T. (2001). Complexity science: The challenge of complexity in health care. *British Medical Journal Quality and Safety, 323,* 625–628.

Polit, D. F., & Beck, C. T. (2012). *Nursing research: Generating and assessing evidence for nursing practice* (9th ed.). Philadelphia, PA: Lippincott Williams & Wilkins.

Shook, J. R. (2006). *Varieties of naturalism.* Retrieved from http://www.naturalisms.org/

Simon, H. (1991). Organizations and markets. *The Journal of Economic Perspectives, 5*(2), 25–44.

Smith, M. J., & Liehr, P. R. (2008). Understanding middle range theory by moving up and down the ladder of abstraction. In M. J. Smith & P. R. Liehr (Eds.), *Middle range theory for nursing* (2nd ed., pp. 13–31). New York, NY: Springer.

Stacey, R. D. (2001). *Complex responsive processes in organizations: Learning and knowledge creation.* New York, NY: Routledge Taylor & Francis.

Swanson, K. M. (1991). Empirical development of a middle range theory of caring. *Nursing Research, 40*(3), 161–166.

Tappen, R. M. (2011). *Advanced nursing research: From theory to practice.* Burlington, MA: Jones & Bartlett Learning.

Trout, D. L. (1977). Max Josef von Pettenkofer (1818–1901): A biographical sketch. *Journal of Nutrition, 107*(9), 1567–1574.

Ullmann, A. (2007). Pasteur-Koch: Distinctive ways of thinking about infectious diseases. *Microbe,* 2(8). Retrieved from http://www.antimicrobe.org/h04c.files/history/Microbe%202007%20Pasteur-Koch.pdf

Vachon, D. (2005). Doctor John Snow blames water pollution for cholera epidemic. I. *Old News, 16*(8). Retrieved from http://www.ph.ucla.edu/epi/snow/fatherofepidemiology.html

Weick, K. E. (1995). *Sensemaking in organizations.* Thousand Oaks, CA: Sage.

CHAPTER 14

Introduction to Evidence-Based Research

■ CLISTA CLANTON ■

■ Objectives:

- Describe the evolution of the evidence-based movement in health care.
- Identify evidence-based models and relevance to evidence-based practice (EBP).
- Relate the various steps in evidence-based methodology to developing an EBP.
- Describe translational research and the link to EBP.

■ The Evolution of the Evidence-Based Movement in Health Care

The integration of research findings into healthcare practice has had some notable historical pioneers who can be traced back hundreds, if not thousands, of years. However, only in the last 70 years or so have research advances, such as the use of randomized controlled clinical trials to demonstrate the safety and efficacy of healthcare services and technologies, made the widespread adoption of research findings into practice possible at both the individual and institutional level. The emphasis on evidence-based health care is thus relatively new despite some historical precedents, and it has been propelled forward by more modern-day champions. David Eddy, MD, submitted a paper to the *Journal of the American Medical Association* (*JAMA*) in 1975 in which he argued, using ocular hypertension as an example, that many widely used treatments and tests were in fact not backed by good evidence or reasoning. Although the editors of *JAMA* were willing to publish the paper, they recommended that the more general points about the widespread lack of good evidence in medicine not be included. Because his main objective was to call attention to the need for better evidence, Dr. Eddy pulled the paper. Continuing his work to push for more formal analyses and integration of research into both practice and the formation of guidelines, Dr. Eddy has used the term "evidence-based" in a series of workshops and talks since at least 1985 (Eddy,

2011). He published a 1990 article in *JAMA* about evidence-based guidelines, thus introducing the term into the clinical literature (Eddy, 1990). The term "evidence-based" received more recognition when David Sackett and colleagues published the seminal article, "Evidence-Based Medicine: A New Approach to Teaching the Practice of Medicine" 2 years later in *JAMA* (Evidence-Based Medicine Working Group, 1992). The British epidemiologist Archie Cochrane (1979) was advocating for critical summaries of randomized controlled trials (RCTs) organized by medical specialties, known now as the systematic review. Recognizing the significance of his views, the Cochrane Collaboration was founded in 1993 and has published over 6200 systematic reviews to date. Clearly, the evidence-based movement in medicine was gaining strength.

■ Evidence-Based Nursing

The field of nursing has adopted and contributed to the evidence-based movement in health care. Research utilization had become a concentrated focus in nursing in the 1970s, although its intent had not been clearly communicated to staff and advanced practice nurses, thus delaying its adoption and slowing the rate at which research findings were incorporated into nursing practice. Furthermore, it was speculated that a lack of understanding of the differences between research utilization and EBP delayed the adoption of EBP by nurses (Melnyk, Stone, Fineout-Overholt, & Ackerman, 2000). Various articles were published in nursing journals in the mid to late 1990s discussing exactly what EBP meant and how to best apply it in the practice of nursing. Efforts by the Agency for Health Care Policy and Research (AHCPR) to develop evidence-based guidelines through an explicit, complex, and rigorous methodology represented one of the first ways that many nurses were exposed to evidence-based terminology (Stetler et al., 1998). Other key drivers for EBP in nursing have been institutions seeking Magnet accreditation, which is awarded to organizations that demonstrate excellence in nursing practice based on 14 key attributes (American Nurses Credentialing Center, 2016) and educational standards for competencies in EBP established by the American Association of Colleges of Nursing (AACN) at the baccalaureate, master's, and doctoral level (AACN, 2008).

Evidence-Based Practice Models

An early and commonly accepted definition of evidence-based medicine (EBM) is "the conscientious, explicit and judicious use of current best evidence in making decisions about the care of individual patients. It means integrating individual clinical expertise with the best available external clinical evidence from systematic research" (Sackett, Rosenberg, Gray, Haynes, & Richardson, 1996, p. 71). This definition was largely physician centric; notably absent in this definition are the patient's values or preferences regarding treatment, but subsequent definitions have included this aspect. The triad of research evidence, the clinician's experience, and the patient's values would then all potentially influence the decisions made regarding the patient's care (see **Figure 14-1**). As evidence-based methodologies developed for medicine have been adopted by other healthcare disciplines, the models have been adapted to better fit those work and research environments.

Nursing has developed multiple EBP models to guide practice. The nursing models are similar to the EBM model in that they contain the three realms of clinical expertise, research evidence, and patient preference to answer clinical questions but may differ in the steps used, level of detail, and types of evidence used in making decisions. The ACE Star Model of Knowledge Transformation developed by Dr. Kathleen Stevens at the University of Texas School of Nursing depicts the relationships between various stages of knowledge transformation as newly discovered knowledge is moved into practice (see **Figure 14-2**). The model illustrates five major stages of knowledge transformation: (1) knowledge discovery, (2) evidence summary, (3) translation into practice recommendations, (4) integration into practice, and (5) evaluation (Stevens, 2004).

Developed at the University of Iowa Hospitals and Clinics, the Iowa Model of Evidence-Based Practice to Promote Quality Care helps clarify the steps needed to put research into practice, with the goal of improving the quality of care (see **Figure 14-3**). This model, organizational and collaborative in nature, contains both problem-focused and knowledge-focused triggers that lead nurses to question current practice and to ask whether patient care could be improved by using research findings. If a review of the current evidence does not show enough of a scientifically sound base on which to make decisions for practice, nurses may then need to conduct their own research (Titler, 2007).

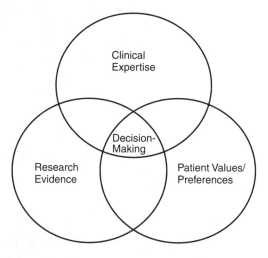

■ **Figure 14-1** Three-Circle Model of Evidence-Based Clinical Decisions

Data from Haynes, R. B., Sackett, D. L., Gray, J. M., Cook, D. J., & Guyatt, G. H. (1996). Transferring evidence from research into practice: 1. The role of clinical care research evidence in clinical decisions. *ACP Journal Club, 125*(3), A14–16.

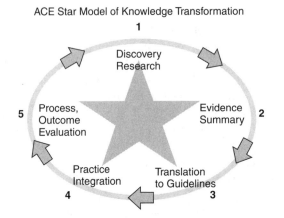

■ Figure 14-2 Ace Star Model of Knowledge Transformation

Reproduced from Copyrighted material Stevens, K. R. (2004). *ACE Star Model of EBP: Knowledge transformation*. Academic Center for Evidence-based Practice, University of Texas Health Science Center at San Antonio. Retrieved from http://www.acestar.uthscsa.edu. Reproduced with expressed permission.

A model that merges both EBP and practice improvement (PI) paradigms is the evidence-based practice improvement (EBPI) model (Levin et al., 2010). The first stage is to describe the practice problem, both internally within the organizational context and externally within disciplinary literature. Once the practice problem area is described, a focused clinical question can then be formed using PICO (defined on page 256). A search for high-quality evidence using leveling schemes and quality ratings is then conducted. The next step, and the last of the traditional EBP functions, is to appraise and synthesize the evidence. The first step of the PI portion of the model is to develop an aim statement to direct attention to the specific outcomes desired, including an operational goal and a measure of achievement. The next step, before implementing a practice innovation, is to engage in small tests of change known as Plan-Do-Study-Act (PDSA) cycles. The last stage of this model involves disseminating the best practices both internally (once pilot projects have shown efficacy) and externally (to the external professional community) when measurable outcomes have been demonstrated.

Transdisciplinary Model of Evidence-Based Practice

Reflecting the fact that a wide range of fields, such as public health, psychology, and social work, have also incorporated evidence-based methods into their practice, a transdisciplinary model of EBP has been proposed (Satterfield et al., 2009). This model has an external frame around three core circles that represents the environment and organizational factors, creating a cultural context that moderates the acceptability and feasibility of an intervention, as well as the balance between adherence and adaptation needed for effective implementation. The three core circles, adapted from

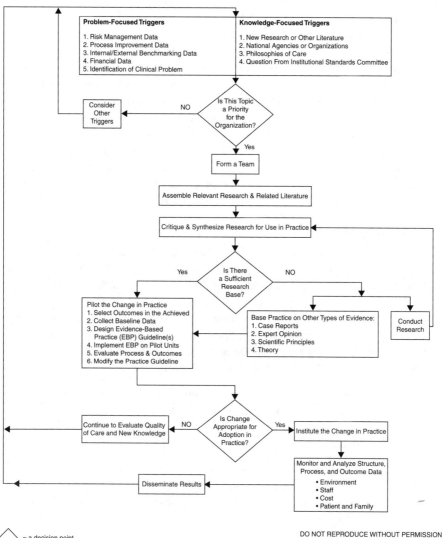

The Iowa Model of
Evidence-Based Practice to Promote Quality Care

Problem-Focused Triggers

1. Risk Management Data
2. Process Improvement Data
3. Internal/External Benchmarking Data
4. Financial Data
5. Identification of Clinical Problem

Knowledge-Focused Triggers

1. New Research or Other Literature
2. National Agencies or Organizations
3. Philosophies of Care
4. Question From Institutional Standards Committee

Is This Topic a Priority for the Organization?

Consider Other Triggers — NO

Yes

Form a Team

Assemble Relevant Research & Related Literature

Critique & Synthesize Research for Use in Practice

Is There a Sufficient Research Base?

Yes — NO

Pilot the Change in Practice
1. Select Outcomes in the Achieved
2. Collect Baseline Data
3. Design Evidence-Based Practice (EBP) Guideline(s)
4. Implement EBP on Pilot Units
5. Evaluate Process & Outcomes
6. Modify the Practice Guideline

Base Practice on Other Types of Evidence:
1. Case Reports
2. Expert Opinion
3. Scientific Principles
4. Theory

Conduct Research

Is Change Appropriate for Adoption in Practice?

Continue to Evaluate Quality of Care and New Knowledge — NO

Yes — Institute the Change in Practice

Monitor and Analyze Structure, Process, and Outcome Data
• Environment
• Staff
• Cost
• Patient and Family

Disseminate Results

◇ = a decision point

Reference

Titler, M. G., Kleiber, C., Steelman, V. J., Rakel, B. A., Budreau, G., Everett, L. Q., Buckwalter, K. C., Tripp-Reimer, T., & Goode C. (2001), The Iowa Model of Evidence-Based Practice to Promote Quality Care. *Critical Care Nursing Clinics of North America, 13*(4), 497–509.

■ Figure 14-3   Iowa Model of Evidence-Based Practice to Promote Quality Care

Reproduced with permission from Marita G. Titler, PhD, RN, FAAN, and the University of Iowa Hospitals and Clinics, Copyright 1998.

the EBM model, consist of the best available research evidence; the client's/population's characteristics, state, needs, values, and preferences; and resources, which include the practitioner's expertise. At the center of the model is decision-making, which the authors defined as "the cognitive action that turns evidence into contextualized evidence-based practices" (Satterfield et al., 2009, p. 383). Decision-making is the center of this model because of four factors: (a) the systematic decisional process, which combines evidence with the client, resources, and context that is required in making decisions; (b) the lack of empirical evidence for the proposition that the practitioner's performance improved with experience (Choudhry, Fletcher, & Soumerai, 2005); (c) demonstration of the difficulties and practical challenges in reconciling the many variables needed to make evidence-based decisions about clinical care, public health, or public policy; and (d) the desire for a collaborative healthcare practice in which health decisions are not solely the practitioner's but are shared among the practitioner(s), clients, and other affected stakeholders.

Formation of Questions

Forming the question is typically the first step in the EBP process, and although it may appear to be simple, it often requires refining to arrive at a well-built question that truly reflects the scenario at hand. Search strategies that are too broad may result in information overload, whereas search strategies that are too specific may exclude relevant articles. Well-built clinical questions should be the starting point of developing a search strategy and therefore should contain all the important aspects involved in the information need at hand. PICO was originally developed to construct clinical questions (Richardson, Wilson, Nishikawa, & Hayward, 1995).

P = The patient or problem being addressed
I = The intervention or exposure being considered
C = The comparison intervention or exposure, when relevant
O = The clinical outcomes of interest

This process of asking questions was slightly modified for nursing usage to PICOT, with the addition of the time it takes for the intervention to achieve the desired outcome, although it is not a required component (Stillwell, Fineout-Overholt, Melnyk, & Williamson, 2010).

P = Patient population
I = Intervention or issue of interest
C = Comparison intervention or issue of interest
O = Outcome(s) of interest
T = Time it takes for the intervention to achieve the outcome(s)

If the information need is a broad what, where, or how background question seeking general knowledge, it can usually be answered by textbooks. Examples of background questions are: At what age should a woman have her first pelvic examination? How often should a woman get a pelvic examination? If the question is a more focused foreground question, PICO or PICOT is useful for framing the question. An example of a foreground question is: In women with an abnormal Pap smear who have also tested positive for human papillomavirus is a loop electrosurgical incision procedure versus a cone biopsy more effective in diagnosing abnormal tissue? Foreground questions will usually require database searches to retrieve research from journal literature. Foreground questions can further be categorized according to type: intervention or therapy, etiology, diagnosis or diagnostic tool, prognosis or prediction, prevention, cost, and meaning. Specific types of research are used to best answer the different categories of questions, and understanding this can help in further refining a search strategy (see **Table 14-1**).

PubMed, the search gateway for over 25 million citations for biomedical literature from MEDLINE, life science journals, and online books, has developed clinical query search filters that can help with this process.

The Preferred Reporting Items for Systematic Reviews and Meta-Analyses statement (PRISMA; Liberati et al., 2009) recommends providing an explicit statement of questions being addressed in a systematic review or meta-analysis. This helps readers to quickly grasp the scope and potential applicability of the review for their setting and purposes. The questions can be developed using PICOS. The first four components are similar to those in PICO and PICOT but also take into consideration important factors that should be reported in the systematic review. Different from PICO or PICOT is the addition of the study design chosen (S).

P = Patient population or the disease being addressed, with a precise definition of the group of participants, their defining characteristics of interest, and, if appropriate, the setting of care being considered.

Table 14-1   Suggested Best Type of Study by Question Type

Type of Question	Suggested Best Type of Study
Therapy	RCT > cohort > case control > case series
Diagnosis	Prospective, blind comparison to gold standard
Etiology/Harm	RCT > cohort > case control > case series
Prognosis	Cohort study > case control > case series
Prevention	RCT > cohort study > case control > case series
Clinical Exam	Prospective, blind comparison with gold standard
Cost	Economic analysis
Meaning	Qualitative

Questions of therapy, etiology, and prevention that can best be answered by RCT can also be answered by a meta-analysis or systematic review.

RCT = randomized controlled trial.

Author.

I = Interventions or exposures under consideration in the systematic review should be reported in a transparent way and with a level of detail sufficient for readers to be able to interpret the review's results and conclusions.

C = Clear reporting of the comparator (control) group intervention(s) is essential for readers to fully understand the selection criteria of the primary studies included in the systematic review. Clear identification of what the intervention is being compared with is important and can have implications for what studies are included in the review.

O = Outcomes of the intervention being assessed should be clearly specified, because they are essential for interpreting the validity and generalizability of the systematic review's results.

S = The type of study design(s) included in the review should be clearly reported (Liberati et al., 2009)

Hierarchies and Ranking of Evidence

The first hierarchy of evidence was developed by the Canadian Task Force on the Periodic Health Examination in 1979, and since then other hierarchies have been developed and used (Canadian Task Force on the Periodic Health Examination, 1979; Cook, Guyatt, Laupacis, & Sackett, 1992; Cook, Guyatt, Laupacis, Sackett, & Goldberg, 1995; Guyatt et al., 1995; Sackett, 1986; Wilson, Hayward, Tunis, Bass, & Guyatt, 1995; Woolf, Battista, Anderson, Logan, & Wang, 1990). The original model for ranking evidence in EBP was a single-hierarchy pyramid that lists the meta-analysis as the highest form of evidence, followed by the systematic review (see **Figure 14-4**). The meta-analysis is "a statistical synthesis of the numerical results of several trials which all addressed the same question" (Greenhalgh, 2006, p. 122). An "ideal" meta-analysis would include studies undertaken in the same setting, use the same design and outcome (measured in the same way and after the same time interval), have no missing data, and include high-quality studies whose effect sizes are similar. Furthermore, when assessing a meta-analysis, it is important to look at the publication date because out-of-date meta-analyses may lead to different conclusions from those in more recent reviews (Holt, 2011). A systematic review is a review of a clearly formulated question that uses systematic and explicit methods to identify, select, and critically appraise relevant research and to collect and analyze data from the studies that are included in the review. Statistical methods (meta-analysis) may or may not be used to analyze and summarize the results of the included studies in the systematic review (Cochrane Collaboration, n.d.). So, although a systematic review also may be a meta-analysis if the corresponding statistical analysis is included, a meta-analysis has always had a systematic review performed to identify the studies being included in the meta-analysis. Because it involves reviewing multiple studies using a rigorous and explicit methodology, a meta-analysis or systematic review is considered a higher form of evidence than a single RCT, although according to Holt (2011), a single RCT may be superior if it is large enough (p. 19). Following the systematic review is the

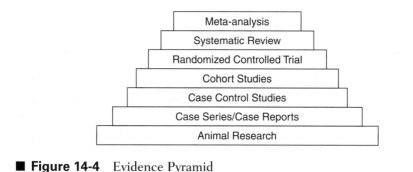

■ Figure 14-4   Evidence Pyramid

RCT, which is considered the gold standard of the individual study types because it is a prospective, analytical, experimental study design that uses primary data generated in a clinical environment. Next is the cohort study, an observational study type that prospectively follows a large group of patients with a specific exposure or treatment and then compares outcomes with an unaffected group. Because cohort studies are observational, they are not considered as reliable as RCTs; the study groups may have variables that affect outcomes other than the ones being studied. After cohort studies are case control studies, which are retrospective studies in which people who have a specific condition or outcome are compared with people who do not. Because researchers are retrospectively relying on patient recall or medical records for their data collection, these studies are considered less reliable than RCTs and cohort studies. Next in the hierarchy are case series and case reports, which are collections of reports on the treatment of individual patients or a single patient. They do not use control groups to compare outcomes and thus have no statistical validity. At the bottom of the pyramid are studies done on animals, and some models include expert opinion in this last level as well.

Not reflected in this original hierarchy of evidence is qualitative research, which explores a deeper understanding of an issue, and other kinds of information that can also be useful in making evidence-based decisions. Noting the limitations of this early model, more recent hierarchies have been proposed to address these lacks. Included in these hierarchies are systematic reviews of descriptive and qualitative studies, single descriptive or qualitative studies, controlled trials without random-ization, physiologic studies, clinical practice guidelines, and opinions of authorities and/or reports of expert committees. There are differences in what is included in these different evidence hierarchies, from the types of research designs to whether to include expert opinion, consensus panels, and unsystematic observations. One of the more comprehensive proposed models originated out of the field of occupational therapy and includes experimental, qualitative, descriptive, and outcome research. The authors maintain that this three-sided pyramid of evidence recognizes that there is no gold standard of research design for answering all questions of importance and that it can better guide research by revealing more comprehensively where the evidence gaps exist (Tomlin & Borgetto, 2011).

Public health practitioners have highlighted the limitations of the single-hierarchy pyramid, noting that frameworks used for quantitative methods answer only some of the public health research questions and that qualitative study designs are needed to find out about all the "what" and "why" questions (Robinson, 2009). In a commentary in *JAMA*, Dr. Donald Berwick (2009) maintained that embracing a wider range of scientific methodologies would help accelerate the improvement of systems in care and practice. According to Berwick (2008):

> Many assessment techniques developed in engineering and used in quality improvement—statistical process control, time series analysis, simulations, and factorial experiments—have more power to inform about mechanisms and contexts than do RCTs, as do ethnography, anthropology, and other qualitative methods. For these specific applications, these methods are not compromises in learning how to improve; they are superior. (p. 1183)

A hierarchy that appears in the text *Evidence-Based Practice in Nursing & Healthcare* (Melnyk & Fineout-Overholt, 2005) has been noted as appearing to be the most relevant hierarchy for nurses practicing in the United States; it is the only one that includes clinical practice guidelines as well as meta-syntheses and qualitative studies that are frequently conducted by nurse researchers (Jones, 2010). Further reflecting the importance that qualitative research is receiving, the Cochrane Collaboration established a Cochrane Qualitative Research Methods Group that advised the Collaboration on developing methods for the integration of qualitative evidence into selected Cochrane intervention reviews. This was a substantial move in position for Cochrane (Noyes, 2010), and the group has since evolved into the Cochrane Qualitative & Implementation Methods Group, with the purpose and focus on methods and processes involved in the synthesis of qualitative evidence and the integration of qualitative evidence with Cochrane intervention reviews of effects. In 2012 the Group's mandate was extended to include methods for undertaking systematic reviews of implementation.

Another way of framing the limitations of current hierarchies is to note that most focus solely on effectiveness, which is concerned with whether an intervention works as intended. This is essential, but it is also important to know whether the intervention is appropriate for its recipient. The evidence on appropriateness looks at the psychosocial aspects of the intervention, which are the questions related to the impact on a person, its acceptability, and whether the consumer would use it. A third dimension of evidence relates to its feasibility, which concerns the impact it would have on an organization or provider, as well as the resources required to ensure its successful implementation. Evidence on feasibility would therefore look at the broader environmental issues related to implementation, cost, and practice change. These three components—effectiveness, appropriateness, and feasibility—provide a more solid base for evaluating healthcare interventions and highlight the range of dimensions that evidence should address for healthcare interventions to be adequately appraised (Evans, 2003). Notably, Evans acknowledged that "the use of any hierarchy is, at best, a guide rather than a set of inflexible rules. A hierarchy provides the end-user of research with a framework to judge the strength of available evidence" (p. 83).

Finally, evidence hierarchies have usually ignored expert opinion or placed it at the bottom level. An obvious barrier to EBP is a situation in which evidence is lacking or nonexistent. Decisions still need to be made, and there is the viewpoint that the development of a locally relevant evidence base using expert consensus is a valuable approach when other evidence is unavailable (Minas & Jorm, 2010). Because there will be instances in health care when there is no evidence, Minas and Jorm maintained that group expert consensus will generally produce better judgments than any single individual's judgment (p. 3). Just as EBP has evolved as different user groups adopt and apply it in their environment, so will the hierarchies used to grade the evidence.

■ Hierarchy of Resources

The efficient retrieval of high-quality evidence to support decisions involves knowing what resources to use. Notable obstacles for implementing evidence-based care range from lack of time because of demanding patient loads to difficulty accessing and assimilating large amounts of research findings from journal literature (Cook, Mulrow, & Haynes, 1997; Sackett, Richardson, Rosenberg, & Haynes, 1997; Shorten & Wallace, 1997). These difficulties have influenced the design of databases used to access the research literature and have led to decision support systems, point-of-care databases, and other tools to help streamline the process of finding relevant information quickly and effectively. The 6S hierarchy of pre-appraised evidence is one way of classifying and approaching the various information systems available (DiCenso, Bayley, & Haynes, 2009) (see **Figure 14-5**). This model is a six-level pyramid of information resource categories. The bottom level of the pyramid contains original studies from the journal literature, which are indexed in databases such as PubMed, CINAHL, Scopus, and PsycINFO. The next level starts the pre-appraised evidence and contains synopses of studies, which provide a brief summary of a high-quality study that can inform clinical practice and that contains value-added commentaries that address the clinical applicability of study findings. These can be found in evidence-based journals such as *ACP Journal Club*, *Evidence-Based Medicine*, *Evidence-Based Mental Health*, and *Evidence-Based Nursing*.

The third lowest level is syntheses, which contains systematic reviews such as those found in the Cochrane Library or Database of Abstracts of Reviews of Effects (DARE). It is worth noting that funding to produce DARE ceased in March 2015, although it can still be accessed via the Cochrane Library. PubMed, CINAHL, and Scopus also index systematic reviews. After syntheses comes the synopses of

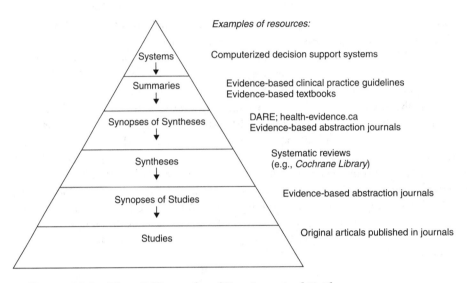

■ Figure 14-5 The 6S Hierarchy of Pre-Appraised Evidence

Reproduced from DiCenso, A., Bayley, L., & Haynes, R. B. (2009). Accessing pre-appraised evidence: Fine-tuning the 5S model into a 6S model. *Evidence-Based Nursing, 12*(4), 99–102. Used with permission.

syntheses level, which summarizes the findings of a high-quality systematic review to provide sufficient information to support clinical action; the advantage of this level is that it provides a convenient summary of the corresponding systematic review and is accompanied by a commentary that addresses the methodological quality of the systematic review and the clinical applicability of its findings. These syntheses can be found in journals such as the *ACP Journal Club, Evidence-Based Medicine, Evidence-Based Mental Health*, and *Evidence-Based Nursing* and are also indexed in databases such as DARE.

Next is the summaries level, which integrates the best available evidence from the lower levels to provide a full range of evidence concerning management options for a particular health condition. These include clinical pathways, textbook summaries, and point-of-care databases that integrate evidence-based information about specific clinical problems and provide regular updating. Resources such as DynaMed, Clinical Evidence, First Consult, the Physicians' Information and Education Resource (PIER), UptoDate, and current evidence-based clinical practice guidelines fall into this category. The top level is systems, or electronic health records (EHRs), which contains individual patient information and links out to the current best evidence that matches the specific circumstances. The goal in using the 6S model is to start at the highest level and work downward if evidence is not available from the upper level resources. Starting at the top levels of the hierarchy saves the clinician time because the resources within these levels have already identified and critically appraised the most relevant research on a particular issue.

An obstacle to using the highest level of the 6S hierarchy is that the implementation of EHRs in most hospitals has yet to happen, and many hospitals that do have EHRs are not currently meeting the federal government's standard of "meaningful use" criteria. The Centers for Medicare & Medicaid Services (CMS) defines the stage 1 criteria for meaningful use as a "focus on electronically capturing health information in a coded format, using that information to track key clinical conditions, communicating that information for care coordination purposes, and initiating the reporting of clinical quality measures and public health information" (CMS, 2010). Data from a 2009 American Hospital Association (AHA) survey of acute care nonfederal hospitals indicated that, of 3101 hospitals that provided information out of 4493 surveyed, only 2% of the 11.9% of hospitals using EHRs met the criteria for meaningful use (Jha, DesRoches, Kralovec, & Joshi, 2010). Although this number had grown to 44% of hospitals using at least a basic EHR system by 2012 and most of those meeting all of the federal stage 1 "meaningful-use" criteria, only 5.1% could meet the broader set of stage 2 criteria (DesRoches et al., 2013). There is also concern of a possible widening of a "digital divide," with smaller, rural, and nonteaching hospitals falling behind other hospitals (DesRoches, Worzala, Joshi, Kralovec, & Jha, 2012). It appears the transition to digital health care will continue to be a drawn out process. If the systems level is therefore not available, start at the summaries level and then work downward as necessary.

■ Translational Research

A little over a decade ago, an initiative by the National Institutes of Health (NIH) called the NIH Roadmap was designed to highlight the need for increased attention to "translating" basic science research more quickly into human studies, leading to treatments or tests for clinical practice that would benefit patients. This led to the formation of translational research centers within NIH institutes and the Clinical and Science Translation Award (CSTA) in 2006, with an expectation that 60 centers would be established by 2012. Indeed, by 2013 the CSTA Consortium had expanded to 62 medical research institutions, also referred to as hubs, located throughout the nation. The goals of the CSTA Program are to (NCATS, 2015):

1. Train and cultivate the translational science workforce
2. Engage patients and communities in every phase of the translational process
3. Promote the integration of special and underserved populations in translational research across the human life span
4. Innovate processes to increase the quality and efficiency of translational research, particularly of multisite trials
5. Advance the use of cutting-edge informatics.

The successful implementation of the translation process requires the crossing of translational barriers. Translational research (TR) emphasizes the importance of different disciplines working together on teams, and although different disciplines, such as epidemiology and bioinformatics, would contribute to the translational process in different ways, all would have the goal of translating research into clinical practice more quickly. T1, T2, and T3, respectively, correspond to translational barriers at the bench-to-bedside, bedside-to-community, and community-to-policy realms (Sarkar, 2010).

An epidemiologic translation model also includes T0 and T4 levels, with T0 being new knowledge and insight into the causes, pathobiology, or natural history of diseases, and T4 focusing on the evaluation of the population-level health impact of interventions (Khoury, Gwinn, & Ioannidis, 2010) (see **Figure 14-6**). At the center of the epidemiology translational model is knowledge synthesis, which Khoury et al. consider an essential role in all phases of TR; it is the "systematic approach to reviewing the evidence on what we know and what we do not know, and how we know it" (p. 521). Meta-analyses and systematic reviews, which help to develop evidence-based recommendations for practice, are examples of knowledge synthesis methods at the T2 level. Because translational teams will be composed of members from various disciplines, the inclusion of biomedical informatics professionals may be essential for enabling the effective translation of concepts between team members with heterogeneous areas of expertise, and various biomedical approaches will be necessary to manage, organize, and integrate the diverse data that will inform decisions from bench to bedside to community to policy (Sarkar, 2010).

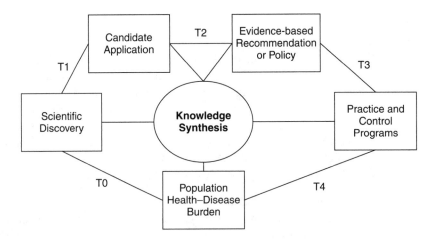

■ **Figure 14-6**   **Epidemiology and the Phases of Translation and Knowledge Synthesis: From Discovery to Population Health Impact**

Reproduced from Khoury, M. J., Gwinn, M., & Ioannidis, P. A. (2010). The emergence of translational epidemiology: From scientific discovery to population health impact. *American Journal of Epidemiology, 172*(5), 517–524. Used with permission.

REFLECTIVE ACTIVITIES

1. Compare and contrast at least three evidence-based models. How are they different? How are they similar?
2. Develop a patient scenario using the PICO and PICOT methods to refine the clinical question.
3. From PICO and PICOT, identify the type of question and databases that would yield satisfactory research evidence to support resolution of the problem.
4. Using information from Reflective Activities 2 and 3, identify the highest level of evidence using a hierarchy of evidence and grading tools.

REFERENCES

American Association of Colleges of Nursing. (2008). *AACN "Essentials" series*. Retrieved from http://www.aacn.nche.edu/Education/essentials.htm

American Nurses Credentialing Center. (2016). *Forces of magnetism*. Retrieved from http://www.nursecredentialing.org/Magnet/ProgramOverview

Berwick, D. M. (2008). The science of improvement. *Journal of the American Medical Association. 299*(10), 1182–2284. doi: 10.1001/jama.299.10.1182

Berwick, D. M. (2009). Measuring physicians' quality and performance. *Journal of the American Medical Association, 302*(22), 2485–2486. doi:10.1001/jama.2009.1801

Canadian Task Force on the Periodic Health Examination. (1979). The periodic health examination. *Canadian Medical Association Journal, 121,* 1193–1254.

Centers for Medicare & Medicaid Services. (2010). *CMS finalizes definition of meaningful use of certified electronic health records (EHR) technology.* Retrieved from http://www.cms.gov/

Choudhry, N. K., Fletcher, R. H., & Soumerai, S. B. (2005). Systematic review: The relationship between clinical experience and quality of care. *Annals of Internal Medicine, 142*(4), 260–273.

Cochrane, A. L. (1979). 1931–1971: A critical review, with particular reference to the medical profession. In *Medicines for the year 2000* (pp. 1–7). London, England: Office of Health Economics.

Cochrane Collaboration. (n.d.). *Frequently asked questions, general: What is the difference between a protocol and a review?* Retrieved from http://www.cochrane.org/faq/general

Cook, D. J., Guyatt, G. H., Laupacis, A., & Sackett, D. L. (1992). Rules of evidence and clinical recommendations on the use of antithrombotic agents. *Chest, 102,* 305s–311s.

Cook, D. J., Guyatt, G. H., Laupacis, A., Sackett, D. L., & Goldberg, R. J. (1995). Rules of evidence and clinical recommendations on the use of antithrombotic agents. *Chest, 108,* 227s–230s.

Cook, C. J., Mulrow, C. D., & Haynes, R. B. (1997). Systematic reviews: Synthesis of the best evidence for clinical decision making. *Annals of Internal Medicine, 126*(5), 376–380.

DesRoches, M., Charles, D., Furukawa, M. F., Maulik, S. J., Kralovec, P., Mostashari, F., Worzala, C., Jha, A. K. (2013). Adoption of electronic health records grows rapidly, but fewer than half of US hospitals had at least a basic system in 2012. *Health Affairs, 32*(8):1478–1485.

DesRoches, C. M., Worzala, C., Joshi, M. S., Kralovec, P. D., Jha, A. K. (2012). Small, non-teaching, and rural hospitals continue to be slow in adopting electronic health record systems. *Health Affairs, 31*(5):1092–1099.

DiCenso, A., Bayley, L., & Haynes, R. B. (2009). Accessing pre-appraised evidence: Fine-tuning the 5S model into a 6S model. *Evidence-Based Nursing, 12*(4), 99–102.

Eddy, D. M. (1990). Practice policies: Where do they come from? *Journal of the American Medical Association, 263*(9), 1265, 1269, 1272, 1275.

Eddy, D. M. (2011). The origins of evidence-based medicine: A personal perspective. *Virtual Mentor, 13*(1), 55–60.

Evans, D. (2003). Hierarchy of evidence: A framework for ranking evidence evaluating healthcare interventions. *Journal of Clinical Nursing, 12,* 77–84.

Evidence-Based Medicine Working Group. (1992). Evidence-based medicine: A new approach to teaching the practice of medicine. *Journal of the American Medical Association, 268*(17), 2420–2425.

Greenhalgh, T. (2006). *How to read a paper: The basics of evidence-based medicine* (3rd ed.). London, England: BMJ Books.

Guyatt, G. H., Sackett, D. L., Sinclair, J. C., Hayward, R., Cook, D. J., & Cook, R. J. (1995). Users guide to the medical literature. IX. A method for grading healthcare recommendations. *Journal of the American Medical Association, 274,* 1800–1804.

Haynes, R. B., Sackett, D. L., Gray, J. M., Cook, D. J., & Guyatt, G. H. (1996). Transferring evidence from research into practice. I. The role of clinical care research evidence in clinical decisions. *ACP Journal Club, 125*(3), A14–A16.

Holt, T. (2011). Evidence-based medicine. I. The power and pitfalls of meta-analysis. *Diabetes & Primary Care, 13*(1), 18–22.

Jha, A. K., DesRoches, C. M., Kralovec, P. D., & Joshi, M. S. (2010). A progress report on electronic health records in U.S. hospitals. *Health Affairs, 29*(10), 1951–1957.

Jones, K. R. (2010). Rating the level, quality, and strength of the research evidence. *Journal of Nursing Care Quality, 25*(4), 304–312.

Khoury, M. J., Gwinn, M., & Ioannidis, P. A. (2010). The emergence of translational epidemiology: From scientific discovery to population health impact. *American Journal of Epidemiology, 172*(5), 517–524.

Liberati, A., Altman, D. G., Tetzlaff, J., Mulrow, C., Gotzsche, P. C., Ioannidis, J. P. A., . . . Moher, D. (2009). The PRISMA statement for reporting systematic reviews and meta-analyses of studies that evaluate healthcare interventions: Explanation and elaboration. *BMJ, 339*(b2700). doi:10.1136/bmj.b2700. Retrieved from http://www.bmj.com/highwire/filestream/381758/field_highwire_article_pdf/0.pdf

Levin, R. F., Keefer, J. M., Marren, J., Vetter, M., Lauder, B., & Sobolewski, S. (2010). Evidence-based practice improvement: Merging 2 paradigms. *Journal of Nursing Care Quality, 25*(2), 117–126.

Melnyk, B. M., & Fineout-Overholt, E. (2005). *Evidence-based practice in nursing & healthcare.* Philadelphia, PA: Lippincott Williams & Wilkins.

Melnyk, B., Stone, P., Fineout-Overholt, E., & Ackerman, M. (2000). Evidence-based practice: The past, the present, and recommendations for the millennium. *Pediatric Nursing, 26*(1), 77–80.

Minas, H., & Jorm, A. F. (2010). Where there is no evidence: Use of expert consensus methods to fill the evidence gap in low-income countries and cultural minorities. *International Journal of Mental Health Systems, 4*(33), 1–6. Retrieved from http://www.ijmhs.com/content/pdf/1752-4458-4-33.pdf

National Center for Advancing Translational Sciences (2015, August 31). *About the CTSA program.* Retrieved from http://www.ncats.nih.gov/ctsa/about

Noyes, J. (2010). Never mind the qualitative feel the depth! The evolving role of qualitative research in Cochrane intervention reviews. *Journal of Research in Nursing, 15*(6), 525–534.

Richardson, W. S., Wilson, M. C., Nishikawa, J., & Hayward, R. S. (1995). The well-built clinical question: A key to evidence-based decisions. *ACP Journal Club, 123*(3), A12–A13.

Robinson, P. (2009). Evidence pyramids, rigour and ethics review of public health research. *Australian and New Zealand Journal of Public Health, 33*(3), 203–204.

Sackett, D. L. (1986). Rules of evidence and clinical recommendations on the use of antithrombotic agents. *Chest, 89,* 2s–3s.

Sackett, D. L., Richardson, S., Rosenberg, W., & Haynes, R. (1997). *Evidence-based medicine: How to practice and teach EBM.* New York, NY: Churchill Livingstone.

Sackett, D. L., Rosenberg, W. M. C., Gray, J. A. M., Haynes, R. B., & Richardson, W. S. (1996). Evidence-based medicine: What it is and what it isn't—It's about integrating individual clinical expertise and the best external evidence. *BMJ, 312*(7023), 71–72.

Sarkar, I. N. (2010). Biomedical informatics and translational medicine. *Journal of Translational Medicine, 8,* 22. doi:10.1186/1479-5876-8-22

Satterfield, J. M., Spring, B., Brownson, R. C., Mullen, J., Newhouse, R. P., Walker, B., & Whitlock, E. P. (2009). Toward a transdisciplinary model of evidence-based practice. *Milbank Quarterly, 87*(2), 368–390.

Shorten, A., & Wallace, M. (1997). Evidence-based practice: When quality counts. *Australian Nursing Journal, 4,* 26–27.

Stetler, C. B., Brunell, M., Giuliano, K. K., Morsi, D., Prince, L., & Newell-Stokes, V. (1998). Evidence-based practice and the role of nursing leadership. *Journal of Nursing Administration, 29*(7/8), 45–53.

Stevens, K. R. (2004). *ACE star model of EBP: Knowledge transformation.* Academic Center for Evidence-based Practice, University of Texas Health Science Center at San Antonio. Retrieved from http://www.acestar.uthscsa.edu

Stillwell, S. B., Fineout-Overholt, E., Melnyk, B. M., & Williamson, K. M. (2010). Evidence-based practice, step by step: Asking the clinical question—A key step in evidence-based practice. *American Journal of Nursing, 110*(3), 58–61.

Titler, M. (2007). Translating research into practice. *American Journal of Nursing, 107*(6), 26–33.

Titler, M., Kleiber, C., Steelman, V., Rakel, B., Budreau, G., Everett, L.,... Goode, C. (2001). The Iowa model of evidence-based practice to promote quality care. *Critical Care Clinics of North America, 13*(4), 497–509.

Tomlin, G., & Borgetto, B. (2011). Research pyramid: A new evidence-based practice model for occupational therapy. *American Journal of Occupational Therapy, 65*(2), 189–196.

Wilson, M. C., Hayward, R. S. A., Tunis, S. R., Bass, E. B., & Guyatt, G. (1995). Users guide to the medical literature. VIII. How to use clinical practice guidelines; B. What are the recommendations and will they help you in caring for your patients. *Journal of the American Medical Association, 274,* 1630–1632.

Woolf, S. H., Battista, R. N., Anderson, G. M., Logan, A. G., & Wang, E. (1990). Assessing the clinical effectiveness of preventative maneuvers: Analytic principles and systematic methods in reviewing evidence and developing clinical practice recommendations. *Journal of Clinical Epidemiology, 43,* 891–905.

CHAPTER 15

Technology Supporting the Search for Evidence

■ Trey Lemley ■

■ Objectives:

- Examine a variety of resources and databases that support best evidence searches.
- Identify steps in determining the appropriate method for keyword searches used by a variety of databases.

Although evidence-based information can be located within a wide variety of sources, the sheer volume of material available can turn any search into a daunting and seemingly unmanageable task. In an effort to bring a sense of order to the process, this chapter includes an examination and description of resources and databases that are useful in finding evidence-based information (Melnyk & Fineout-Overholt. 2011).

The 6S hierarchy of pre-appraised evidence (DiCenso, Bayley, & Haynes, 2009) will be used as a framework for this chapter. The 6S hierarchy of pre-appraised evidence serves as a means for classifying and approaching searches. This six-level pyramid is categorized as follows (starting from the bottom and going to the tip of the pyramid): (a) studies, (b) synopses of studies, (c) syntheses (e.g., systematic reviews), (d) synopses of syntheses, (e) summaries, and (f) systems. (Chapter 14 of this text contains a detailed explanation of the hierarchy with graphics.)

The resources in the upper levels of the 6S hierarchy of pre-appraised evidence contain only evidence-based materials; in contrast, databases in the bottom rung (the *studies* level) are more comprehensive in scope and contain a wider variety of health-related information, drawn from thousands of journals and scholarly sources. Because of their size and variety of content, these databases are more complicated to search than are resources in the upper levels of the hierarchy.

There are two major methods of searching in the studies level. First is by *natural language,* more commonly called *keyword searching*—for example, the method used to search Google. To perform a keyword search on the phrase *heart attack,* the user would simply enter the phrase *heart attack* into the search box, click the search button, and obtain results. Second is by means of a *controlled vocabulary,* also called a thesaurus, in which all articles and citations in the database have been indexed and then categorized by different subject headings. Examples of controlled vocabularies include the Medical Subject Headings (MeSH) of MEDLINE, CINAHL Headings, the Thesaurus of PsycINFO, and the Emtree thesaurus of Embase.

Both keyword and controlled vocabulary searching have advantages. Keyword search does not require any knowledge of data organization or storage (Cappellari, 2012, p. 632). Keyword searching is useful when a concept is new: to illustrate, currently, CINAHL is the only database with a controlled vocabulary subject heading for *meta synthesis;* as a result, a keyword search would be the most efficacious means of locating information on the topic of *meta synthesis* in MEDLINE and other health-related databases (other than CINAHL).

A major advantage of a controlled vocabulary system is its ability to *map* search terms to the subject heading in the controlled vocabulary that is most relevant to the search terms entered. To illustrate, the search phrase *collapsed lung,* when entered in CINAHL is mapped to the CINAHL Heading *Pulmonary Atelectasis.* (CINAHL Headings, the controlled vocabulary system of CINAHL, are accessed via a link on the top sidebar of the main search page in CINAHL.) (See **Figures 15-1** and **15-2**.)

Mapping gathers related terms and topics under one subject heading. This can provide the user with overview and context information about the search term, which is especially useful when researching a new topic or when the search is unfocused (Hall, 2014, p. 353). In contrast, keyword searching can fail to retrieve literature that uses synonyms, variant phrases, and keywords other than those specified by the researcher (Beall, 2008, p. 439). For instance, a search in PubMed using the phrase *cerebral vascular accident* will not return as many results as a search using the MeSH heading *stroke.* Using the preceding examples, a search on the phrase *collapsed lung* might not find articles about pulmonary atelectasis.

■ Single Studies

The Single Studies layer is the bottom layer of the 6S hierarchy of pre-appraised evidence. It includes single studies from the research literature that are indexed and made searchable by the following databases.

Cumulative Index to Nursing and Allied Health Literature
Website: http://www.ebscohost.com/cinahl

CINAHL is a comprehensive database that indexes more than 5000 journals from the fields of nursing and allied health. Although CINAHL is not limited to evidence-based information, it is a useful place to find studies from the lower level of the

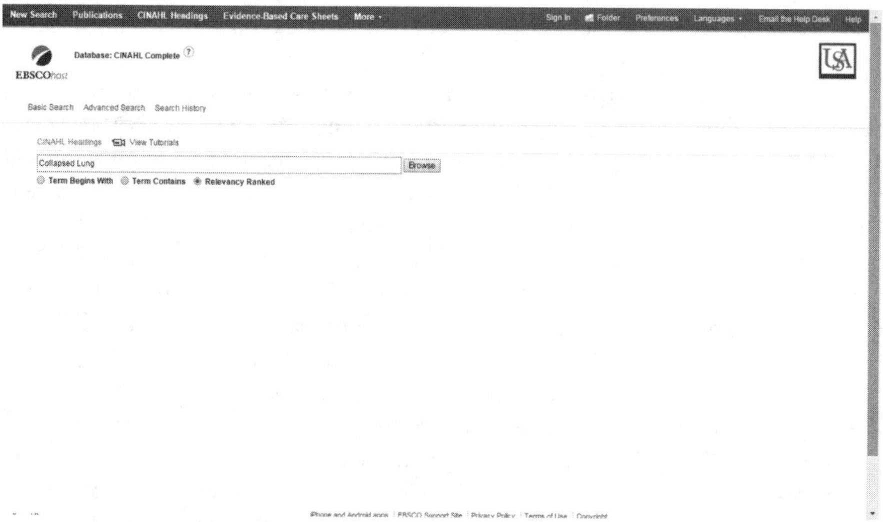

■ Figure 15-1 The CINAHL Headings Search Page With Search Phrase *Collapsed Lung* Entered in the Search Box

Reproduced from EBSCO (https://www.ebsco.com/).

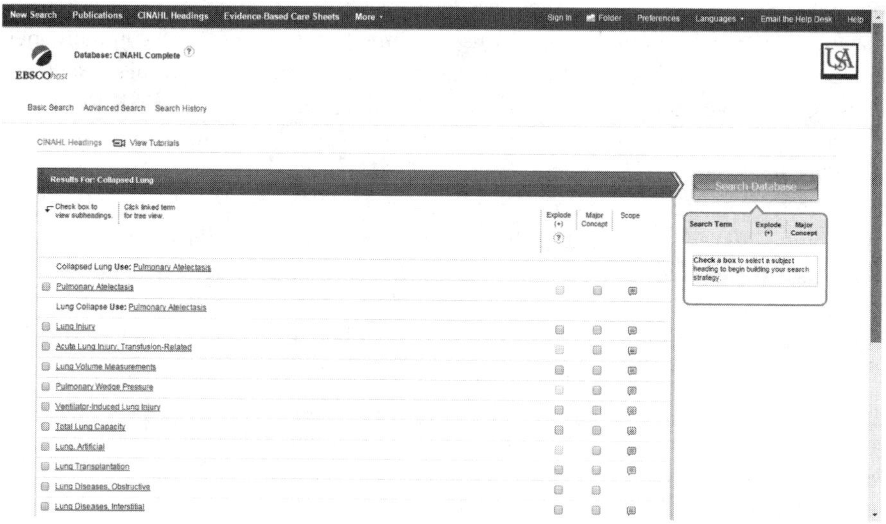

■ Figure 15-2 Results of Search from Figure 15-1, Showing the Search Phrase *Collapsed Lung* Mapped to *Pulmonary Atelectasis*, the Most Relevant CINAHL Heading

Reproduced from EBSCO.

evidence-based hierarchy, including randomized controlled trials, systematic reviews, and meta-analyses.

CINAHL has two major search functionalities: Basic Search and Advanced Search. Both allow searching via keyword (*natural language*) and via CINAHL Headings. On its main search page, CINAHL Basic Search has one search box (or *find fields* to use the terminology of EBSCO, the parent company of CINAHL), whereas CINAHL Advanced Search allows for up to 12 search boxes. In addition, CINAHL Advanced Search has a larger number of limiters, plus the added functionality of Guided-Style Find fields, a means of searching by field codes, such as AU-Author or TI- Article Title. Because of these extra search capabilities, CINAHL Advanced Search can produce a more focused, refined, and specific search result.

CINAHL Headings, as described earlier, are a controlled vocabulary system (or thesaurus) similar in function and structure to the US National Library of Medicine's MeSH. CINAHL Headings incorporate MeSH as the standard vocabulary for disease, drug, anatomical, and physiological concepts. Developed to reflect the research needs of nursing and allied health professionals, the approximately 15,000 CINAHL Headings that index the literature contained in the CINAHL database provide a more effective and thorough search than a keyword search. In addition, there are thousands of cross-references that assist in finding the most appropriate subject heading.

To search by CINAHL Headings, the searcher types a search term in the search box, which is then mapped to the most relevant CINAHL Heading. Search results may be narrowed by a number of very useful limits/limiters, the more common ones being date, author, publication (e.g., *Journal of Advanced Nursing*), journal subset (e.g., nursing), and age group. Several CINAHL Headings are related to evidence-based practice, including *Professional Practice, Evidence-Based,* which includes *Medical Practice, Evidence-Based, Nursing Practice, Evidence-Based, Occupational Therapy Practice, Evidence-Based,* and *Physical Therapy Practice, Evidence-Based.* Furthermore, linked to the top sidebar of the main search page in both Basic and Advanced Search are the *Evidence-Based Care Sheets,* which are short, practical summaries on various topics.

In addition, CINAHL has several limiters that are very helpful in finding evidence-based materials, including *clinical trial, randomized controlled trial, systematic review, meta-analysis, meta synthesis, evidence-based care sheet, case study,* and *practice guideline,* among others. These limiters are found under the Publication Type box on the Limits page. Recently, CINAHL has developed a CINAHL Heading for *meta synthesis.*

▪ Example of a Search in CINAHL

To demonstrate the search capabilities of CINAHL, the same search was performed in two different search functionalities of CINAHL: CINAHL Advanced Search using CINAHL Headings and CINAHL Advanced Search using keywords.

The search:

In elderly patients, does supplementation with vitamin D reduce the risk of accidental falls? Results should be from the last 5 years, representing the highest level of evidence possible.

Because the question is in Patient Intervention Comparison Outcome (PICO) format, it is helpful to break it down into its elements—for example, elderly (P), supplementation with vitamin D (I), and fall reduction (O). Accordingly, each of the three search terms (*elderly, vitamin d,* and *falls*) was entered individually in the CINAHL Headings search box. *Elderly* mapped to the CINAHL Heading *Aged,* (which included three subheadings: *Aged, 80 and Over, Aged, Hospitalized,* and *Frail Elderly*). *Vitamin D* mapped to the CINAHL Heading *Vitamin D,* and finally, *Falls* mapped to *Accidental Falls.* All three resulting CINAHL Headings were *exploded,* added to the search, and connected by the Boolean connector AND. (Exploding a term means that the search will retrieve all references indexed to that term, in addition to all references indexed to any narrower term. To illustrate, exploding the CINAHL Heading *Aged* will add the three subheadings, as described earlier, to the search.) A total of 248 results were retrieved; however, after limiting the date to the last 5 years and the publication type to *Meta-analysis,* three results were retrieved, as demonstrated in **Figure 15-3**. For the keyword search, the three search terms (*elderly, vitamin d,* and *falls*) were each entered into a separate search box on the main CINAHL search page, as demonstrated in **Figure 15-4**. A total of 128 results were retrieved; however, with the two limiters used previously (i.e., last 5 years, meta-analysis publication type), the total number of results was only 1. To conclude, this search demonstrates the advantage of the controlled vocabulary search using CINAHL Headings over a simple keyword search, which resulted in a much smaller number of relevant results.

MEDLINE
Website: http://www.ncbi.nlm.nih.gov/pubmed/
MEDLINE is one of the world's leading databases for biomedical research. It is developed by the U.S. National Library of Medicine (NLM), which also provides free access via PubMed. MEDLINE is a comprehensive database, with more than 22 million references from over 5600 journals in the fields of life science and health, including medicine, nursing, dentistry, veterinary medicine, healthcare systems, public health, and preclinical sciences. Although MEDLINE is not limited to evidence-based information, it is possible to limit a search to retrieve results with an evidence-based focus. Similar to CINAHL, MEDLINE is a good place to find studies from the lower level of the hierarchy of resources, including randomized controlled trials, systematic reviews, and meta-analyses.

MEDLINE provides coverage for materials from 1946 to the present, adding from 2000 to 4000 references each day. For citations published in 2010 or later, over 90% are published in English (although MEDLINE provides citations for articles in

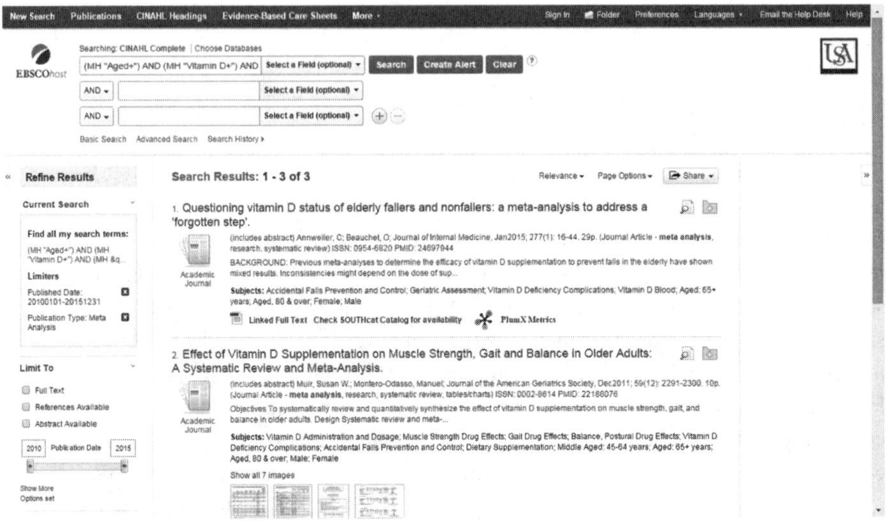

■ Figure 15-3 Results of CINAHL Subject Heading Search
Reproduced from EBSCO.

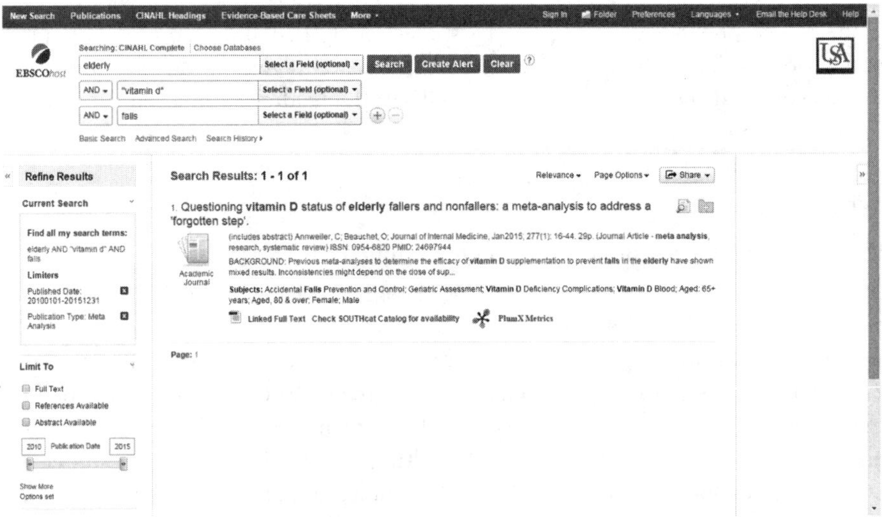

■ Figure 15-4 Results of CINAHL Keyword Search
Reproduced from EBSCO.

40 languages), and approximately 40% of the citations are for articles published in the United States.

The majority of the publications covered in MEDLINE are searchable via PubMed, a free database also produced by the NLM. Using PubMed, MEDLINE can be searched in several different ways, both by keyword (*natural language*) and by the MeSH (*MEdical Subject Heading*) controlled vocabulary/thesaurus system developed by the NLM. With a MeSH search, the search term (*user query*) is matched to the most relevant MeSH heading via automatic term mapping, thus improving retrieval performance.

PubMed provides mainly citations and abstracts but does not include full-text electronic access to many articles. However, the option for institutions such as libraries to link out to the full text content of subscribed journals is available. In addition, numerous vendors provide a fee-based subscription to MEDLINE in which the electronic full-text version for many of the journals and articles indexed in MEDLINE are included. For example, EBSCO's MEDLINE with Full Text provides the electronic full-text versions for more than 1400 indexed journals. Ovid, Web of Knowledge, and Proquest are additional databases that provide full-text access to many of the citations in MEDLINE, for a fee. Finally, individual journal articles can be ordered for a fee per article through the Loansome Doc Article Ordering Service, provided by the NLM.

Like CINAHL, PubMed has several limits, or *filters*, that are very useful in locating evidence-based materials, including *Clinical Trial, Meta-Analysis, Practice Guideline, Randomized Controlled Trial, Systematic Review, Controlled Clinical Trial,* and *Guideline.* These filters are all found under the *Article Types* heading on the left sidebar of the search results page, as shown in **Figure 15-5**. At this time, there is not a filter for *Meta-synthesis;* however, the following search string is very effective in returning results: **"meta synthesis" OR metasynthesis OR meta-synthesis**. If, for example, the user is trying to find a meta-synthesis on mental illness, a productive search strategy in PubMed is as follows: **Mental Disorders [MeSH] AND ("meta synthesis" OR metasynthesis OR meta-synthesis),** which returned 51 results (see **Figure 15-5**).

PubMed Clinical Queries

Website: http://www.ncbi.nlm.nih.gov/entrez/query/static/clinical.shtml

PubMed Clinical Queries is an efficient and useful means of locating evidence-based materials in PubMed. Using preset filters developed by R. Brian Haynes of McMaster University, Clinical Queries restricts searching to specific clinical research topics. Clinical Queries has three search engines, two of which are especially useful for locating evidence-based materials: *Clinical Study Categories* enables searching by one of five clinical categories: etiology, diagnosis, therapy, prognosis, and clinical prediction guide (see **Figure 15-7**), whereas *Systematic Reviews* displays citations for systematic reviews, meta-analyses, reviews of clinical trials, evidence-based medicine, consensus development conferences, guidelines, and citations to articles from journals specializing in review studies of value to clinicians.

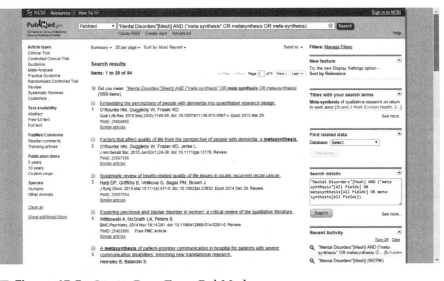

■ **Figure 15-5** Limits Page From PubMed
Reproduced from PubMed.

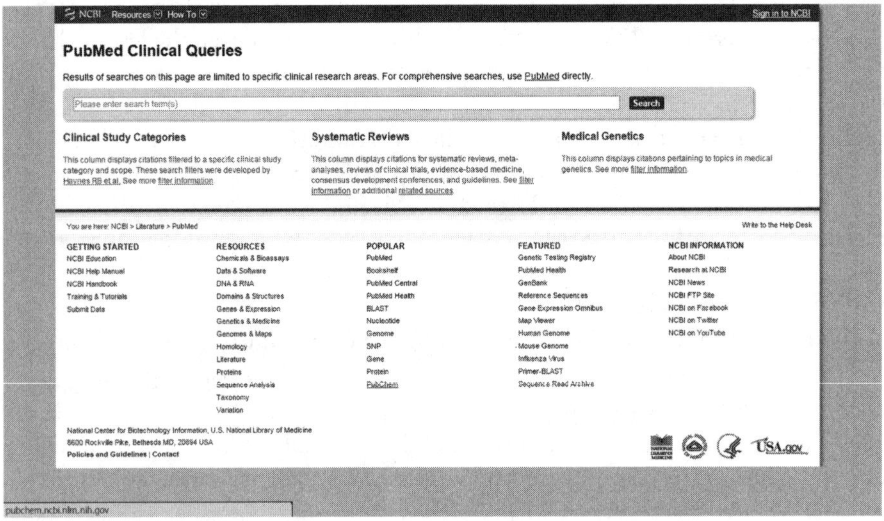

■ **Figure 15-6** Results of PubMed Search, Combining MESH and Keywords, Showing Filter Display
Reproduced from PubMed.

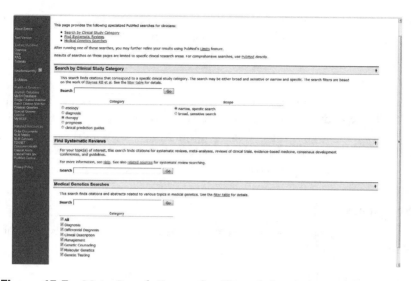

■ **Figure 15-7** Main Search Screen for Clinical Queries

Reproduced from PubMed.

Scopus

Website: http://www.scopus.com/home.url

Scopus is a large citation and abstract database of peer-reviewed research literature (scientific journals, books, conference proceedings) in the sciences, health sciences, life sciences, physical sciences, social sciences, and arts and humanities, providing coverage for more than 21,000 titles. Scopus allows searching both by keyword (via the Document Search tab) and by a system called *indexterms* (via the Advanced Search tab), which are terms assigned to a document by a controlled vocabulary system, such as MeSH from MEDLINE or Emtree from Embase; however, Scopus will not explode MeSH or Emtree terms.

Scopus contains numerous search fields that make it easy to refine a search in order to obtain a narrower, more focused result. As an illustration, a search on the phrase *systematic review* with the search field restricted to *all fields* resulted in 1,092,949 results. Performing the same search with the search field restricted to *article title, abstract, keywords* resulted in 129,402 results, whereas performing the same search with the search field restricted to *keywords* resulted in 95,235 results. Using indexterms, the controlled vocabulary feature available in the Advanced Search tab, performing the search on the word phrase *systematic review* resulted in 89,444 results.

Scopus is another useful resource to locate evidence-based literature, whether searching by keyword or by indexterms. For example, there are indexterms for *meta-analysis, systematic review, randomized controlled trial,* and *clinical trial.* Furthermore, Scopus allows a search to be narrowed via a left-hand sidebar that limits search results by up to 10 categories, including year, author name, subject area, document type, source title, keyword, affiliation, country, source type, and language. Scopus can provide metrics via its excellent citation analysis feature.

■ Synopses of Studies

Synopses of studies summarize well-designed studies in order to be useful to clinical practice. These studies can be located in evidence-based journals, for example, *ACP Journal Club,* (a monthly feature of the *Annals of Internal Medicine,* http://annals.org/journalclub.aspx), *Evidence-Based Medicine* (ebm.bmj.com), *Evidence-Based Nursing* (ebn.bmj.com), and *Evidence-Based Mental Health* (ebmh.bmj.com).

■ Syntheses

Syntheses are systematic reviews. There are several excellent resources for locating studies in this level of the 6S hierarchy.

The Cochrane Library

Website: http://www.cochrane.org/

The Cochrane Library is a collection of databases that contain high-quality evidence designed to be of use in healthcare decision-making. Produced by the Cochrane Collaboration, the Cochrane Library contains the following seven components:

1. Cochrane Database of Systematic Reviews (CDSR)
2. Cochrane Central Register of Controlled Trials (CENTRAL)
3. Cochrane Methodology Register (CMR)
4. Database of Abstracts of Reviews of Effects (DARE)
5. Health Technology Assessment Database (HTA)
6. NHS Economic Evaluation Database (EED)
7. About the Cochrane Collaboration

The primary output of the Cochrane Collaboration, the CDSR, is a preeminent and authoritative resource for systematic reviews in the healthcare field. Reviews included in the CDSR answer a particular research question and are developed using methods found in the *Cochrane Handbook for Systematic Reviews of Interventions.* Reviews are produced by review author teams working in coordination with 1 of the 52 Cochrane Review Groups located around the world, with each group devoted to a particular area of health care. There are five types of reviews, including intervention reviews, diagnostic test accuracy reviews, methodology reviews, qualitative reviews, and prognosis reviews. Some of the reviews contain meta-analyses as well. The CDSR has a very easy to use search interface. Because it is limited to systematic reviews, the CDSR does not have the large number of citations as databases such as MEDLINE or Scopus.

Turning to the other components of the Cochrane Library, the Cochrane Central Register of Controlled Trials contains records of randomized and quasi-controlled trials taken from bibliographic databases such as MEDLINE and Embase. Although it has not been updated since 2012, the Cochrane Methodology Register is a bibliography of publications (articles, books, conference proceedings) that reports on methods used to conduct controlled trials. The Health Technology Assessment Database contains assessments about technology innovations in health care from around the world. DARE contains abstracts of systematic reviews developed outside the Cochrane Collaboration that have been quality assessed. (Although funding both for EED and DARE ended in 2015, DARE can still be accessible via numerous databases.)

Joanna Briggs Institute
Website: http://www.joannabriggs.org

The Joanna Briggs Institute (JBI) is a major resource in the field of evidence-based health care. Based at the University of Adelaide in Australia, the JBI is an international collaboration of clinicians, academics, quality managers, and researchers from nursing, medical, and allied health fields. Its goal is to connect the best available evidence to the point of care through the processes of evidence translation, evidence transfer, and evidence utilization. In a manner similar to the Cochrane Database of Systematic Reviews, JBI has developed a rigorous, standardized framework to appraise and synthesize evidence.

The JBI EBP Database contains over 3000 records across seven publication types (JBI Library of Systematic Reviews, Systematic Review Protocols, Consumer Information Sheets, Evidence Based Recommended Practices, Evidence Summaries, Technical Reports, and Best Practice Information Sheets). In addition, the JBI has resources to develop organizational policy and practice manuals based on the best available evidence.

The Joanna Briggs Institute Thematic Analysis Program (JBI TAP) is available for primary researchers and practitioners in fields such as health, social sciences, and humanities, to assist in the analysis of qualitative research data. In addition, as of 2014, JBI Levels of Evidence and Grades of Recommendation are now being used for all JBI documents. JBI also provides modules to facilitate various evidence-based practice (EBP) studies, including SUMARI (System for the Unified Management, Assessment and Review of Information), QARI (Qualitative Appraisal and Review Instrument), MAStARI (Meta Analysis of Statistics Assessment and Review Instrument), ACTUARI (Analysis of Cost, Technology and Utilisation Assessment and Review Instrument) and NOTARI (Narrative, Opinion and Text Assessment and Review Instrument).

■ Synopses of Syntheses

Synopses of Syntheses summarize and integrate resources from the syntheses level—that is, systematic reviews, and are searchable by keyword in a straightforward and accessible manner. Because they contain neither the large number of resources nor the controlled vocabularies of large databases like CINAHL or PubMed, they do not require complex search strategies to optimize access to information. Synopses of syntheses include the following journals: *ACP Journal Club,* (a monthly feature of the *Annals of Internal Medicine,* http://annals.org/journalclub.aspx), *Evidence-Based Medicine* (ebm.bmj.com), *Evidence-Based Nursing* (ebn.bmj.com), *Evidence-Based Mental Health* (ebmh.bmj.com), and *Evidence-Based Child Health: a Cochrane Review Journal* (http://childhealth.cochrane.org/cochrane-child-health-evidence).

■ Summaries

Summaries include point-of-care resources such as Dynamed (http://www.dynamed .com), UpToDate (http://www.uptodate.com/), Clinical Evidence (http://clinicalevi dence.bmj.com/), and ACP Smart Medicine, plus clinical practice guidelines from the National Guideline Clearinghouse (see later), the Registered Nurses' Association of Ontario (see later), NICE, the National Institute for Health and Care Excellence (http://www.nice.org.uk/guidance), the Canadian Diabetes Association (https://www .diabetes.ca/), and Clinical Key, which includes guidelines.

National Guideline Clearinghouse
Website: http://www.guideline.gov
The National Guideline Clearinghouse (NGC) is a database of evidence-based clinical practice guidelines, guideline syntheses, expert commentaries, and other relevant resources. Guidelines are based on recent systematic reviews. NGC is an initiative of the Agency for Healthcare Research and Quality, US Department of Health & Human Services.

In addition to the resources listed here, there are resources that search across the various levels of the 6S hierarchy. As mentioned earlier, databases such as CINAHL, MEDLINE, and Scopus index and abstract systematic reviews and meta-analyses, for example. Other helpful databases include SUMSearch (http://sumsearch.org/), Epistemonikos (http://www.epistemonikos.org/), MacPLUS (http://plus.mcmaster.ca/Mac-PLUSFS), and TRIP, *Turning Research into Practice* (https://www.tripdatabase.com).

■ Selected Organizations That Support Evidence-Based Practice and Research

Institute of Medicine of the National Academies
Website: http://www.iom.edu
The Institute of Medicine (IOM) of the National Academies of Sciences, Engineering, and Medicine is an independent, nongovernmental organization with the stated goal of improving the nation's health by providing guidance to governmental entities, the private sector, and the public. Specifically, the IOM sponsors activities (forums, roundtables, and standing committees) and prepares studies designed to facilitate discussion on health-related issues. Many IOM studies are prepared at the request

or mandate of Congress and federal agencies. The IOM is very influential in the development of public policy.

The IOM has devoted much of its output to the topic of evidence-based health care, as evidenced by these resources profiled herein.

- *Psychosocial Interventions for Mental and Substance Use Disorders: A Framework for Establishing Evidence-Based Standards* (2015) offers recommendations for those who provide care to individuals with various psychological conditions.
- *Clinical Practice Guidelines We Can Trust* (2011) recommends eight standards to develop trustworthy clinical practice guidelines.
- *IOM: Military Psychological Interventions Lack Evidence* (2014) examines the quality and evidence basis of programs offered by the Department of Defense to prevent negative psychological health outcomes for veterans.
- *A National Model for Developing, Implementing, and Evaluating Evidence-Based Guidelines for Prehospital Care* (2012) discusses a model to improve the quality of EMS care.
- *Evidence-Based Medicine and the Changing Nature of Healthcare* (2008) is a summary of the 2007 IOM annual meeting, which called for a more systematic approach to the role of evidence and its implementation in order to increase the quality and efficiency of medical care.
- *Finding What Works in Health Care: Standards for Systematic Reviews* (2011) is a result of the Medicare Improvement for Patients and Providers Act of 2008, in which Congress directed the IOM to develop standards for conducting both systematic reviews and clinical practice guidelines. In response, the IOM developed 21 standards to ensure objective, transparent, and scientifically valid reviews. The resulting standards address the entire systematic review process, from screening and selecting the lower level studies for review, to addressing how findings are to be synthesized and assessed, to producing the final report.

Other examples of organizations that support evidence-based practice and research include the following organizations.

Agency for Healthcare Research and Quality
Website: http://www.ahrq.gov/

Registered Nurses Association of Ontario: Nursing Best Practice Guidelines
Website: http://rnao.ca

McMaster University, Health Information Research Unit
Website: http://hiru.mcmaster.ca/hiru/

Grey Literature
In performing a search on a topic, a researcher should not overlook *grey literature* that might be useful and relevant to a search. One study estimated that approximately 10%

of all literature cited in scholarly journals tends to be grey literature (Oermann et al., 2008, p. 583). Grey literature includes reports, policy briefs, newsletters, conference proceedings, theses, and dissertations produced by governmental entities, academics, business and industry but not published commercially (Schöpfel, 2011).

The use of grey literature is problematic, however. Because it is not created by commercial publishers and does not tend to find its way into established commercial outlets for publication (such as scholarly journals), grey literature is difficult to locate and, thus, remains hidden, or *fugitive* (Turner, Liddy, Bradley, & Wheatley, 2005, p. 488). As a result, databases such as MEDLINE and CINAHL are unable to index grey literature and provide reliable access (Turner et al., 2005, p. 488).

However, for many scientists, especially in fields in which knowledge changes rapidly, grey literature is often a primary means of communication and an important source of information. Even though it is not peer reviewed, grey literature is critical in helping researchers keep current with developments in their areas of expertise, with one reviewer noting that all literature is grey literature before undergoing the peer-review process and publication (Hooper, 2014, p. 182). In a survey at CERN (the European Organization for Nuclear Research in Geneva, Switzerland), many physicists preferred using grey literature sources and open-access repositories over journal articles or information from commercial databases because these traditional means of scholarship were considered to be too slow to be useful (Hawkins, 2008, p. 28). In addition, omitting grey literature from a meta-analysis might produce a result that is biased, producing a skewed result and possibly overestimating intervention effect (McAuley, Pham, Tugwell, & Moher, 2000, p. 1230).

There are numerous resources for finding grey literature. The Grey Literature Report in Public Health (http://www.greylit.org/), maintained by the New York Academy of Medicine, contains information about grey literature publications and has a searchable database. The System for Information on Grey Literature in Europe (http://www.opengrey.eu/) provides access to 700,000 bibliographical references of grey literature from European sources. The Canadian Agency for Drugs and Technologies in Health (https://www.cadth.ca/) produces *Grey Matters: A Practical Tool for Evidence-Based Searching*, while GreySource is a web portal that provides links to a wide variety of information about grey literature, in addition to producing *The Grey Journal*. (http://www.greynet.org/greysourceindex.html).

■ **Case Study: Dilemma of the Decision Domino Effect**

Created by Susan J. Garpiel, RN, MSN, C-EFM, Director of Perinatal Clinical Practice, Trinity Health

Eileen is an experienced director of a busy labor and delivery unit in a large urban hospital that provides care for more than 5000 births per year. She is an actively engaged leader involved in a multidisciplinary perinatal safety and quality council within a five-hospital consortium. Eight months ago, the leaders made a decision to standardize the concentration and dosing of the oxytocin solution that is used for inducing and augmenting labor. Their decision was based on a review of the perinatal safety literature, recommendations from external consultants, and a thoughtful, unified purpose to reduce high-alert medication errors and improve patient outcomes. Furthermore, the literature identified the potential newborn outcomes of improving newborn Apgar scores, reducing perinatal morbidity and admission to the special care nursery or neonatal intensive care unit.

The decision to standardize the oxytocin concentration provided the hospitals an added benefit to reduce supply costs through high-volume purchasing. However, there were a number of clinical processes that needed to be realigned for a smooth transition from the current solution of 20 units of oxytocin in 1000 milliliters of normal saline to the new solution of 30 units of oxytocin in 500 milliliters of normal saline. The pharmacy processes included reprogramming the infusion pump libraries with the new concentration and replacing the premixed solution stock with the new premixed infusion solution. Clinician labor order sets and policies required revision to accommodate the new standardized concentration. The anticipated implementation date would occur approximately 9 months after the original decision.

As the implementation date was approaching and Eileen was preparing her nursing team to launch the practice change, she began hearing concerns about the new solution's downstream impact on the administration of oxytocin after delivery. Nurses were concerned about the impact of a higher concentration on their postpartum administration practices and the patients' risk for complications from a higher dosage of the drug. Anesthesia providers were unaware that they would not have access to the current premixed solution, and they would need to change their practices. Pharmacy colleagues and the obstetrical providers noted that the postdelivery order sets did not reflect the new solution concentration. Eileen recognized that these concerns were more than the natural cultural response to change; they were valid concerns about patient safety! Reflecting upon the consortium leaders' original decision, Eileen realized that the team's decision to improve the safe administration of oxytocin during labor created a domino effect of increasing the safety risk for the patient after delivery.

Eileen contacted the consortium leaders from the multidisciplinary perinatal safety and quality council to identify if they were encountering the same issues during the implementation of the practice change. The leaders confirmed that their teams had similar concerns about the potential impact on postdelivery workflow processes and patient safety outcomes. Unfortunately, the implementation date could not be delayed further as the solution supply had replaced the previous stock, and the medical record changes were ready to launch in production. This dilemma created an urgent need to develop and implement a short-term plan to mitigate the forecasted risk.

In order to develop a comprehensive plan to address the patient safety and practice concerns, Eileen developed a practice survey to identify the prevalent current processes and practices during the postdelivery period. She believed that the most effective plan would need to take into consideration current workflows and potential bottlenecks and project additional potential downstream impact. The survey results highlighted that there was significant variability among the nursing staff and practitioners regarding the medication bolus and maintenance doses for vaginal and cesarean deliveries. She was concerned that the variability was based on the individual's workflow rather than the current evidence and the patient's clinical condition. In addition, registered nurses (RNs) were operating outside of their scope of practice. In many cases, RNs were determining the oxytocin bolus and maintenance doses and volume of the intravenous infusion because of the lack of standardization and orders to drive patient care. It was evident that continuing their current postpartum management practices with both the current and the new solution concentrations posed significant risk to the patient. This would require immediate action to finalize and communicate a plan before the practice change was operationalized in 2 weeks.

Eileen and the multidisciplinary team considered the data regarding practitioner and nursing workflows and the best available evidence regarding postdelivery oxytocin management. From their analyses, the best solution for the dilemma was to recommend a standardized oxytocin bolus and maintenance dosage for the low-risk postdelivery patients. These dosages would be adjusted if clinically necessary by an obstetrical/gynecological provider order. In addition, these dosages were hard-wired into the postdelivery order sets, thus closing the variability gap revealed in the practice survey. Further, the team determined that postpartum oxytocin would be administered via an infusion pump consistent with high-alert medication practices and the solution and pump settings would require a nurse witness to validate the correct administration of the drug. The implementation plan was well received by the clinical practitioners and nursing staff, with one unforeseen downstream impact. The new practice of using an infusion pump did affect the current supply utilization and cost. However, the risks of not using an infusion pump outweighed the supply cost concern.

Overall, the team was satisfied that the action plan completely addressed the patient safety and practice concerns. They were confident that the new practice would be sustainable with the process changes. The evaluation plan included performing quality monitoring of the process measure "oxytocin order utilization," and the patient clinical outcome measure "postpartum hemorrhage rate" to evaluate the change and the impact. Despite the daunting dilemma that the new safety standardization labor practice created, Eileen and the team believed that it illuminated an unsafe postpartum safety practice that they were able to successfully resolve.

Questions to consider:

1. From the chapter, select an additional tool that may assist a leader in the identification of the downstream impact of the new action plan. What are the benefits of this tool over the practice survey?
2. Which process model or tool would facilitate the leaders in developing the most effective action plan in this scenario? What are the advantages and disadvantages of using this particular model or tool?
3. How would the leaders measure the outcomes and sustainability of this change?
4. What leadership qualities would Eileen need to possess and foster in her team to successfully transition this dilemma into an opportunity for improving quality and safety?

REFLECTIVE ACTIVITIES

1. Why are comprehensive bibliographic databases (such as CINAHL, PubMed, and Scopus) more complicated to search than databases such as DynaMed and the Cochrane Database of Systematic Reviews?
2. Given that grey literature is not peer reviewed, why would researchers want to use it?

REFERENCES

Beall, J. (2008). The weaknesses of full-text searching. *Journal of Academic Librarianship, 34*(5), 438–444.

Cappellari, P., Virgilio, R., & Roantree, M. (2012). Path-oriented keyword search over graph-modeled Web data. *World Wide Web, 15*(5/6), 631–661. doi:10.1007/s11280-011-0153-1

DiCenso, A., Bayley, L., & Haynes, R. B. (2009). Accessing pre-appraised evidence: fine-tuning the 5S model into a 6S model. *Evidence-Based Nursing, 12*(4), 99–102.

EBSCO (https://www.ebsco.com/)

Hall, M., Fernando, S., Clough, P., Soroa, A., Agirre, E., & Stevenson, M. (2014). Evaluating hierarchical organisation structures for exploring digital libraries. *Information Retrieval Journal, 17*(4), 351–379. doi:10.1007/s10791-014-9242-y

Hawkins, D. (2008). Gray literature: what's new on the information landscape. *Information Today, 25*(2), 27.

Hooper, J. (2014). Investigation into the use of grey literature in evidence-based medicine: The role of the NHS Library and Information Services Professional. *Grey Journal (TGJ), 10*(3), 182–183.

McAuley, L., Pham, B., Tugwell, P., & Moher, D. (2000). Does the inclusion of grey literature influence estimates of intervention effectiveness reported in meta-analyses? *Lancet, 356*(9237), 1228.

Melnyk, B. M., & Fineout-Overholt, E. (2011). *Evidence-based practice in nursing & healthcare.* 2nd ed. Philadelphia, PA: Lippincott Williams & Wilkins.

Oermann, M., Nordstrom, C., Wilmes, N., Denison, D., Webb, S., Featherston, D., & Striz, P. (2008). Information sources for developing the nursing literature. *International Journal of Nursing Studies, 45*(4), 580–587.

Schöpfel, J. (2011). Towards a Prague definition of grey literature. *Grey Journal (TGJ), 7*(1), 5–18.

Turner, A., Liddy, E., Bradley, J., & Wheatley, J. (2005). Modeling public health interventions for improved access to the gray literature. *Journal of the Medical Library Association, 93*(4), 487–494.

CHAPTER 16

A Doctor of Nursing Practice Systems Change Project: Educating for Early Intervention in Methamphetamine-Exposed Children and Families

■ SARA C. MAJORS ■

■ Objectives:

- Provide an example of a doctor of nursing practice (DNP) systems change project illustrating integration of research, evidence-based practice, and system change.
- Identify how collaboration yields sustained change and improvement.

This chapter provides an example of how being grounded in clinical practice, knowing how to recognize and appraise research evidence, understanding improvement science, and collaborating yield sustainable quality improvement. Many educational programs, such as clinical nurse leader, executive nurse administrator, and the DNP, provide learning opportunities and experiences in project planning, management, and evaluation. The doctoral project example in this chapter, Educating for Early Intervention in Methamphetamine-Exposed Children and Families, offers an illustration of a synthesis of principles and concepts described throughout this text.

■ Background

When working with children exposed to methamphetamine (meth), I noted ongoing concerns of children in families exposed to meth. Disabilities include lower scores in vision integration, attention, verbal memory, and long-term spatial memory compared to nonexposed children. Children living in violent and neglectful situations experience neglect and stress that negatively affect their growth and physical development, as well as their safety and emotional development (Bauer, 2003). These children often have low self-esteem, poor social skills, and a sense of shame. It is typical for parents of these children to fail to protect these children from harm and to fail to provide the essentials of life including food, shelter, medical and dental care, and hygiene (Anglin, Burke, Perrochet, Stamper, & Dawud-Noursi, 2000; Breslin & McCampbell, 2009; Winslow, Voorhees, & Pehl, 2007). Children's needs include crisis intervention, a medical examination, and placement in a foster home where foster parents are trained to take care of a child affected by meth.

Meth is a dangerous drug, and the threat is rising. The strength of meth has become greater because of refining the development of the drug. Meth is administered via injection, snorting, smoking, or ingesting. It is usually a white, odorless, bitter-tasting powder that melts. The drug is known as "crank, speed, go fast, ice or crystal" (Swetlow, 2003, p. 2). The meth user experiences a quick rush followed by a feeling of euphoria that could last up to 8 hours. Meth stimulates the central nervous system and is made with chemicals from easily accessible products (e.g., medication for cold, weight loss pills, lithium batteries, matches, hydrogen peroxide, gasoline, kerosene, paint thinner, and rubbing alcohol) (Swetlow, 2003).

Dean Max Michael described crystal meth as "a home-grown, do-it-yourself affair" different from cocaine and heroin, which are transported to the United States from other countries (The University of Alabama at Birmingham [UAB] School of Public Health, 2006, p. 2). Meth costs less than other drugs; however, the highs obtained from meth are more powerful and dangerous. The addiction from meth is extreme (UAB School of Public Health, 2006). Meth is a central nervous system stimulant, and its use results in dependence. Health effects of meth use include stroke, cardiac arrhythmia, shaking, anxiety, insomnia, paranoia, hallucinations, and structural changes to the brain (Breslin & McCampbell, 2009; Winslow et al., 2007).

Federal meth lab seizures in the state of Alabama increased from 2 seizures in 1995 to 165 seizures in 2001 (Kraman, 2004). Law-enforcement officials raided approximately one home meth lab per year in the 1990s in a three-county area located in North Alabama. In 2003, officials raided 98 home meth labs in the same area, which is more than raids occurring in eight combined New England states (UAB School of Public Health, 2006).

Meth is the largest drug threat in the state of Alabama. Marijuana remains the drug of choice; however, methamphetamine has exceeded cocaine in abuse throughout the state. An effort of intelligence and enforcement has been introduced in Alabama to recognize key drug trafficking establishments involved in the import of methamphetamine, and the manufacture and distribution as well. Meth labs are located mainly in remote communities. EPIC statistics reported that in 2004 there were 297 meth labs seized, 280 in 2003, and 207 in 2002 (Friends of Narconon, 2016).

In 2005, a law was passed in Alabama that required presenting identification and signing a register to purchase ephedrine and pseudoephedrine (Office of National Drug Control Policy, 2006). Congress passed the Combat Methamphetamine Epidemic Act, and former President George W. Bush signed the act into law under the USA Patriot Improvement and Reauthorization Act (H.R. 3199) on March 9, 2006

(The White House, 2006). Meth made with allergy medication that contains ephedrine and pseudoephedrine, which can be purchased over the counter, is the target of this act. If children are present in the setting where the meth is made, the individual could face time in prison up to 20 years (U.S. Library of Congress, 2006).

From 2002 to 2005, 0.84% of individuals 12 years of age or older residing in the state of Alabama reported the use of meth in the past year. Nearly 3% of individuals aged 18–25 residing in the state of Alabama reported using meth in the past year (Substance Abuse and Mental Health Services Administration, 2006) (see **Figures 16-1** and **16-2**). In 2008, the Drug Enforcement Administration (DEA) reported meth as the number one drug risk in the state of Alabama for the second consecutive year even though the meth lab development has decreased secondary to the sales restriction of pseudoephedrine. However, meth is the most significant drug threat to the state of Alabama. Drug trafficking organized by Mexican drug trafficking organizers has increased the meth supply to Alabama. Meth in Alabama is called "ice," an uncontaminated type of the drug transported from Mexico and Texas. In addition, meth is being transported over the state lines from Georgia by independent dealers (Meth Lab Homes, 2008). The Alabama Department of Human Resources (DHR) is aware of the meth problem in the state and is aggressively working to find solutions.

The percentage of intakes of children from homes in Alabama where meth was used or made increased at an alarming rate from 2005 to 2006. My quest to understand the

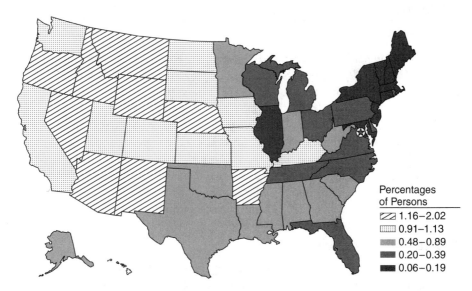

Percentages
of Persons
▨ 1.16–2.02
▦ 0.91–1.13
▨ 0.48–0.89
▨ 0.20–0.39
▨ 0.06–0.19

■ **Figure 16-1** Percentages of Persons Aged 12 or Older Reporting Past Year Methamphetamine Use, by State: 2002, 2003, 2004, and 2005

Reproduced from Substance Abuse and Mental Health Services Administration. (2006). State estimates of past year methamphetamine use. *The National Survey on Drug Use and Health (NSDUH) Report*, 37. Retrieved from http://www.samhsa.gov/data/2k6/stateMeth/stateMeth.htm

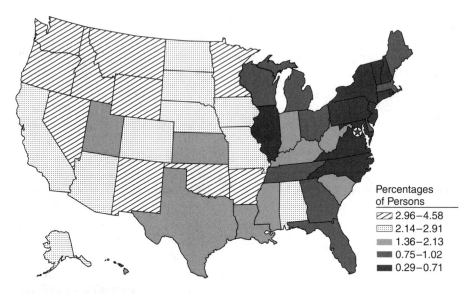

■ **Figure 16-2** Percentages of Young Adults Aged 18 to 25 Reporting Past Year Methamphetamine Use, by State: 2002, 2003, 2004, and 2005

Reproduced from Substance Abuse and Mental Health Services Administration. (2006). State estimates of past year methamphetamine use. *The National Survey on Drug Use and Health (NSDUH) Report,* 37. Retrieved from http://www.samhsa.gov/data/2k6/stateMeth/stateMeth.htm

meth epidemic in northern Alabama led to visits to the counties where meth use figures were high (2006 total/percentage because of meth): Blount (60/25%), DeKalb (72/27%), Cullman (189/22%), Bibb (31/39%), and Marshall (184/40%). Common users identified are low-income, Caucasian, young, old, men, and women. For this project I communicated with A. Jackson, a DHR foster care program specialist employed with the Alabama DHR. The following data were provided: (a) 1492 child welfare staff members in Alabama, and this number included supervisors, directors, and secretarial staff; (b) approximately 1000 social workers and 225 supervisors were employed; (c) approximately 70% female and 30% male among social workers; and (d) more than 5000 children are currently in foster care in Alabama (A. Jackson, personal communication, September 2006).

■ **Selected Evidence**

The inability of a meth-dependent parent to act as a responsible parent and caregiver increases the child's risk for injury or ingesting harmful chemicals. (In one instance, a baby developed cortical blindness from sucking on a bag of crystal meth.) Children of meth abusers may be abused and neglected, and the use of meth by pregnant women leads to a host of developmental disorders in neonates and long-term cognitive deficits in children (Anglin et al., 2000; Breslin & McCampbell, 2009; Winslow et al., 2007).

Meth-exposed children have lower scores compared with nonexposed children in terms of vision integration, attention, verbal memory, and long-term spatial memory. Exposed children have a reduction in brain structures that is correlated with poorer performance on sustained attention (Breslin & McCampbell, 2009; Winslow et al., 2007).

Meth use has tremendous effects on the child welfare system (Breslin & McCampbell, 2009). In a study of 6000 Californian mothers entering treatment, 60% of those active with child protective services cited meth as their primary drug abused (Shillington, Hohman, & Jones, 2001). Additionally, in California children were found in 176 meth lab seizures from 1997 to 1999. From these homes nearly 500 children were removed by child welfare officials. Of the nearly 500, more than one-third of these children tested positive for illicit drugs secondary to their exposure in the home environment. Dependency petitions were filed for 386 of the children and sustained in juvenile court (Oishi, West, & Stuntz, 2000).

The Methamphetamine Interagency Task Force provided several recommendations to improve intra-agency work. The Task Force suggested that jurisdictions share information and promote collaboration in prevention, treatment, education, and law enforcement. Agencies were encouraged to work together, standardize guidelines, and ensure that consideration of the safety of the children, families, and responding personnel was reflected in the procedures (California Governor's Office of Criminal Justice Planning, 2003). When law enforcement officials seize meth labs, healthcare personnel should be immediately available to take care of children when their parents are taken to jail. More foster parents who are willing to function in an emergency are needed. Children's needs include crisis intervention, medical examination, and placement in a foster home (Messina, Jeter, Casey, West, & Rawson, 2014).

Meth may decrease a child's immune defense system, resulting in increased susceptibility to a variety of opportunistic infections. Meth has been known to impair gross motor skills (Winslow et al., 2007; Zickler & Notes, 2002). The process of cooking meth produces a powder-like cloud of drug dust that spreads through the house. Children living in these labs exhibit the same effects they would if they had taken the drug directly (Breslin & McCampbell, 2009; California Governor's Office of Criminal Justice Planning, 2003).

Meth exposure on a developing child's brain was documented by Chang et al. in 2004. The researchers examined the neurotoxic effects of prenatal meth exposure. Using magnetic resonance imaging (MRI), children who were exposed to meth (n = 13) compared to the unexposed control group (n = 15) were evaluated. Quantification of global brain volumes and regional brain structures were completed. Additionally, 10 meth-exposed children and 9 unexposed children were evaluated using neurocognitive assessments. Although no significant difference was found in the children of either group on motor skills, short-delay spatial memory, or measures of nonverbal intelligence, other differences were noted. Specifically, the meth-exposed children scored lower on measures of visual-motor integration, attention, verbal memory, and long-term spatial memory. Additionally, exposed children had smaller putamen bilaterally (−17.7%), smaller globus pallidus (left: −27%, right: 30%), smaller hippocampus volumes (left: 19%, right: −20%), and a trend for a smaller caudate bilaterally (−13%). These findings correlated with associated neurocognitive deficits. The researchers posit that although their findings are preliminary, there is evidence of the possibilities of meth influencing neurotoxicity to the developing brain and the need to investigate further (Chang et al., 2004). Roos, Jones, Howells, Stein, and Donald (2014) conducted a study with children (n = 18) known to have prenatal meth exposure and children not exposed to meth (n = 18) who were matched for age, sex, socioeconomic profile, birth conditions, gestation, and education. The findings suggested significant variations in brain structure. These changes were mostly in the striatal, parietal, and temporal regions in 6-year-old meth-exposed children compared to children in the control group (Roos et al., 2014).

■ Aim of the Project

The aim of this DNP project was to provide education on meth to social workers employed by DHR in the state of Alabama working in foster care.

Purpose

The purpose of this project was to provide educational presentations on meth in five areas chosen by the Alabama DHR to train social workers focused in foster care. The five areas included (1) meth abuse and risks to the community; (2) precautions for persons working with meth users; (3) children exposed to meth: signs, symptoms, and recommendations; (4) adolescents and meth; and (5) family counseling for meth abuse and treatment recommendations.

The five presentation areas served to inform social workers of critical information necessary to work with meth-exposed children to add to the social worker's intake of the children, to better assess the situation, and to offer appropriate treatment alternatives for these children.

Intervention

The first stage of the project included focus groups to gather valuable data, which resulted in understanding that DHR social workers felt helpless and uninformed on how to deal with meth use in families. The educational intervention included face-to-face workshops in the five areas identified by the Alabama DHR. In addition to the five workshops, a compact disc (CD) was developed as a toolkit for these presentations, which served as guide for the social workers to continue improving their efforts to assist these children. This project provided a useful package of summarized evidence to clients in a form that suited time, cost, and care standards. Recommendations were generically termed "clinical practice guidelines" and were provided as presentations in this project. In addition, the project included best strategies for working with and within community resources, as well as best treatment options for the drug user. The important aspects of behavior, cognition, and emotional liability of children exposed to meth were detailed, and the best evidence-based interventions were included.

The proposed outcome of this project was for social workers to have the tools necessary for early intervention and to improve outcomes for children exposed to meth, including school readiness, cognition, and behavior.

■ Conceptualization

Kitson, Harvey, and McCormack (1998) described criteria involved in putting evidence-based research into practice: "(1) the nature of the evidence; (2) the context in which the proposed change is to be implemented; and (3) the mechanisms by which the change is facilitated" (p. 150). Current research is inconclusive as to whether one step is more important than the other two, so they stand as equally essential to the process. Although this is the current standing, the effectiveness of most evidence-based literature is judged by the level and rigor of evidence. When considering useful evidence to make, change, or improve a health practice, there seems to be an imbalance. It is clear that the process that researchers use when putting empirical evidence into practice is complex. It is important to look for a variety of ways of representing the complexity of the process of change and implementing findings. Through their research and development team, the Royal College of Nursing Institute proposed a conceptual framework that demonstrated the interplay of many factors, influencing the way evidence integrates into practice.

■ Implementation

Many steps were included in the implementation of this project: a meeting, focus groups, development of presentations and CD, and evaluation. A meeting was held at the DHR state headquarters on February 7, 2007. At that time, I made a presentation proposing to offer educational programs for social workers in Alabama. Following the meeting, DHR committed to the project, stating that it had not yet begun to educate about meth and wanted the doctoral project for Alabama's care of foster children. The DHR was in the beginning stages of developing educational guidelines for social workers' self-protection. This was the first stage of approaching the meth problem, and the DHR was eager to partner with me.

Focus groups served in understanding the status of DHR employees' knowledge of how to address the meth problems they faced and how this could be used to inform the process. Specific counties were invited to participate in the focus groups secondary to the percent of increase from 2005 to 2006 in the intake of children from homes where meth was made or used. Focus groups were held in the following counties in Alabama: Marion (100%), Franklin (65%), Baldwin (60%), Cherokee (58%), Marshall (40%), and Bibb (39%).

The state office of the DHR took a 2-week period to ask counties what topics should be covered and then agreed that five topics were clearly needed. DHR requested that the information be delivered in the form of live presentations to be offered at different times in four areas of the state. Four podium presentations were given in the following areas in the state of Alabama: Mobile, Huntsville, Birmingham, and Montgomery. A total of 423 participants attended the presentations (see **Table 16-1**). A CD of the presentations was professionally packaged and delivered to each county in Alabama. The evaluation of this project was ongoing and continues today.

It was anticipated that the new educational offerings presented strategies that allowed for early identification of Alabama children exposed to meth. As a result of this project, a change was expected in the manner in which these children and families were managed. For example, frequent drug testing of previous meth abusers was recommended. Drug testing of women delivering in hospitals would be carried out when any drug use was suspected. Children with known exposure would receive early assessment and intervention as needed.

Alabama foster care providers needed sufficient information to be safe when working with families using meth. The presentations informed DHR case workers

Table 16-1   Final Outcomes: Alabama Department of Human Resources Presentations

Location of Presentation	Counties Included	Dates/Times	Participants
Mobile	Mobile, Baldwin, Clarke, Choctaw, Washington, Escambia, Monroe	September 16 9:30 and 1:30	75
		September 18 9:30 and 1:30	62
		October 10 10:30	28 (foster parents)
Huntsville	Cullman, Cherokee, DeKalb, Madison, Limestone, Morgan, Lauderdale, Colbert, Jackson, Marshall	October 16 9:30	32
		1:30	27
Birmingham	Jefferson, Shelby, Bibb, Tuscaloosa, St. Clair, Blount, Talladega, Etowah, Cleburne, Walker, Winston	October 30 9:30	87
		1:30	52
Montgomery	Chilton, Autauga, Dale, Elmore, Bullock, Barbour, Coffee, Lee, Montgomery, Dallas, Lowndes, Chambers, Butler, Houston, Henry, Conecuh	November 1 9:30	35
		1:30	25
			Total 423

to call in law enforcement officers before entering the home of a suspected meth user. DHR case workers were informed about the importance of decontamination for children and themselves. DHR workers were educated on the common problems and challenges faced by exposed children.

Workers learned the danger of approaching a meth user and how to protect themselves when confronted—by retreating and calling officials. Children would be assessed medically and emotionally during the intake period. Families using meth would be referred for drug treatment. Children would be assessed and recommended for early intervention as needed, especially in terms of speech issues, cognitive delays, aggression, and various other symptoms.

Mentor and Team

An interdisciplinary team was identified to assist in the planning, developing, implementation, and evaluation phases of this project. Margaret Bonham, director of the Office of Interagency Planning and Collaboration of the Alabama DHR, served as the candidate's mentor. Andy Jackson and Marie Fain of the DHR participated on the team. They reviewed the project for appropriateness with the goals of the DHR and attended the candidate's presentation. Dr. Teena McGuinness served as faculty advisor. Julie Bellcast of Mobile Mental Health Department and the current president of Mobile County DHR Quality Assurance served as health advisor for drug treatment. Jay M. Wurscher, Alcohol & Drug Services Coordinator in Portland, Oregon, served on the team through email in the same role as Ms. Bellcast. Ms. Rive Ward, MSN, who is an adolescent and child therapist dealing with foster children, evaluated presentations. The interdisciplinary team members collaborated and evaluated the educational presentations as they were written and served as advisors.

■ Impact and Outcomes

Outcome data revealed that 6073 foster children were affected by this evidence-based quality improvement system change focused on early intervention in meth-exposed children and family systems. Alabama foster parents and grandparents also benefitted from this intensive educational offering, which included hands-on conferences and follow-up CDs with screening tools and evidence-based practice guidelines (2017 Alabama foster parents; 2922 grandparents [Kinship Care]). Eleven Alabama children residences were involved, further spreading the intensive educational training. Child welfare staff members (1492) were the target population. Social workers and case workers were coached and counseled using presentations and CDs for further reinforcement of risk factors of meth exposure and strategies to improve safe care for workers, children, and families.

DHR social workers received new information and recommendations for care from the five presentations. It was anticipated that education would lead to social workers being informed, thereby leading to the appropriate referral and treatment of families affected by meth abuse. Secondary to this project, children were assessed and recommended for early intervention as needed, specifically in terms of speech issues, cognitive delays, and aggressive behaviors. Social workers were able to identify the need for early intervention promoting school readiness for meth-exposed children. The project and distribution of the information on a CD to counties in Alabama promoted new awareness of meth and fostered a change in intervention in meth-exposed children, leading to organizational change.

■ Evaluation Plan

The final stage in knowledge transformation is evaluation. Evaluation of the project led to success by providing value-added services to the stakeholders. Evaluation contributes to identifying program risks and reporting findings in a complete and transparent manner. Cultivating and maintaining a strong client service orientation were keys to the evaluation. To do this, this author communicated on an ongoing basis with the counties adopting the guidelines.

The specific needs addressed by the program included the need for greater understanding of meth effects, understanding of decontamination procedures, knowledge of managing children who have been exposed to meth, and information about treatment guidelines. The program sought to improve understanding of the meth problem in Alabama and how to manage it. The program focused on increasing the use of evidence-based teaching and resources in working with meth-exposed children and adults. During the evaluation period, I maintained a partnership with the DHR to facilitate the assessment of the program.

In collaboration with stakeholders and review of evidence on children and meth exposure, evidence-based clinical guidelines were developed and presented face-to-face in five presentations. After the workshops were held, clinical guidelines were adapted and used as local standards for practice. This project represented a beginning effort to change a system for the purpose of educating social workers to better outcomes of children and families exposed to meth. It is anticipated that with this foundational work, the benefits of education related to best practices will improve the protocols across the state of Alabama.

■ Conclusion

This chapter offered an example of a DNP systems change project that incorporated the use of evidence-based guidelines, educational strategies, and interdisciplinary collaboration. Without feedback and input from social workers, families, and state department stakeholders, this project would have fallen short of having an impact on at-risk children with meth exposure. Disseminating results of the project also further spread the information and knowledge and included the following presentations: Doctors of Nursing Practice conference, National Association of Pediatric Nurse Practitioners (NAPNAP) conference, National Association of Neonatal Nurses

(NANN) conference, seminars with the public health department in Mobile and Baldwin Counties, and the Mobile Teachers Conference. I served on the board for the Alabama DHR, Mobile County Foster Care Quality Assurance, and had a faculty practice through the Alabama Department of Human Resources, Mobile County Foster Care. I have continued to work with at-risk foster kids and have completed screens for drug-exposed children since completing this doctoral project. I work 1 day per week with the DHR, screening and interviewing children, families, foster parents, teachers, and social workers to obtain a complete picture of children's delays and problems and then make recommendations related to the children's care. Using my DNP project as a springboard, I continue to fine-tune the screening process, using several mental health instruments. In 2011, I completed a residency at Arizona State University that prepares nurse practitioners in mental health and pediatrics.

REFLECTIVE ACTIVITIES

1. Describe the association among the need for change (background), the aim of the project, and the purpose for undertaking an improvement change.
2. Identify the tools and population necessary to determine the need for a project.

REFERENCES

Anglin, M., Burke, C., Perrochet, B., Stamper, E., & Dawud-Noursi, S. (2000). History of the methamphetamine problem. *Journal of Psychoactive Drugs, 32*(2), 137–141.

Bauer, L. (2003). Work to keep families together: Expert will tell Missouri leaders to focus on parents' strengths, not weaknesses. *News-Leader.* Retrieved from http://springfield.news-leader.com

Breslin, D., & McCampbell, M. (2009). Annotated bibliography on clandestine methamphetamine labs. Community Oriented Policing Services, U.S. Department of Justice. Retrieved from http://www.cops.usdoj.gov/pdf/Annotated-Bibiography.pdf

California Governor's Office of Criminal Justice Planning. (2003). Multi-agency partnerships: Linking drugs with child endangerment. National Criminal Justice Reference Service, U.S. Department of Justice. Retrieved from https://www.ncjrs.gov/App/Publications/abstract.aspx?ID=201359

Chang, L., Smith, L., LoPresti, C., Yonekura, M., Kuo, J., Walot, I., & Ernst, T. (2004). Smaller subcortical volumes and cognitive defects in children with prenatal methamphetamine exposure. *Psychiatry Research, 132*(2):95–106.

Friends of Narconon. (2016). Alabama Fact Sheet. Retrieved from http://www.friendsofnarconon.org/drug_distribution_in_the_united_states/alabama_drug_facts/alabama_factsheet/

Kitson, A., Harvey, G., & McCormack, B. (1998). Enabling the implementation of evidence based practice: A conceptual framework. *Quality in Health Care, 7,* 149–158.

Kraman, P. (2004). Drug abuse in America: Rural meth—Trends alert. The Council of State Governments. Retrieved from http://www.csg.org/knowledgecenter/docs/TA0403RuralMeth.pdf

Messina, N., Jeter, K., Marinelli-Casey, P., West, K., Rawson, R. (2014). Children exposed to methamphetamine use and manufacture. *Child Abuse Neglect, 38*(11), 1872–1883. doi:10.1016/j.chiabu.2006.06.009

Meth Lab Homes. (2008). Meth lab statistics in Alabama. Retrieved from http://methlabhomes.com/meth-lab-statistics-alabama/

Office of National Drug Control Policy. (2006). Pushing back against meth: A progress report on the fight against methamphetamine in the United States. Executive Office of the President of the United States. Retrieved from http://www.nattc.org/resPubs/meth/FINALPushingBackAgainstMethReport.pdf

Oishi, S. West, K., & Stuntz, S. (2000). *Drug endangered children resource center safety manual.* Los Angeles, CA: Drug Endangered Children Resource Center.

Roos, A., Jones, G., Howells, F. M., Stein, D. J., & Donald, K. A. (2014). Structural brain changes in prenatal methamphetamine-exposed children. *Metabolic Brain Disease, 29*(2), 341–349.

Shillington, A. M., Hohman, M., & Jones, L. (2001). Women in substance use treatment: Are those involved with the child welfare system different? *Journal of Social Work Practice in the Addictions, 1*(4), 25–46.

Substance Abuse and Mental Health Services Administration. (2006). State estimates of past year methamphetamine use. *The National Survey on Drug Use and Health (NSDUH) Report, 37.* Retrieved from http://www.samhsa.gov/data/2k6/stateMeth/stateMeth.htm

Swetlow, K. (2003, June). Children at clandestine methamphetamine labs: Helping meth's youngest victims. *Office for Victims of Crime Bulletin.* U.S. Department of Justice. Retrieved from http://www.ojp.usdoj.gov/ovc/publications/bulletins/children/197590.pdf

The University of Alabama at Birmingham School of Public Health. (2006). Crystal meth use soars. *The Handle: The Magazine of the UAB School of Public Health, 5*(1), 2. Retrieved from http://www.soph.uab.edu/media/SOPHpubs/handle_spring2006.pdf

The White House. (2006). USA Patriot Act. Retrieved from http://georgewbush-whitehouse.archives.gov/infocus/patriotact/

U.S. Library of Congress. (2006). Public Law 109–177: USA Patriot Improvement and Reauthorization Act of 2005. Retrieved from http://thomas.loc.gov/cgi-bin/cpquery/?&dbname=cp109&sid=cp109djs6R&refer=&r_n=hr333.109&item=&sel=TOC_358801&>

Winslow, B. T., Voorhees, K. I., & Pehl, K. A. (2007). Methamphetamine abuse. *American Family Physician, 76*(8), 1169–1174.

Zickler, P., & Notes, N. (2002, April). Methamphetamine abuse linked to impaired cognitive and motor skills despite recovery of dopamine transporters. *National Institute on Drug Abuse, 17,* 1. Retrieved from https://archives.drugabuse.gov/NIDA_Notes/NNVol17N1/Methamphetamine.html

CHAPTER 17

Integrating Research-Based Evidence Into Clinical Practice

■ LINDA A. ROUSSEL, ELIZABETH S. PRATT,
AND HEATHER R. HALL ■

■ Objectives:

- Describe the process of securing research-based evidence that supports scholarly practice.
- Identify strategies for creating a culture of inquiry.
- Outline challenges to creating a culture of safety.
- Describe steps in the project planning process that lead to successful implementation.
- Provide a scholarly project exemplar that incorporates the best of strategic project planning, implementation, and evaluation and integrates research-based evidence.

In healthcare settings, evidence-based practice (EBP) implementation is essential to ensuring that research is utilized by clinical staff. EBP, the problem-solving approach that integrates research into practice, allows clinicians to identify problem questions and process improvement needs. With appropriate resources, clinicians may do research studies and synthesize the evidence to determine intervention strategies based on sound science. Using an EBP approach, clinicians may effectively initiate an outcomes-based best practice project, measure the impact of the change, and hardwire it for sustainability.

In 2010, the Institute of Medicine (IOM) published *The Future of Nursing: Leading Change, Advancing Health,* which identified a need to support research for evidence-based educational practices in order to challenge existing norms (Committee on the Robert Wood Johnson Foundation, 2010). The IOM Committee noted that front-line teams must be empowered to make best practice changes that are patient centered and add value to the workplace. Leaders in health care must support value-added, cost-effective, innovative ways within an interdisciplinary framework that integrates research into practice.

■ Evidence for Implementation of Best Practice

Clinical leaders must be knowledgeable about EBP as a methodology for project planning and implementation. Newhouse (2006) examined the support for evidence-based nursing practice and found that EBP increases knowledge and supports freedom to act autonomously. Being involved in EBP leads clinical staff to develop a sense of professionalism and growth. It also may result in improved job satisfaction and a perception of higher quality of delivered care. Utilizing EBP as a method to improve patient care provides not only optimal patient outcomes but also optimal staff outcomes. Empowering nurses to know and change practice based on the best-known research only leads to a greater sense of ownership in that practice change.

The American Nurses Credentialing Center (ANCC) provides healthcare organizations with standards and resources for promoting practice excellence in nursing. ANCC's Magnet Recognition Program highlights the generation of new knowledge and improvements, in addition to empirical quality results (ANCC, 2011). Employing EBP results in quality care and promotes professional responsibility among nurses. Cronenwett et al. (2007) stated that when nurses are able to describe and demonstrate the use of sound research evidence in their practice and they value the concept, EBP becomes integral to determining best clinical practice and positive patient outcomes. Cronenwett et al. also noted that as nurses become involved in the steps of EBP, they value the need for continuous quality improvement based on the evidence and a sound process improvement system.

■ A Culture of Clinical Inquiry

To successfully implement and sustain EBP in the clinical setting, the culture must support clinical inquiry. The setting must be open for all clinicians to ask the clinical questions. Mutual respect and open communication are essential among all interdisciplinary team members. Collaborative practice among the disciplines leads to improved and sustained outcomes. The environment must be open to change. For example, a nursing division with high staff turnover would not be a preferred pilot study unit. The environment must support resources for clinicians to seek out information and disseminate results. The leadership also must support lifelong learning, to include resources and time for continuing education and implementation of EBP.

To determine the status of the clinical culture and the spectrum of understanding and supporting EBP, consider Evans's (2008) four steps in the culture's language development. The first step is *hearing* the language. When staff hear the language, they begin discussing how EBP is defined and translated into practice in staff meetings, the clinical setting, and leadership meetings. The next step is *recognizing* the process of creating an EBP environment and the implications of sound practice evidence at the point of care, which is essential to improving patient care. Recognizing also includes valuing that research evidence supports scholarly practice. The third step involves *understanding* the new language. In this step, staff and clinicians acknowledge the ramifications of EBP and are interested in translating research at the point of care. Finally, the culture in which we want to implement best practice begins *speaking* the language and actively uses the steps of EBP in daily practice. If the culture is such that staff members are in the hearing or recognizing stage, the charge of implementing research evidence is likely on its way to being a culture of inquiry. Those who are in the understanding and speaking EBP stage are ready to implement into clinical practice the research that has been synthesized and analyzed (Evans, 2008).

An example of understanding and discussing EBP is illustrated in the research study conducted by Walker et al. (2012). The researchers suggested that the use of interactive e-learning to improve capacity for EBP is also an effective strategy. The method consisted of a face-to-face educational intervention converted to a 10-week interactive e-learning program. Commercial software was used and hosted on a learning management system of a local university. Over the 10 weeks, participants completed coursework that integrated didactic content and mentored EBP project development. Two phases were completed during the study. In the first phase, 10 clinical staff members and 2 intervention e-learning mentors participated. The clinical staff completed seven online modules and assignments, including interactive forums using discussion boards. Participants developed projects with their assigned mentor. In phase two, the numbers increased to 14 clinical staff and 13 e-learning intervention mentors. Collected data consisted of demographics, focus groups, and quantitative measures. The quantitative measures and EBP Beliefs and Implementation Scales were completed in a prepost, immediately post, and 6-months post course completion. The results of this study suggested that participants' capacity for EBP increased through e-learning, and most importantly, patient outcomes were improved (Walker et al., 2012). The results of this study provide evidence that a culture of clinical inquiry can be developed using different strategies for improvement.

Evans (2008) developed the following questions to guide the discussion of readiness for change toward creating a culture of clinical inquiry:

1. What do we need to know to safely care for patients?
2. Why do we perform the skills we do?
3. How are the outcomes related to my practice?

A thoughtful reflection on responses from questions related to patient safety in a safe, nonthreatening way goes far in creating a culture of openness and engagement. With an open and therapeutic milieu, the didactics of staff competencies and skill acquisition can be addressed with candor. This provides the opportunity to drill down on the steps in the process and gives staff the ability to carry out the tasks. This approach also provides staff with the opportunity to eliminate unnecessary steps that do not add value to patient outcomes. Connecting value-added practice to patient outcomes underscores the importance of carrying out evidence-based protocols that support quality care. Engaging front-line staff in the process by sharing feedback and acting on the feedback is also critical to creating a culture of safety. By linking EBP to the clinical questions and interest of staff, the project leader can begin to engage staff in a project focused on practice improvement.

■ Addressing Challenges in the Culture

Identifying challenges with implementation prior to the project allows the team to prevent barriers, rather than react to them. A realistic approach to these challenges allows for an honest look at the project feasibility and likelihood of success. The initiative must have appropriately trained EBP mentors who have been educated in all steps of EBP. These individuals will lead the project through all the phases of EBP with confidence. The culture of the environment must support EBP, and the individuals participating in the clinical steps must believe in the project itself, value the process, and support EBP as a method of problem-solving. A lack of resources may deter the implementation of costly initiatives; additional staff and support may be required. All the appropriate stakeholders must be involved as early as possible to ensure that support and resources are available for the EBP project; without appropriate interdisciplinary stakeholders, a project can be successfully initiated but not sustained.

Fink, Thompson, and Bonnes (2005) demonstrated in a descriptive presurvey/postsurvey design that nurses' perceptions of barriers in the organizational culture have an impact on the utilization of research. Findings from the survey included barriers to supporting changing clinical practice, lack of administrative support and mentoring, insufficient time allowed for staff, and a lack of education regarding research utilization. Fink et al. noted that to implement research and EBP in the clinical setting, the environment must make an organizational commitment to providing the time and resources needed to make the practice change. When preparing for project implementation, the leader should assess the culture, considering the following elements:

1. Supportive leadership
2. Organizational infrastructure
3. Resources to implement the project, including clinical staff
4. Communication strategies in the clinical setting
5. Incentives for participating in the project
6. Benefit of project outweighing the risk of implementation

■ Project Site Assessment

A strong clinical department is essential to the success of a project. A department with quality infrastructure but a clear need for improvement is ripe for project implementation. The environment should have energetic staff engaged in quality improvement and EBP changes. Implementing the project on a strong, enthusiastic, and resourceful unit facilitates successful implementation in other clinical settings and further enhances sustained change.

The key to success is building a strong infrastructure and ensuring a just culture before implementing a change. Before implementing the project, the team must ensure that the project aligns with the facility's mission, vision, and values. Knowing the facility's strategic priorities, goals, and resources, as well as conflicts that may occur with other projects, is essential to the success of the project. Helpful tools of evaluation are discussed in Advisory Board's *Leading Change: Implementing Improvements in the Health Care Organization* (2008). Reviewing the possible impact, assessing personal conviction and stakeholders, and building a communication plan allow best practice teams to assess the project environment prior to implementation.

Before project implementation, the project leader needs to assess the capability of the team. The project leader should consider the following questions:

1. Does the team have a clear leader with an outlined time frame and roles and responsibilities of project management?
2. Do the team members have the time and commitment available to implement this project?
3. What sort of outcomes measurement is expected?
4. Will this make an impact, whether positive or negative?
5. What are the expectations of communication during and after the project implementation?

■ Project Planning

Project planning involves a number of components, including interdisciplinary team development. Lewis (2011) described steps in the project planning process and considered strategy as an overall approach to a project. This is the "playbook" or template that details exactly how the work will be accomplished. Without strategic planning, work may be duplicative and redundant, thereby increasing costs of material and personnel resources. Project strategy and technical strategy are aligned, yet different from a theoretical and didactic perspective. The project strategy identifies the "what" that needs to be done (project aim), whereas the technical strategy describes the "how to" of the project planning process. Risk analysis and an assessment of the strengths, weaknesses, opportunities, and threats (SWOT) are part of the hierarchy in this stage of the planning. Process maps and work breakdown structures are excellent tools in this phase of project plan development (Lewis, 2011). Cost-benefit analysis of alternative strategies within the project plan are also considered in the process. Developing a budget aligned with the strategic plan and resources available is the cornerstone of successful project implementation. Considering contingencies and possible barriers and planning accordingly give the team a stronger sense of successful project planning; thus, implementation and overall positive outcomes are more likely to follow. This approach involves creating a timeline of the processes and delegating responsibilities up front and along the way as the project evolves over time.

As the team develops the strategic plan and maps out the steps based on analytical processes, roles are assigned based on competencies, skill sets, and positioning within the organizational system. The use of research-based evidence that is critically appraised with an eye toward implementation within an interdisciplinary team perspective further validates the value-added dimension of the project plan.

▪ Project Implementation

Selecting a theoretical framework to implement a practice project is important to the scientific underpinnings of a professional practice. It is important to use the EBP steps in the process and focus on sound research on the topic. Improvement science incorporates a scholarly approach to performance. Lean strategy, Six Sigma, and a Plan-Do-Study-Act (PDSA) improvement cycle are essential to the holistic approach to improvement change and sustainability of a best practice (Langley, Nolan, Nolan, Norman, & Provost, 2009; Simmons, 2002).

Additional project management tools and strategies include the following (Melnyk & Fineout-Overholt, 2005; Newhouse, 2006; Stevens, 2004):

1. Developing the clinical or practice question based on the aim(s) of the project. The team may want to use an evidence-based model perspective with a patient/population, intervention, comparison, and outcomes (PICO) framework that will likely guide the team in reflective thinking, problem-solving, and decision-making (Langley et al., 2009).

2. Using the PICO or other evidence-based framework moves the team into determining the gaps or variations in the practice. Understanding quality improvement and improvement science methodology strengthens the case to be built for proceeding with project development, implementation, and evaluation.

3. Reviewing existing standards and evidence-based protocols requires an extensive (or selected) review of the research literature. Critically appraising the research evidence and synthesizing the strongest evidence support credibility of the project.

4. Once the research evidence is provided in a succinct, user-friendly way (evidence-based guidelines, protocols, policy/procedures), the team moves to the next phase of implementation. Using PICO, the team considers outcomes and strategies to evaluate (analyze) indicators for successful implementation.

5. Assessing the organization's culture, structure, communication channels, and systems in place is crucial to successful implementation. Assessing the organization's readiness for change and readying the environment for change must involve the stakeholders, change champions, and opinion leaders and consider how the organization has managed change in the past. Considering the context of the change, the change itself, and the individuals involved in the change goes far in successful implementation and, more important, spread and sustainability (Gladwell, 2000).

6. Incorporating strategic interventions with outcomes that are measurable is a cornerstone of mapping out the process. Establishing responsibilities and accountabilities for the various stages in the process ensures consistency in implementation. Additionally, determining methods of collecting data and setting up data points along the way provide the depth and breadth of information necessary to understand the gestalt of the change. Determining a timeline for ongoing monitoring and check-ins is important in removing barriers that may arise despite the most careful planning (Lewis, 2011). Institutional review board approval will be necessary if the team wishes to disseminate its work outside the organizational system. This is strongly advised because lessons learned about the collaborative efforts and changes made along the way are invaluable to the team and others wishing to pursue similar outcomes within their practice systems.

7. Outcomes and other indicators of the project's success (practice change) are developed in tandem with the performance improvement cycle. The use of valid and reliable tools and instruments—for example, fall and pressure ulcer screening tools, quality-of-life surveys, and patient and staff satisfaction questionnaires—is essential to the credibility of the team's work. The evaluation of the project must hold up to scrutiny and involve the use of rigorous statistical tools and methods; patient care safety and quality depend on these very important components of project planning.

8. Team members must be able to share their results in a clear, succinct, and comprehensive way, thus affording others the opportunity to benefit from the wisdom and efforts of this important work.

9. Spreading the change, hardwiring the processes, and sustaining improvement over time are the hallmarks of the ultimate success of the quality improvement project initiative (Langley et al., 2009; Studer, 2005).

An exemplar of a scholarly doctoral project is provided. The preceding tools and strategies were used as a guide to integrate research-based evidence into clinical practice. The doctoral student integrated all components of project planning from a theoretical, evidence-based, and quality improvement perspective.

Brainstorming

In 2007, the TCAB program was started on the pilot unit at the target facility, one of 67 hospitals in the United States chosen to participate. Brainstorming new ideas for quality improvement, a key component of TCAB (Rutherford, Moen, & Taylor, 2009), encouraged the front-line staff to make observations and formulate strategies for decreasing the incidence of MDROs transmitted via cross-contamination on the unit. The "snorkel" (deep-dive) sessions generated a creative possible solution to the problem: as a rapid test of change, staff decided on the idea of an isolation kit for use when patients are placed on transmission-based precautions. The staff were instrumental in drilling down the contents of the kit based on identified barriers: ordering isolation precaution equipment individually caused delays in necessary items making it to the bedside; writing pens were used in isolation rooms and then put in the uniform pocket; "pain" boards (a sustained result of the TCAB initiative) in all patient rooms required use of a whiteboard marker to communicate vital information regarding pain management and list the care providers for the shift; and antibacterial wipes were noted to be in short supply and were not always readily available for decontamination of medication computers, vital sign machines, and other items between patients. After the discussions, finalized contents of the isolation kit were a disposable stethoscope, disposable thermometer, disposable blood pressure cuff, whiteboard marker, writing pens, Clorox wipes, patient/family teaching materials, and an isolation door sign for the patient room. All items in the kit were designated for disposal following patient discharge.

Staff Education

Prior to project implementation, education regarding transmission and prevention of MDROs, review of hospital infection control policies, and the procedure for use of the kit was provided for the staff of the target unit. The staff included registered nurses (RNs), licensed practical nurses (LPNs), PCAs, and student nurses. The staff on all shifts were given a PowerPoint presentation at a time during the shift that allowed for the greatest participation. The nurses were awarded one continuing education unit for program attendance.

Tools

A preeducational and posteducational intervention test was developed to measure staff knowledge related to MDROs. The test included questions about transmission, prevention, and isolation procedures at the target facility. Not included in the original project plan but added to the posttest were additional questions related to TCAB principles such as value-added processes, patient-centered care, safe and reliable care, vitality of teamwork, and staff satisfaction with the project (Stefancyk, 2009a, 2009b, 2009c, 2009d). The answer response was displayed on a 6-point Likert scale. The purpose of the questions was to elicit staff satisfaction with the systems change and to evaluate the TCAB aims. The answer responses were offered on a 6-point Likert scale, in which 0 was *strongly disagree* and 6 was *strongly agree*. The scores ranged from 5 to 5.6, indicating a strong staff satisfaction related to the rapid test of change.

A tool for measuring patient satisfaction was developed that adhered to the requirements established by the National Quality Measures Clearinghouse. The survey was formatted based on the recommendations of the Clinician & Group Survey and Reporting Kit 2007 using Arial 12-point font, a specific type of column design, and a 6-point scale to increase readability (Consumer Assessment of Healthcare Providers and Systems, 2007). The survey consisted of six questions. An additional tool was crafted for monitoring staff compliance related to the use and placement of the isolation kits.

The target facility collects data that reflect patient satisfaction using the Hospital Consumer Assessment of Healthcare Providers and Systems (HCAHPS) system. The focus of HCAHPS is the measurement of patient perception that uses a standardized survey tool and data collection method related to care provided in hospitals (HCAHPS, 2010). HCAHPS survey results are available on a quarterly basis. A survey reflecting HCAHPS was constructed to obtain timely data for manuscript completion.

Analysis/Results

Project Aim I: Decrease in Hospital-Acquired Methicillin-Resistant *Staphylococcus aureus*—Safe and Reliable Care and Value-Added Processes

The target facility reports data related to HAIs to the NHSN. Using MRSA as marker data from July 2010 through December 2010, 18% of the patients with MRSA on the target unit were victims of cross-contamination. From January 2011 through March 2011, the incidence rate of HAI MRSA was 10%. Data displayed on a run chart revealed a tight control of the incidence of HAI MRSA. The lines were straight, with no spike above or below the upper or lower control. A steady state of zero incidence of HAI MRSA, moving closer to the lower control, would be the goal. The isolation kits were implemented on the target unit April 11, 2011. The time period following project implementation through the end of May 2011 yielded a HAI MRSA cross-contamination rate of 0%.

Initially, daily rounding for process evaluation was performed to determine compliance in an effort to delineate the effect of the DNP project on infection and cross-contamination rates. The frequency of rounding decreased as the project continued and staff buy-in increased. Overall compliance was 100%; every patient admitted or placed on isolation precautions during the project period had the isolation kit placed in the patient isolation room. During rounding, the patient rooms were audited to determine if all items in the isolation kit were available in the patient room for use. Periodically, items were missing from the patient room. The compliance data on individual items ranged from 91% to 99%, indicating early and sustained stakeholder participation. The data related to each item are displayed in **Figure 17-1**.

Project Aim II: Increase in Staff Knowledge—Vitality and Teamwork

Prior to project implementation, education was provided to the staff of the target unit. The staff were given a pretest for knowledge assessment. Education continued throughout the implementation process; the PowerPoint presentation was made available to all staff via email, flyers were posted on the unit, and a copy was placed in the unit staff communication book. The posttests were made available via the change champions for a 2-day period to allow access for all staff members. The staff members who completed the pretest consisted of 19 RNs, 9 certified nursing assistants, 1 LPN, and 1 unknown. The return rate on the posttest was 42%. The mean score

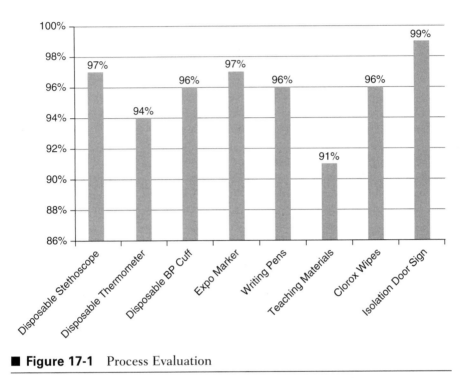

■ **Figure 17-1** Process Evaluation

on the pretest was 77%, and the mean score on the posttest was 93%, representing a 22% increase in staff knowledge. The plan for tracking pretest and posttest scores was to have a self-assigned identifier entered on each test. On the posttest, the staff did not use the self-assigned identifiers, rendering the data unsuitable for significance calculations. **Figure 17-2** depicts the increase in staff knowledge.

Overall, staff reported strong agreement with all points addressed. The scores ranged from 5 to 5.6, indicating strong staff satisfaction related to the rapid test of change—notably, statements indicating delivery of a higher quality of patient care, more time available for direct patient care, the perception of value given to staff suggestions, and increased compliance with isolation precautions.

Project Aim III: Increase in Patient Satisfaction— Patient-Centered Care

Before and after, patient satisfaction data were collected, analyzed, and compared using a one-tailed t-test with determination of significance levels. No significant improvement was noted for overall healthcare rating or trust for doctors and nurses to provide the best care possible. Areas that significantly increased were patient education, inclusion in decision-making, taking an active role in care, and feeling that the doctors and nurses were concerned with patient feelings regarding isolation.

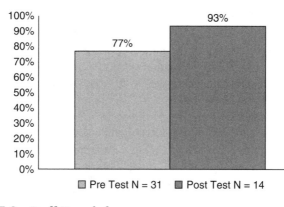

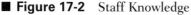

■ **Figure 17-2** Staff Knowledge

■ Discussion

The project was effective in achieving the aims of a decrease in HAI MRSA transmitted via cross-contamination. Prior to the systems change project, obtaining items necessary for adherence to isolation precautions required arduous searching on the part of busy staff and was therefore likely not done consistently. Because no policy was in place for patient-dedicated writing pens, whiteboard markers, or antibacterial wipes, the items were often transferred, along with the resident organisms. The isolation kit provided a convenient method for obtaining items for adherence to isolation precautions, streamlining workflow processes. Nurses found the isolation kits easy to access and use, making adherence to isolation precautions very convenient. This led to high levels of compliance with best practices for the prevention of cross-contamination.

Staff overall compliance with use of the kits was high. Initial daily rounding and frequent presence on the unit maintained high visibility for the project coordinator. The front-line staff members, two change champions per shift, and managers were engaged. The pilot unit never depleted the supply of kits because the project coordinator ensured sufficient quantity.

The writing pens were custom ordered in a distinct color and shape and were stamped with the project title and instructions not to remove them from the room; no pens were ever discovered outside of patient isolation rooms and were in the room 96% of the time. The Clorox wipes were often found nearly empty and subsequently replaced, giving credence to the assumption that availability of supplies increases compliance with isolation precautions.

The staff satisfaction with the change was evidenced by positive scores on the staff satisfaction survey completed. TCAB principles, including brainstorming, snorkeling, and rapid test of change, engaged the front-line staff and improved staff perceptions of importance and worth, leading to compliance that exceeded expectations.

The increase in staff pretest and posttest scores indicates an increase in staff knowledge related to transmission and prevention of MDROs. The 42% return rate on posttests may be a result of the nurses' apprehension regarding testing, perhaps because they feared punitive measures. The pilot unit was an extremely busy unit, and heavy workload on posttesting days may have been a contributing factor as well.

Patient overall satisfaction with care provided and with trust in healthcare providers to provide the best care did not significantly increase; the scores were favorable before project implementation, with little room for improvement. Patients and family members frequently commented on the high-quality care provided by the target unit staff. Scores increased with significance in the education, decision-making, and patient participation in care areas.

A substantial savings may be incurred with a reduction in HAI MDROs. From July 2010 through December 2010, the target unit reported seven cases of HAI MRSA. Using the cost estimate range—$6000 to $40,000 for treating a single patient with MRSA—the savings would range from $42,000 to $280,000 if cross-contamination had been prevented on a single unit for a 6-month period. The negligible cost of an individual isolation kit for the project was $18.46. The unit was able to perform a rapid test of change with fast, time-saving evaluation regarding the decision to adapt, adopt, or abandon the project. The project effectively addressed the IOM aims of safe and reliable care by showing a decrease in the incidence of HAI MRSA. Patient-centered care was improved, as evidenced by increased patient satisfaction scores. Efficient, timely, and effective care was achieved in part by providing a streamlined process of obtaining items necessary for adherence to isolation precautions, decreasing the rate of HAIs and extrapolating to a decrease in cost and patient length of stay.

■ Conclusion

Contact precautions are necessary for all patients suspected of MRSA infection/colonization. Processes and tools for enhancing best practice guidelines for preventing the spread of infection via cross-contamination, such as the rapid test of change and isolation kit implementation, should become a part of the total system culture. In a time when more is demanded of fewer staff, tools to improve workflow processes must be implemented.

Nurses caring for patients with existing or new-onset MRSA must communicate to patients and family members the measures necessary for preventing the spread of the infection. Educational materials for patients should be conveniently placed to improve workflow and nurse compliance. Educated patients will become empowered to take an active part in preventing the spread of MDROs in healthcare facilities and the community (Noble, 2009; Romero, Treston, & O'Sullivan, 2006).

The findings from the project have implications for the nurse executive. Indirect costs associated with increased retention rates alone are substantial. Savings can be compounded by decreasing length of stay and treatment costs. With the current movement by third-party payers to withhold payment for preventable events, the time is coming when HAI MDRO infection will no longer be reimbursed.

This chapter described integrating research-based evidence into clinical practice within quality improvement and project planning frameworks. The creation of a culture of inquiry focused on EBP methods further enhances interdisciplinary collaboration and team development.

■ Exemplar One: The Bug Stops Here: Preventing the Spread of Multidrug-Resistant Organisms via Cross-Contamination

Debra Swanzy

Background

The National Nosocomial Infections Surveillance (NNIS) System Report (National Nosocomial Infections Surveillance System, 2004) reported that the number of infections among hospitalized patients caused by organisms resistant to traditionally used antibiotics has risen in spite of extensive efforts to control the spread of such organisms. Multidrug-resistant organisms (MDROs) at one time affected only the most critically ill patients in hospitals, but MDROs are increasingly identified as the cause of infections among a large number of hospitalized patients who are significantly less ill (Weber & Soule, 2009). The leading cause of death in the world and the third leading cause of death in the United States is infectious disease. Of the organisms that cause healthcare-associated infections (HAIs), 70% are resistant to one or more commonly prescribed antimicrobials (Muto et al., 2003). An estimated 250,000 patients in the United States experience bacteremia related to HAIs annually, of which the rate of mortality is 35% and length of patient stay is increased by 24 days. The general cost of care for a patient who has developed methicillin-resistant *Staphylococcus aureus* (MRSA) is approximately $6000 to $40,000 higher than for patients with antibiotic-susceptible infections (Aragon, Sole, & Brown, 2005; Cosgrove, 2006). If the patient requires isolation precautions, nursing hours are increased and further costs are incurred. The estimated financial burden of treating HAIs in the United States is between $17 and $29 billion annually (Aragon et al., 2005).

Two factors have been identified as the major driving force behind the proliferation of MDROs. The first factor is physician or other prescriber misuse or overuse of antibiotics. The effect of misuse or overuse of antibiotics is the formation of strains of organisms that are able to avoid the killing mechanisms of the drugs, allowing for continued reproduction of the organism. The transmission of MDROs from patients, either colonized or infected, to others is the second factor

(continues)

contributing to the explosion of MDROs. The most common site for the transmission of the organisms is healthcare facilities, in which the number of individuals carrying the resistant organisms is higher than in the population at large (Weber & Soule, 2009).

Trials have been conducted on many measures aimed at preventing transmission of MDROs, including campaigns to improve hand hygiene compliance, addressing contaminated equipment, appropriately identifying isolation precautions, and implementing aggressive surveillance interventions (Creamer et al., 2010; Cummings, Anderson, & Kaye, 2010; Davis, 2009; Harbarth, Pittet, Grady, & Goldmann, 2001; Henderson, 2006; Lederer, Best, & Hendrix, 2009; Lowe, 2004; Muto et al., 2003; Walker, 2007). However, the incidence of MDROs continues to increase (National Nosocomial Infections Surveillance System, 2004).

Purpose

The purpose of the systems change project was to decrease the number of hospital-acquired MDROs transmitted by cross-contamination in a 406-bed acute care teaching hospital in Mobile, Alabama. The aims of the project were a decrease in hospital-associated MDRO infections on the target unit, an increase in staff knowledge regarding MDROs and the modes of transmission and prevention methods, and an increase in patient satisfaction with care provided. The pilot unit was the sixth floor, a 35-bed medical-surgical unit with a population consisting mainly of orthopedic, trauma, and surgical patients.

Unit Processes

The nurses on the pilot unit administer medications using a computerized cart. The cart is moved from room to room regardless of whether the patient is on isolation precautions. Additionally, the patient care assistants (PCAs) and nurses use portable machines for vital sign assessment from room to room. Policies are in place for the cleaning of the equipment.

When a patient is admitted or placed on transmission-based isolation precautions, the nurse or PCA obtains the items necessary for adherence to isolation precaution procedures. Patients who require transmission-based isolation at the time of admission have an indicator flagged on the admitting or face sheet of the patient chart. Patients who are placed on isolation precautions after admittance are reclassified after the nurse receives a phone call from either the laboratory or the infection control nurse. The single-patient–dedicated disposable stethoscopes, disposable blood pressure cuffs, gowns, goggles, and masks (if indicated) recommended by the facility infection control policies must be obtained from the clean supply cart or ordered from central supply. Gloves are readily available in all patient rooms and care areas. Hand sanitizer is available in each patient room as well as several stations in the hallways and medication preparation areas. Teaching materials for the patient and family must be obtained from the hospital intranet and printed for use.

Methods

Needs Assessment

The target facility reports data related to HAIs to the National Healthcare Safety Network (NHSN). The NHSN compiles data on infection rates from more than 300 hospitals that participate on a voluntary basis (Centers for Disease Control and Prevention, 2011). The infection control nurse at the target facility tracks the MDROs *Acinetobacter baumannii,* vancomycin-resistant *Enterococcus, Pseudomonas aeruginosa,* and MRSA. The majority of MDROs at the target facility are MRSA, hence the focus of the data from the pilot unit. From July 2010 to December 2010, 33 patients were admitted to the pilot unit with an existing infection/colonization of MRSA. During the same period, the pilot unit reported seven cases of HAI MRSA. The infection control department had a surveillance system in place for the purpose of monitoring hand hygiene compliance and isolation precaution compliance. Despite high compliance rates, MDROs resulting from cross-contamination occurred. For example, during the month of July and November 2010, hand hygiene compliance was 100% and isolation precaution compliance was 100%, yet two cases of hospital-associated MRSA were reported in each of those months. Juxtaposed, in December 2010, hand hygiene compliance was observed at 100%, isolation precaution compliance was observed at 100%, and no cases of MRSA were reported. The data expose a concern related to the process, given that cases of MRSA were reported when hand hygiene compliance and isolation precaution compliance were at 100%.

■ Exemplar One: Guiding Frameworks

Transforming Care at the Bedside

The principles from Transforming Care at the Bedside (TCAB), an initiative of the Robert Wood Johnson Foundation, are distinguished from other quality improvement models. TCAB seeks engagement from front-line staff and managers, promotes transformative change, and places emphasis on a continual process of learning and discovery with the goals of increasing safe and reliable care, patient-centered care, value-added care, and vitality and teamwork (Bolton & Aronow, 2009; Rutherford et al., 2009). TCAB principles served as the mechanism of action for the quality improvement project.

Transtheoretical Model of Change

The transtheoretical model (TTM) of change integrates concepts from other theories and demonstrates how individuals modify problem behaviors or form new

(continues)

behaviors. The TTM is organized by three constructs: change stages, change processes, and change levels (DiClemente & Prochaska, 1998). According to the TTM, change is deliberate and develops through five stages (Velicer, Prochaska, Fava, Norman, & Redding, 1998). Change is staged to follow progression through the well-defined steps of the process. Progression through the steps of change, however, is not linear, but dynamic (DiClemente & Prochaska, 1998). The staff of the target unit were initially in the precontemplative stage of change but moved dynamically through contemplation, preparation, action, and maintenance via application of TTM in project execution.

Institute of Medicine Aims

Six aims or domains were identified by the IOM in an effort to improve quality of care to patients. The aims for safe, timely, effective, efficient, equitable, and patient-centered quality health care appear throughout by the Doctor of Nursing Practice (DNP) project plan (IOM, 2001).

Iowa Model

Developed by Titler and colleagues in 1994 and revised in 2001, the Iowa model of EBP was utilized as a framework to provide direction for the project, blending the underpinnings of TCAB, TTM, and the IOM aims (Titler et al., 2001). The problem or trigger of hospital-acquired MDROs was identified as a priority at the target facility, and a review of the literature was performed. A comprehensive search of the Cumulative Index to Nursing and Allied Health Literature (CINAHL), Scopus, and PubMed revealed evidence to support the project. In an effort to provide high-quality and reliable evidence from systematic reviews, the Cochrane Collaboration was utilized. National guidelines from the Centers for Disease Control and Prevention, National Guidelines Clearinghouse, Society for Healthcare Epidemiology of America, and the World Health Organization were reviewed. The Strength of Recommendation Taxonomy (SORT) was the tool selected for the project to rate the level and strength of the evidence. The SORT taxonomy and leveling grid is straightforward, broad, and easily used. Clear and strong recommendations receive an A, moderate recommendations receive a B, and weak recommendations receive a C (Ebell et al., 2004). Data from all levels were included in the literature review. Data at the highest level provided strong support for the project. The Iowa model provides a guide for discovering and using the best evidence available to guide the provision of quality care (Titler et al., 2001).

The project facility has processes in place that target the prevention of HAIs caused by MDROs, but the problem is compliance on the part of the healthcare workers (T. Aikens, personal communication, August 25, 2010). Noncompliance with hand hygiene guidelines has been identified as the major modifiable cause of HAIs (Aragon et al., 2005; Boyce & Pittet, 2002; Pittet et al., 2000). Failure to properly comply with isolation precaution procedures for patients infected with MDROs has been associated with the cross-contamination and subsequent infections of other patients (Aragon et al., 2005). Evidence has tethered the structural problem of nurse understaffing and downsizing driven by cost reduction interventions to negative patient outcomes such as HAIs from MDROs (Hugonnet, Harbarth, Sax, Duncan, & Pittet, 2004). Additionally, transmission is significantly increased by healthcare workers' failure to comply with the simplest methods of the spread of infection—handwashing and adherence to isolation precautions, for example (Weber & Soule, 2009). Blood pressure cuffs, computer keyboards, mobile communication devices, pulse oximeter probes, pens, and neckties have been identified as potential sources for cross-contamination (Brady, Verran, Damani, & Gibb, 2009; Davis, 2009; de Gialluly, Morange, de Gialluly, Loulergue, & Quentin, 2006; Dixon, 2000; Fukada, Iwakiri, & Ozaki, 2008; Sim, Feasey, Wren, Breathnach, & Thompson, 2009).

■ Exemplar Two: A Doctor of Nursing Practice Systems Change Project: The Effect of a Basal Bolus Insulin Protocol on Inpatient Glucose Levels

Mary Therese Callens, Donna Stevens, and Lenora Wade

Background

In 2011, 25.9 million people in the United States had a diagnosis of diabetes. Of these individuals, 90–95% had type 2 diabetes mellitus with a threefold greater chance of hospitalization (Centers for Disease Control and Prevention [CDC], 2011; Australian Diabetes Society, 2012). Thirty percent of these individuals will require two or more hospitalizations in any given year compared to those without diabetes (CDC, 2011; Draznin, Gilden, Golden, & Inzucchi, 2013).

Poor glycemic control is associated with poor immune response, increased cardiovascular events, thrombosis, inflammatory changes, delayed healing, and other problems (Qaseem, Humphrey, Chou, Snow, & Shekelle, 2011). In the hospitalized patient, hypoglycemia and hyperglycemia are associated with increased morbidity, mortality, and overall hospital costs (Eiland, Goldner, Drincic, & Desouza, 2014; McCulloch, 2013; Australian Diabetes Society, 2012).

There has been much debate over the lab values that indicate ideal glycemic control. According to the American Diabetes Association (Inzucchi et al., 2012) the optimal range for glucose in hospitalized patients is 140–180 mg/dL (7.8–10 mmol/L). Achieving glycemic control safely in inpatients may be complicated by a multitude of factors, especially when considering variability among patients. Physiologic stress responses, comorbid conditions such as renal insufficiency, medications associated with insulin resistance such as steroids, and changes in nutritional schedules have the potential to increase the difficulty of maintaining euglycemia in the noncritical inpatient (Inzucchi et al., 2012).

There are no published research studies indicating the fluctuation of blood glucoses associated with meals. However, differences can be attributed to the amount

(continues)

of carbohydrates consumed and other physiologic issues associated with insulin production and glucose metabolism such as circadian rhythms (Boden, Ruiz, Urbain, & Chen, 1996). The potentially life-threatening complication of endogenous glucose control, such as insulin administration, is hypoglycemia. As with hyperglycemia, hypoglycemia is an independent risk factor for poor outcomes in the hospitalized patient (Eiland, Goldner, Drincic, & Desouza, 2014).

The outcome of rigorous treatment to achieve strict glycemic control in noncritical hospitalized patients remains uncertain (Furnary, Wu, & Bookin, 2004). Historically, studies have focused on the critically ill, such as those patients who have experienced myocardial infarctions or strokes or have undergone cardiac surgery (Malmberg et al., 1995; Furnary, Wu, & Bookin, 2004; Boris et al., 2013; Moghissie, et al., 2009; Murad, et al., 2012). These findings are not generalizable to noncritical patients because they are vastly different.

Prior to implementation of the basal bolus insulin protocol (BBIP), the primary treatment of hyperglycemia at the hospital was sliding scale insulin. This practice involved insulin dosage based on a specific blood glucose value. In agreement with current research (Apsey et al., 2013), sliding scale insulin was found to be ineffective in managing inpatient hyperglycemia and represented a safety concern for patients. Therefore, in 2012 the hospital implemented BBIPs to maximi patient safety. The objective of this project is to determine if the use of a BBIP improves glycemic control while simultaneously decreasing the incidence of hypoglycemia in noncritical adult inpatients with hyperglycemia when compared to traditional methods such as sliding scale insulin when observed over a calendar year.

Methodology

For success of this quality improvement project, the hospital administration empowered an interdisciplinary task group known as the Inpatient Glycemic Task Force (IGTF). The goal was to develop interventions to address the following objectives: improve patient care and outcomes, increase staff awareness and knowledge, standardize care where possible based on evidence based protocols, provide ongoing performance-feedback to providers, optimize electronic health record (EHR) capabilities, proactively identify patients at risk for poor clinical outcomes or readmission, optimize interprofessional team work and economical use of staff training and licenses, and use inpatient resources more effectively (Shapiro, 2013).

This led to the development of weight-based BBIPs to address hyperglycemia of noncritical hospital patients. Prior to the development of the protocols, mechanical changes were initiated to support the program. This included altering the EHR with input-guided order entry insulin protocols with dosing calculators, system-generated consults, creation of a permanent training system apparatus, creation of a structure for monitoring, and a tiered diabetes management assistance system.

The first priority of implementation was to educate and engage healthcare providers in the success of the BBIP. Major issues addressed were fear of inducing hypoglycemia and illustrating the deficits of current practices. These included use of sliding scale insulin for the treatment of hyperglycemia. A phased approach was utilized to implement the use of the BBIP. With this strategy, individual departments in the hospital were allowed to observe the successful results of glycemic control and fears were allayed. This methodical implementation was instrumental in the success of such a major change in practice.

General overview of the process includes monitoring food intake and insulin administration. Meals are served on-demand to each patient by room service between the hours of 07:00 and 19:00. Prior to the meal, the patient's capillary glucose is checked at the bedside and recorded. No more than 60 minutes after the meal, bolus as part insulin is administered. The dose is derived from the ordered nutritional insulin, which is specified to be given if at least 50% of the meal is ingested and correctional insulin, based on the premeal glucose reading. These two insulin dosages are administered in one injection. Finally, the glucose is checked prior to bedtime and glargine insulin (the basal insulin) is given. After the dinner meal no bolus correction insulin is administered unless the glucose reading is above 420 mg/dL (23.3 mmol/L).

The BBIP involves a stepwise approach. On admission, the patient's history of diabetes and the current treatment regimen is assessed. If on insulin therapy, the Home Conversion Protocol is ordered with 70% of the patient's total daily home regimen dose administered, 50% basal and 50% bolus insulin given in three divided doses. If on oral therapy, medications are held and a weight-based insulin protocol is initiated with pharmacy titration.

Alternatively, if there is no history of diabetes and hyperglycemia occurs, the Information Glucose Management Team (IGMT) receives a system-generated consult. After assessing whether the patient is on the appropriate oral diet, it is determined whether insulin therapy is needed. An order is placed for a weight-based protocol with pharmacy titration if appropriate.

When ordering a BBIP, there are three different options: low, moderate, and high dosing. The choice depends on hypoglycemia risk factors. These risk factors include age over 70 years, glomerular filtration rate less than 50%, insulin-naïve, type of diabetes, and liver function.

The low-dose protocol is appropriate for those with two or more risk factors for hypoglycemia. Basal insulin (glargine) of 0.1 unit/kg is given nightly. Bolus insulin is given three times per day with the correctional insulin, based on the premeal glucose reading, of 0–5 units plus a bolus of 0.03 units/kg for the meal (if at least 50% of the meal is ingested). The moderate-dose protocol is given to those with one risk factor for hypoglycemia and 0.15 units/kg of basal insulin is administered with a moderate correction scale of 0–8 units of insulin and a bolus insulin dose of 0.05 units/kg. The high-dose protocol is appropriate for those with no risk factors for hypoglycemia or those who are morbidly obese. The basal insulin dose is 0.2 units/kg nightly with a high correction scale of 0–16 units and a bolus for the meals of 0.07 units/kg.

The efficacy of the BBIP was evaluated using a retrospective chart review method. Data were gathered to compare glycemic control 1 year before and 1 year

(continues)

after implementation of the BBIPs. The project directors endeavored to show that hyperglycemia, defined as a glucose reading greater than 300 mg/dL (16.7 mmol/L), was improved from the baseline by at least 20% and severe hypoglycemia, defined as glucose of less than 40 mg/dL (2.2 mmol/L), was simultaneously reduced by at least 10% by use of the basal bolus insulin protocols. They also intended to determine the effectiveness of the basal bolus protocols in managing glycemic control.

After institutional review board approval was obtained, a computer-generated list of patients meeting the inclusion and exclusion criteria from January through December 2011 (the preimplementation phase) and from January through December 2013 (the postimplementation phase) was utilized to identify the sample. Each patient's record underwent a second review from the computer-generated list to validate inclusion and exclusion criteria because the list was generated based on ICD-9 coding and there were some coding discrepancies. Data, including age, sex, length of stay, and average glucose for the hospital stay, were obtained. In addition, to evaluate any extremes in blood glucoses (>300 mg/dL or 16.7 mmol/L) or (<40 mg/dL or 2.2 mmol/L), all blood glucose values from the hospital stay were evaluated. Information was extrapolated and placed in the Statistics Package for Social Sciences (SPSS) database. No additional tools were used for data collection. After data collection was completed, an independent t-test was performed to compare the nominal data for evaluation of outcomes of the BBIPs.

The study population was selected from patients cared for by the Hospitalist Service, a team responsible for the delivery of care to general medicine patients and the first Service to introduce the BBIPs.

Inclusion and Exclusion Criteria

Inclusion criteria for the retrospective study of 100 preimplementation and 100 postimplementation patients included those:

- Admitted to the hospitalist service
- Younger than 75 years of age
- With at least one serum or capillary glucose reading of greater than 180 mg/dL (10 mmol/L)
- 2013 patients treated with the BBIP for at least 48 hours

Criteria that would exclude participation in the study include:

- A previous or current diagnosis of type 1 diabetes
- Receiving steroid medication
- Receiving enteral or total parental nutrition
- Diagnosed with diabetic ketoacidosis during current admission
- Current use of a subcutaneous insulin pump
- Taking oral hyperglycemia agents
- Diagnosed with any of the listed comorbidities of cystic fibrosis or chronic kidney disease (glomerular filtration < 35%)
- History of a solid organ transplantation or pancreatectomy

Evaluation

Initially, the methodology to be used for this project was to perform a t-test to compare the mean glucose for the hospital stay for the preimplementation and postimplementation groups. However, it was noted that the variability of glucoses were not assessed using this method. Extremes in glucose readings that occurred in a day would average out to be comparable to those that remained in a constant acceptable range.

The average age of all of the patients for 2011 was 58.14 and for 2013 was 56.08. Of the participants, 53% were female in 2011 and 63% of the participants were male in 2013. The average length of stay for 2011 and 2013 was 5.64 and 5.65, days, respectively. The average glucose for the hospital stay for 2011 was 193.27 and for 2013 was 179.86. The percentage of glucose values below 40 mg/dL (2.2 mmol/L) for 2011 and 2013 were 0.5% and 0.3%, respectively. In 2011, 46.7% of the glucose values were in target range (80–140), and 58.4% were in target range in 2013. The percentage of glucose values above 300 mg/dL (16.7 mmol/L) in 2011 and 2013 were 9.9% and 6.4%, respectively.

It would be easy to decrease the rate of hypoglycemia at the expense of having higher rates of hyperglycemia. However; it is much more difficult to improve hypoglycemia while simultaneously improving hyperglycemia; narrowing the range of extremes (Davis & Alonso, 2004). The p-value for both the average glucose value for the stay and also for every glucose reading recorded was 0.070. Although not significant, goals of the project were met as the extremes of blood glucoses were narrowed. The initial goals set by the IGTF were met when there was a noted simultaneous 40% improvement in severe hypoglycemia and a 30% improvement in hyperglycemia. Additionally, the glucose range improved from 321.30 mg/dL (17.8 mmol/L) to 224.35 mg/dL (12.4 mmol/L).

Strengths and Limitations

Strengths and limitations of the project were noted. The major strengths of the project included having standardized protocols for insulin therapy and management of hypoglycemia, daily titration of insulin by trained pharmacists, and an expert team of nurse practitioners for management of high-risk patients. Having strong administrative support was another strength. Administrators gave the necessary support to make the project happen. A third strength was the checks and balance system that was incorporated. Auto-referrals through the EHR helped ensure that those with hyperglycemia were captured.

The major weakness of the project was related to care coordination. Timing of the glucose check, meal intake, and insulin administration was imperative in maintaining good glycemic control. Use of ancillary personnel to perform bedside glucose monitoring (on all units except two general medicine units) and delivery of self-service ordered meals made it difficult to coordinate appropriate timing with insulin administration by nursing personnel A great deal of communication

(continues)

between and among the staff and patient was required. At times, communication was lacking resulting in sub-optimal results.

Second, dietary issues caused some limitations. The system for food ordering was set up to allow ordering of one additional carbohydrate serving before the dietary staff is flagged. Theoretically, someone limited to four carbohydrate servings could eat a five carbohydrate meal. Some patients ate food obtained from family members or vending machines, despite an order to not eat outside food. Finally, the protocols called for administration of nutritional insulin only if at least 50% of the meal was consumed. It could be difficult to ascertain whether insulin should be administered, according to what the patient ordered. For example, someone on a full liquid diet who only ordered oatmeal and juice receive insulin if they ate half the meal?

Third, there were limitations associated with physicians ordering and use of the protocols. Some physicians did not want to administer basal bolus insulin to those who could not afford to fill these medications after discharge. Additionally, the protocols were intentionally designed to be conservative to avoid hypoglycemia and to facilitate the paradigm shift that needed to occur. Despite this, some were cautious about maintaining glycemic control at a lower range and were resistant to using the protocols initially. Finally, it was the primary medical teams' responsibility to order the insulin protocols at the time of admission. Often, protocols were not ordered and the patient became hyperglycemic. An automated consult was triggered through the electronic medical record, but valuable time was lost before insulin was administered. At times, glycemic control was not attainable prior to discharge.

Recommendations

Recommendations for improvement include planning and implementation of additional education, implementation of changes that will be used to gain glycemic control in a more timely fashion, and additional protocol changes for targeted special populations. To implement additional education, the team will continue to provide monthly small group education, continue to present at Medical and Nurse Practitioner Grand Rounds annually, work with the Advanced Nursing Coordinators to provide education to new staff, and streamline education on the online learning system for the hospital as a refresher course that will be completed annually. The plan to gain glycemic control more aggressively and in a more timely fashion will be accomplished by increasing the dose of insulin by 0.1 units/kg in each of the BBIPs. To meet the goal of improving glycemic control in special populations, the IGTF will complete data analysis hospital-wide to identify special populations who need protocol additions or changes. Small work groups will be formed that will identify the needs and develop a plan for improvement.

Conclusion

Randomized trials have noted the effectiveness of insulin basal bolus protocols in the treatment of hyperglycemia in hospitalized patients. (Umpierrez, 2011;

Umpierrez, 2012). However, the authors wanted to determine the efficacy of BBIPs in an actual hospital setting. Hyperglycemia remains a problematic issue across the nation; however, compelling data support optimal glycemic control. By improving glycemic control, the hospital has the potential to decrease length of stay, decrease overall hospital costs, and improve patient safety. This quality improvement project will add to the foundation of knowledge of optimizing glycemic control of noncritical inpatients using a BBIP.

References

Apsey, H. A., Coan, K. E., Castro, J. C., Jameson, K. A., Schlinkert, R. T., & Cook, C. B. (2013). Overcoming clinical inertia in the management of postoperative patients with diabetes. *Endocrine Practice, 20*(4), 1–25.

Australian Diabetes Society. (2012). *Guidelines for routine glucose control in hospital.* Retrieved from https://www.diabetessociety.com.au/documents/ADSGuidelinesforRoutineGlucoseControlinHospitalFinal2012_000.pdf

Boden, G., Ruiz, J., Urbain, J., & Chen, X. (1996). Evidence for a circadian rhythm of insulin secretion. *American Journal of Physiology, 271*(2), E246–E252. Retrieved from http://www.ncbi.nlm.nih.gov/pubmed8770017

Boris, D., Gilden, J., Golden, S.H., Inzucchi, S. E. (2013). Pathways to quality inpatient management of hyperglycemia and diabetes: A call to action. *Diabetes Care, 36*(7), 1807–1814. doi:10.2337/dc12-2508

Centers for Disease Control and Prevention. (2011). *National diabetes fact sheet.* Retrieved from http://www.cdc.gov/diabetes/pubs/pdf/ndfs_2011.pdf

Davis, D., & Alonso, M. D. (2004). Hypoglycemia as a barrier to glycemic control. *Journal of Diabetes and Its Complications, 18,* 60–68. doi:10.1016/S1056-8727(03)00058-8

Eiland, L., Goldner, W., Drincic, A., & Desouza, C. (2014). Inpatient hypoglycemia: A challenge that must be addressed. *Current Diabetes Reports, 14*(1), 1–9.

Furnary, A. P., Wu. X. Y., & Bookin, S. O. (2004). Effect of hyperglycemia and continuous intravenous insulin infusions on outcomes of cardiac surgical procedures: The Portland diabetic project. *Endocrine Practice, 10*(2), 21–33.

Inzucchi, S. E., Bergenstal, R. M., Buse, J. B., Diamant, M., Ferrannini, E., Nauck, M., . . . Matthews, D. R. (2012). Management of hyperglycemia in type 2 diabetes: A patient-centered approach. Position statement of the American Diabetes Association (ADA) and the European Association for the Study of Diabetes (EASD). *Diabetes Care, 35*(6), 1364–1379.

Malmberg, K., Ryden, L., Efendic, S., Herlitz, J., Nicol, P., Waldenström, A., . . . Welin L. (1995). Randomized trial of insulin-glucose infusion followed by subcutaneous insulin treatment in diabetic patients with acute myocardial infarction (DIGAMI Study): Effects on mortality at 1 year. *Journal of the American College of Cardiology, 26*(1), 57–65.

McCulloch, D. (2013, May). Glycemic control and vascular complications in type 2 diabetes mellitus. *UpToDate.* Retrieved from http://www.uptodate.com/contents/glycemic-control-and-vascular-complications-in-type-1-diabetes-mellitus

Moghissi, E. S., Korytkowski, M. T., DiNardo, M., Einhorn, D., Hellman, R., Hirshch, Irl,.B., . . . Umpierrez, G. E. (2009). American Association of Clinical Endocrinologists and American Diabetes Association consensus statement on inpatient glycemic control. *Diabetes Care, 32*(6), 1119–1131.

(continues)

Murad, M. H., Coburn, J. A., Coto-Yglesias, F., Dzyubak, S., Hazem, A., Lane, M. A., . . . Montori, V. M. (2012). Glycemic control in non-critically ill hospitalized patients: A systematic review and meta-analysis. *The Journal of Clinical Endocrinology and Metabolism, 97*(1), 49–58. doi:10.1210/jc.2011-2100

Qaseem, A., Humphrey, L. L., Chou, R., Snow, V., & Shekelle, P. (2011). Use of intensive insulin therapy for the management of glycemic control in hospitalized patients: A clinical practice guideline from the American College of Physicians. *Annals of Internal Medicine, 154*(4), 260–267.

Shapiro, R. (2013). *Inpatient glycemic control in an academic medical center: A new approach to care management.* Alabama, AL: University of Alabama at Birmingham, Office of the Chief Quality and Safety Officer.

Titler, M. G., Kleiber, C., Steelman, V. J., Rakel, B. A., Budreau, G., Everett, L. Q., Buckwalter, K. C., . . . Goode, C. J. (2001). The Iowa model of evidence-based practice to promote quality care. *Critical Care Nursing Clinics of North America, 13*(4), 497–509.

Umpierrez, G. E., Smiley, D., Jacob, S., Peng, L., Temponi, A., Mulligan ,P., Umpierrez, D., . . . Rizzo, M. D. (2011). Randomized study of basal bolus insulin therapy in the inpatient management of patients with type 2 diabetes undergoing general surgery. (RABBIT 2 Surgery). *Diabetes Care, 34*(2), 256–261. doi:10.2337/dc10-1407

Umpierrez, G., Hellman, R., Korytkowski, M., Kosiborod, M., Maynard, G. A., Montori, V. M., . . . Van den Berghe (2012). Management of hyperglycemia in hospitalized patients in non-critical care setting: An Endocrine Society clinical practice guideline. *Journal of Clinical Endocrinology Metabolism, 97*(10), 16–38. doi:10.1210/jc.2011-2098

REFLECTIVE ACTIVITIES

1. Select at least one EBP method, beginning with the clinical questions.
2. Using your clinical question, outline a plan for developing a project idea to improve clinical practice.
3. Guided by the tools and strategies offered in this chapter, use the scholarly project exemplar to critique the practice improvement.

REFERENCES

Advisory Board Academies. (2008). *Leading change: Implementing improvements in the health care organization.* Washington, DC: The Advisory Board Company.

American Nurses Credentialing Center. (2011). *Magnet Recognition Program.* Retrieved from http://www.nursecredentialing.org/Magnet.aspx

Aragon, D., Sole, M. L., & Brown, S. (2005). Outcomes of an infection prevention project focusing on hand hygiene and isolation practices. *AACN Clinical Issues, 16*(2), 121–132.

Bolton, L. B., & Aronow, H. U. (2009). The business case for TCAB: Estimates of cost savings with sustained improvement. *American Journal of Nursing, 109*(11), 77–80.

Boyce, J. M., & Pittet, D. (2002). Guideline for hand hygiene in health-care settings. *MMWR, 51*(16), 1–45.

Brady, R. R., Verran, J., Damani, N. N., & Gibb, A. P. (2009). Review of mobile communication devices as potential reservoirs of nosocomial pathogens. *Journal of Hospital Infection, 71*(4), 295–300.

Centers for Disease Control and Prevention. (2011). *National Healthcare Safety Network (NHSN).* Retrieved from http://www.cdc.gov/nhsn

Committee on the Robert Wood Johnson Foundation Initiative on the Future of Nursing, at the Institute of Medicine. (2010). *The future of nursing: Leading change, advancing health.* Washington, DC: National Academies Press.

Consumer Assessment of Healthcare Providers and Systems. (2007). Preparing a questionnaire using the CAHPS® Clinician & Group Survey. *CAHPS® Clinician & Group Survey and Reporting Kit 2007.* Retrieved from http://www.cahps.ahrq.gov/

Cosgrove, S. E. (2006). The relationship between antimicrobial resistance and patient outcomes: Mortality, length of hospital stay, and health care costs. *Clinical Infectious Diseases, 42*(Suppl. 2), S82–S89.

Creamer, E., Dorrian, S., Dolan, A., Sherlock, O., Fitzgerald-Hughes, D., Thomas, T., . . . Humphreys H. (2010). When are the hands of healthcare workers positive for methicillin-resistant *Staphylococcus aureus? Journal of Hospital Infection, 75*(2), 107–111.

Cronenwett, L., Sherwood, G., Barnsteiner, J., Disch, J., Johnson, J., Mitchell, P., . . . Warren, J. (2007). Quality and safety education for nurses. *Nursing Outlook, 55*(3), 122–131.

Cummings, K. L., Anderson, D. J., & Kaye, K. S. (2010). Hand hygiene noncompliance and the cost of hospital-acquired methicillin-resistant *Staphylococcus aureus* infection. *Infection Control and Hospital Epidemiology, 31,* 357–364. doi:10.1086/651096

Davis, C. (2009). Blood pressure cuffs and pulse oximeter sensors: A potential source of cross-contamination. *Australasian Emergency Nursing Journal, 12*(3), 104–109.

de Gialluly, C., Morange, V., de Gialluly, E., Loulergue, J., & Quentin, R. (2006). Blood pressure cuff as a potential vector of pathogenic microorganisms: A prospective study in a teaching hospital. *Infection Control and Hospital Epidemiology, 27,* 940–943.

DiClemente, C. C., & Prochaska, J. O. (1998). Toward a comprehensive, transtheoretical model of change: Stages of change and addictive behaviors. In W. R. Miller & N. Heather (Eds.), *Treating addictive behaviors* (2nd ed., pp. 3–24). New York, NY: Plenum Press.

Dixon, M. (2000). Neck ties as vectors for nosocomial infection. *Intensive Care Medicine, 26*(2), 250.

Draznin, B., Gilden, J., Golden, S. H., Inzucchi, S. E. (2013). Pathways to quality inpatient management of hyperglycemia and diabetes: A call to action. *Diabetes Care, 36*(7): 1807–1814. doi:10.2337/dc12-2508

Ebell, M. H., Siwek, J., Weiss, B. D., Woolf S. H., Susman J., Ewigman B., & Bowman M. (2004). Strength of recommendation taxonomy (SORT): A patient-centered approach to grading evidence in the medical literature. *American Family Physician, 69,* 548–556.

Evans, H. (2008). *Winning with accountability: The secret language of high-performing organizations.* Dallas, TX: CornerStone Leadership Institute.

Fink, R., Thompson, C., & Bonnes, D. (2005). Overcoming barriers and promoting the use of research in practice. *Journal of Nursing Administration, 35*(3), 121–129.

Fukada, T., Iwakiri, H., & Ozaki, M. (2008). Anaesthetists' role in computer keyboard contamination in an operating room. *Journal of Hospital Infection, 70*(2), 148–153.

Gladwell, M. (2000). *The tipping point.* New York, NY: Little, Brown.

Harbarth, S., Pittet, D., Grady, L., & Goldmann, D. A. (2001). Compliance with hand hygiene practice in pediatric intensive care. *Pediatric Critical Care Medicine, 2*(4), 311–314.

HCAHPS. (2010). *CAHPS® hospital survey.* Retrieved from http://www.hcahpsonline.org/home.aspx#aboutsurv

Henderson, D. K. (2006). Managing methicillin-resistant staphylococci: A paradigm for preventing nosocomial transmission of resistant organisms. *The American Journal of Medicine, 119,* 545–552. doi:10.1016/j.amjmed.2006.04.0002

Hugonnet, S., Harbarth, S., Sax, H., Duncan, R., & Pittet, D. (2004). Nursing resources: A major determinant of nosocomial infection? *Current Opinion in Infectious Diseases, 17*(4), 329–333.

Institute of Medicine. (2001). *Crossing the quality chasm: A new health system for the 21st century.* Retrieved from http://www.nap.edu/html/quality_chasm/reportbrief.pdf

Langley, G. L., Nolan, K. M., Nolan, T. W., Norman, C. L., & Provost, L. P. (2009). *The improvement guide: A practical approach to enhancing organizational performance.* San Francisco, CA: Jossey-Bass.

Lederer, J. W., Jr., Best, D., & Hendrix, V. (2009). A comprehensive hand hygiene approach to reducing MRSA health care-associated infections. *Joint Commission Journal on Quality and Patient Safety, 35*(4), 180–185.

Lewis, J. (2011). *Project planning, scheduling and control* (5th ed.). New York, NY: McGraw-Hill.

Lowe, J. R. (2004). The effectiveness of alcohol based hand rubs and compliance with hand hygiene. *Kentucky Nurse, 52*(1), 22–22.

Melnyk, B., & Fineout-Overholt, E. (2005). *Evidence-based practice in nursing and healthcare.* Philadelphia, PA: Lippincott Williams & Wilkins.

Muto, C. A., Jernigan, J. A., Ostrowsky, B. E., Richet, H. M., Jarvis, W. R., Boyce, J. M., & Farr, B. M. (2003). SHEA guideline for preventing nosocomial transmission of multidrug-resistant strains of *Staphylococcus aureus* and *Enterococcus. Infection Control and Hospital Epidemiology, 24,* 362–386.

National Nosocomial Infections Surveillance System. (2004). National Nosocomial Infections Surveillance (NNIS) System report, data summary from January 1992 through June 2004, issued October 2004. *American Journal of Infection Control, 32*(8), 470–485.

Newhouse, R. (2006). Examining the support for evidence-based nursing practice. *Journal of Nursing Administration, 26*(7/8), 337–340.

Noble, D. B. (2009). Patient education on MRSA prevention and management: The nurse's vital role. *MEDSURG Nursing, 18,* 375–378.

Pittet, D., Hugonnet, S., Harbarth, S., Mourouga, P., Sauvan, V., Touveneau, S., & Perneger, T. V. (2000). Effectiveness of a hospital-wide programme to improve compliance with hand hygiene. Infection Control Programme. *Lancet, 356*(9238), 1307–1312.

Romero, D. V., Treston, J., & O'Sullivan, A. L. (2006). Hand-to-hand combat: Preventing MRSA. *Nurse Practitioner, 31*(3), 16–18, 21–23.

Rutherford, P., Moen, R., & Taylor, J. (2009). TCAB: The "how" and the "what": Developing an initiative to involve nurses in transformative change. *American Journal of Nursing, 109*(11), 5–17.

Sim, D. A., Feasey, N., Wren, S., Breathnach, A., & Thompson, G. (2009). Cross-infection risk of felt-tipped marker pens in cataract surgery. *Eye, 23,* 1094–1097.

Simmons, J. C. (2002). Using Six Sigma to make a difference in health care quality. *The Quality Letter for Healthcare Leaders, 14*(4), 2–10, 1.

Stefancyk, A. L. (2009a). Improving processes of care: Making changes that hit and miss. *American Journal of Nursing, 109*(6), 36–37.

Stefancyk, A. L. (2009b). Placing the patient at the center of care: Making changes in one of four focus areas. *American Journal of Nursing, 109*(5), 27–28. doi:10.1097/01.naj.0000351501.24262.09

Stefancyk, A. L. (2009c). Safe and reliable care. *American Journal of Nursing, 109*(7), 70–71.

Stefancyk, A. L. (2009d). Vitality and teamwork: Continuing to make changes and final thoughts on our progress. *American Journal of Nursing, 109*(8), 70–71. doi:10.1097/01.naj.0000358507.31582.31

Stevens, K. R. (2004). *ACE Star Model of EBP: Knowledge transformation.* Academic Center of Evidence-Based Practice, University of Texas Health Science Center at San Antonio. Retrieved from http://www.acestar.uthscsa.edu/

Studer, Q. (2005). *Hardwiring excellence: Purpose, worthwhile work, making a difference.* Gulf Breeze, FL: Fire Starter Publishing.

Velicer, W. F., Prochaska, J. O., Fava, J. L., Norman, G. J., & Redding, C. A. (1998). Smoking cessation and stress management: Applications of the transtheoretical model of behavior change. *Homeostasis, 38,* 216–233.

Walker, B. W. (2007). New guidelines for fighting multidrug-resistant organisms. *Nursing, 37*(5), 20.

Walker, L., Green, A., Huett, A., Boateng, B., Jeffs, D., Lowe, G., & Pate, B. (2012, April). *Improving capacity for EBP using interactive e-learning.* Poster session presented at The New Frontier: Pediatric Nurses Embracing Our Changing Environment, 22nd Annual Convention of the Society of Pediatric Nurses, Houston, TX.

Weber, S. W., & Soule, B. M. (2009). Antibiotic resistance: Patients and hospitals in peril. Why is the issue of antibiotic resistance important to you and your organization? In S. W. Weber & B. M. Soule (Eds.), *What every health care executive should know: The cost of antibiotic resistance* (pp. 1–12). Oakbrook Terrace, IL: Joint Commission Resources.

CHAPTER 18

Evidence-Based Practice in the Global Community: Building Bridges

■Gordana Dermody■

■ Objectives:

- Describe the relevance of evidence-based nursing practice in the global community.
- Outline the challenges of integrating principles of evidence-based nursing practice in the global community.
- Discuss strategies and models for framing experiences learning, translating, and applying evidence-based nursing practice within a global context.

■ Evidence-Based Practice in the Global Community

Ongoing health inequities, sub-optimal patient outcomes, and the existence of inefficient and fragmented healthcare services around the globe is a sign that the chasm between evidence and practice is a continual problem. Evidence-based practice (EBP) is necessary to promote individual and population health. The gap to translating evidence into practice is estimated to be a staggering 10–17 years in the United States (Titler, 2008). This lag time is significant because if a country with an advanced healthcare system struggles to translate evidence into practice, other countries in our global community with unique challenges could experience even longer lag times, which could result in continued health inequities (Egerod & Hansen, 2005; Green, Ottoson, Garcia, & Hiatt, 2009; Köpke, Koch, & Balzer, 2013; Thorsteinsson, 2013). The global collective of nursing professionals can work together to integrate EBP into nursing curricula, healthcare policy, institutional policy, and practice settings across the world (World Health Organization [WHO], 2016; International Council of Nurses [ICN], 2012). Nurses need to lead the integration of evidence-based nursing practice because they have always been population health leaders (Savage & Kub, 2009). The overarching purpose of this chapter is to empower nurses in the global community to become bridge-builders to facilitate and expedite the translation of evidence into practice. Literature describing the integration of evidence-based nursing practice in various countries will be discussed, and barriers and strategies will be described. Finally, two exemplars of nurses who have undertaken bridge-building activities will be presented.

■ Nurses as Bridge Builders to Harness the Power of Knowledge

Knowing that the integration of evidence-based research is a slow and cumbersome process could contribute to feelings of powerlessness among nurse researchers and clinicians. It can feel overwhelming to think about the enormous amount of work that needs to be accomplished to cross the decade-long evidence-to-practice chasm (Green et al., 2009). This is why it is important for nurses practicing within the global community to share best practices. Although the EBP movement has been credited to Dr. Cochrane and the medical profession, history shows that nurses have been frontrunners in promoting best nursing practices that foster the health of individuals, families, and populations (Hegge, 2011; Fineout-Overholt, Melnyk, & Schultz, 2005).

In the late 1800s Florence Nightingale, a pioneering and neophyte nurse scientist, was the one of the first nurses to systematically advocate for improved care on the behalf of her patients (Hegge, 2011). Nightingale (1860) used basic research and statistics to generate epidemiologic evidence that nursing care based on her recommendations was effective in saving the lives of wounded soldiers in the Crimea (Keith, 1988; Kopf, 1978; Nightingale, 1860). Nightingale discovered that patient outcomes were not only based on the quality care provided by nurses but were negatively influenced by a variety of barriers to nursing practice (Keith, 1988; Kopf, 1978; Nightingale, 1860). Beginning as a vocation, nursing has grown into a formidable scientific discipline, with a social responsibility to promote quality health care for individuals and populations (ANA, 2001). A hallmark of nursing as a discipline is nursing advocacy, which is underpinned by moral values and ethics (ANA, 2001; 2010a; 2010b).

The commitment to population health drives nurses to serve in the midst of a variety of population health concerns such as shifts in population aging in developed countries, man-made and environmental-related disasters, economic woes, conflicts, and the related migration of peoples to other countries. Using moral and ethical principles to guide their efforts, nurses could influence policy-makers in various countries to address existing health disparities through EBP (Matthews, 2012). In their publication *Closing the Gap: From Evidence to Action,* the ICN made a case for nurses everywhere to embrace evidence-based nursing practice. The ICN is a federation of more than 130 national nurses associations that represent nurses around the globe (ICN, 2012). Understanding EBP concepts and critically appraising research-generated evidence are key steps in identifying the relevance and strength of the evidence (Melnyk & Fineout-Overholt, 2015).

■ Challenges to Integrating Evidence-Based Practice in the Global Community

As in the days of Nightingale, the readiness and feasibility for change in nursing practice is influenced by sociopolitical and economic challenges, culture, and existing educational health systems and structures (Hudson, 2014; ICN, 2012). From the available literature it can be assumed that most research-generated nursing knowledge tends to be developed by a cadre of nurse scientists and advanced clinicians in higher income countries and new nursing knowledge seems to be more readily implemented in affluent countries where access to funding, supplies, and organizational support facilitates implementation (Hall & Roussel, 2014; Melnyk & Fineout-Overholt, 2015). Translating research into action in a global context is a complex process requiring careful consideration of the impact on nurses, physicians, and other members of the interdisciplinary team. A change in practice also may have an impact on health care–providing agencies, policies and policy-makers, and educators (Ditlopo, Laauw, Penn-Kekana, & Rispel, 2014; ICN, 2012; Berkowitz, 2012).

■ Unique Challenges to Implementing Evidence-Based Practice in the Global Community

It is challenging to integrate evidence-based nursing practice in developed countries, developing countries, and countries in conflict. Some challenges may include weak or complex healthcare infrastructures, nursing shortages, nursing work environment issues, cultural factors, policy and political factors, qualified nurse educator shortages, limited career advancement for nurses, and lack of resources (ICN, 2012; WHO, 2010). For instance, the nursing shortage in various countries is staggering. Canada will need 60,000 more nurses by 2022. India is short 2.4 million nurses, and the Caribbean and Latin American countries will need 10,000 more nurses by 2025. Because many developing nations have limited career or professional opportunities and less optimal nursing work conditions, nurses migrate to work in more developed nations. For example, a pattern of global migration of Caribbean nurses shows that between 2002 and 2006 approximately 1800 Caribbean nurses migrated to work in other nations (WHO, 2010). The migration of nurses also could have an impact on the presence of qualified nursing educators in countries with a great need for nurses and advancing best-practice nursing care. Nations who are in conflict may have even greater challenges because of elevated migration, keeping progress in evidence-based nursing at a stand-still.

To respond to the nursing shortage and limited nursing education opportunities, the ICN in collaboration with the National League for Nurses developed the International Nursing Education Network (INEN). This network provides a forum for nurse educators who are interested in addressing the role of nurse educators worldwide, improving the quality of nursing education, and responding to international nursing and nursing faculty shortages (ICN Fact sheet).

■ Attitudes, Knowledge, and Skills of Nurse Educators and Organizational Support

Some studies suggest that the beliefs of nurses about EBP could have implications on how effectively it is implemented (Stokke, Olsen, Espehaug, & Nortvedt, 2014). This could be due to barriers that nurses may encounter when attempting to implement EBP (Boström, Ehrenberg, Gustavsson, Wallin, 2009; Boström, Rudman, Gustavsson, & Wallin, 2013; Brown, Wickline, Ecoff, & Glaser, 2008; Eizenberg, 2010; Stokke et al., 2014). In a descriptive study of 540 Icelandic nurses, researchers examined their beliefs and perceptions about EBP, as well as their skills in accessing to resources to implement EBP. A lack of skills to search for and appraise the evidence was identified as the primary barrier to utilizing research-based evidence in clinical practice (Thorsteinsson, 2013). This finding is congruent with another study in which increased scores in nurse knowledge and EBP skills was associated with higher practice scores (Brown et al., 2008). Having the skills to access and appraise research-based information and the capacity to garner organizational support for change enhance nurses' ability to use EBP in their clinical practice (Brown et al., 2008; Eizenberg, 2010; Köpke, et al., 2013).

Although technology has promoted greater accessibility to research-generated evidence, in some developing nations limited access to evidence may be a stumbling block to EBP. Developing countries frequently have less than optimal internet connection, making the retrieval of articles challenging or impossible. In addition, much of the evidence is reported in the English language, which makes the available evidence inaccessible to nurses, nurse administrators, and nurse educators who may not possess English language skills. However, there is limited knowledge regarding how lacking technology infrastructure and non-English speaking affect the integration of evidence-based nursing practice in lower income or developing countries.

Nurse educators are important contributors in teaching nurses EBP, yet a paucity of literature exists about the attitudes of nurse educators in the global community toward EBP. It has been reported that nurse educators may not have sufficient knowledge of EBP or the skills necessary to teach nurse-clinicians how to integrate EBP into their practice (Stichler, Fields, Kim, & Brown, 2011). Some issues may include difficulty integrating EBP into nursing curriculum, the appropriate use of models and frameworks, and limited skills and knowledge to appraise research literature (Stichler et al., 2011). To be optimally effective, nursing curricula need to show students that EBP is congruent with the nursing needs in both developed and resource-poor developing nations (ICN, 2012; WHO, 2010). A contextual approach—rather than an overlay of westernized EBP standards—could enable nurse-educators to convey to students the relevance of EBP in a variety of practice settings. There are other factors that could have an impact on the education of nurses on EBP decision-making, such as the state of nursing research capacity and the level of autonomous practice of nurses holding advanced specialty degrees (Ditlopo, et al., 2014; Weston, 2008, 2010).

To make the translation of research-generated evidence into the practice setting a reality in the global context, a paradigm shift in nursing care delivery is necessary. This paradigm shift requires wider systemic support for nursing education and practice. Given their knowledge and experience, nurses need to lead the development of innovative approaches and models of nursing care delivery. The expertise of nursing scientists lends credibility to their efforts to advocate for EBP (Feetham & Doering, 2015). The involvement of nurse scientists in policy development and change provides an opportunity to educate key political stakeholders on issues related to evidence-based nursing care practice in the global community (Ditlopo, et al., 2014). Ultimately, scientific investigation by nurse researchers should influence the development and promotion of policy goals (Abood, 2007; Hinshaw & Grady 2011; Price, 2012).

■ Building Bridges to Evidence-Based Practice in a Global Community: Useful Strategies

It is important for nurses in all settings to recognize that there is a synergistic relationship between EBP and the healthcare outcomes for individuals and populations. International collaboration among nurses, nurse educators, and nursing scientists, as well as with other health professionals, is key to improving education, research, and clinical practice in the global setting (Hern, Vaughn, Mason, & Weitkamp, 2005; Levine, 2009; Moten, Schafer, & Montgomery, 2012; Sherwood & Liu, 2005).

One strategy is to collaborate with local leaders, both governmental and nongovernmental, to create a wide system of support for the delivery of health care (Moten et al., 2012; Sherwood & Liu, 2005). For example, a chief of a fishing village in Ghana with 4500 residents collaborated with village community leaders, local government, families, and social service organization to improve access to primary care services. Chief Nana Akousa Mfrasie II was instrumental in establishing a community-based health planning and service in this Western Ghana fishing village to bring primary care from sub-districts to the local community (Vikpeh-Lartey, Nkansah-Baidoo, & Furlane, 2016). This example shows that establishing collaborative relationships promotes evidence-based education and sustains EBP.

The advancement of nursing education is critical to the integration of evidence-based nursing practice and the promotion of innovative approaches to healthcare delivery (Hall & Roussel, 2014; ICN, 2012; Melnyk & Fineout-Overholt, 2015). A variety of programs that develop educational infrastructures for nursing education have been shown to be successful (Moch, Cronje, & Branson, 2010). For example, a partnership to advance nursing education between the United States and China by The Committee on Graduate Nursing Education (COGNE) was one of two initiatives of the China Medical Board in New York to build an infrastructure for graduate nursing education in China (1988–1992). The goal of this program was to bring Chinese nurses to the United States to provide them a master's education so they could return to China and contribute to nursing education development there.

However, the retention rate for Chinese nurses to return to China after receiving their degree was low. The second more successful initiative was the Program of Higher Nursing Education Degrees (POHNED) designed to develop opportunities for higher education in China through collaboration and assistance from the international community. Eighty-four master's prepared nurses graduated from this program in China in 7 years (Sherwood & Liu, 2005).

Short-term immersion experiences for nursing students represent another strategy for nursing collaboration and knowledge exchange. Immersion experiences have been considered useful in helping students develop a global perspective (Hern et al., 2005; McAuliffe & Cohen, 2005). Students are immersed in a different sociocultural context while collaborating with their counterparts, and these programs facilitate discussion and reflection on that experience (Levine, 2009). Bridges are designed for two-way crossing. Although developed nations have much to share in regard to the integration of evidence-based nursing practices, it is vital to foster a dual exchange of knowledge. Nurses who are working in settings in which evidence-based nursing practices are not integrated or are minimally integrated, may be able to offer useful insights about the challenges of evidence-based integration in their setting. When access to resources are lacking and nurses in advanced nursing roles have limited function in their healthcare systems, creative strategies emerge. These resourceful nurses could and should share important information with nurses practicing in settings that may be more conducive to evidence-based integration (Egerod & Hansen, 2005; Eizenberg, 2010; Stokke et al., 2014; Thorsteinsson, 2013).

■ Theoretical Framework and Models

A model to initiate sustainable partnerships begins with relationship-centered dialogue between and among cross-national dwelling nurses (**Table 18-1** and **Figure 18-11**). This dialogue should encompass all levels of nursing practice, education, and research. Although culture, language differences, and geographic location play an important role in dialogue, they need to be embraced as part of the collaborative process in the global context. Change often begins with discontentment of the status quo. Nightingale believed that without discontentment, individuals will not reach out for change (Poovey, 1992). The recognition for change needed leads to participate in dialogue with other, like-minded individuals. The subsequent development of cross-national partnerships could create a shared vision and the development of goals that can lead to change.

The development of nursing as a profession, its evolution as a science, and the strengthening of health-system infrastructures are three important components that support implementation of evidence-based nursing practice in the global setting. Further, nursing education, nursing research, and clinical practice are dependent community and national support for these nursing endeavors.

Table 18-1 Content and Nature of Relationship-Centered Dialogue

Dialogue Content	*The Nature of Dialogue*
■ Identification of the need for change	■ Exchange of experiences, ideas, and concerns
■ Assessment of barriers, and strengths	■ Mentorship
■ Exchange of ideas and strategies for change	■ Collaborative, verbal, and nonverbal
■ Articulation of a shared vision common goals for change	■ Dialogue that transcends culture and sociopolitical structure
	■ Relational, respectful, and development of trust

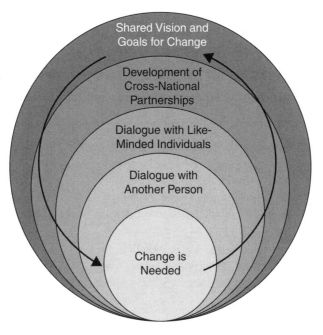

■ **Figure 18-1**

■ Kotter's Change Management Theory

The most effective bridge builders use theoretical frameworks to underpin their efforts to frame the learning, translation, and application of evidence-based nursing practices. Kotter's Change Management Theory (**Table 18-2**) has been used successfully to facilitate change in the healthcare context (Campbell, 2008; Clark, 2010). The first step in Kotter's Framework is to counteract existing complacency by establishing a sense of urgency (Kotter, 1996). Providing analytic data such as statistics, cost of

Table 18-2 Kotters' 8-Step Process for Change (Kotter, 1996)

Creating a Climate for Change
1. Establishing a sense of urgency
2. Creating the guiding coalition

Engaging and Enabling the Organization
3. Developing and communicating a vision and strategy
4. Communicating the change vision
5. Empowering broad-based action
6. Generating short-term wins

Implementing and Sustaining the Change
7. Consolidating gains and producing more change
8. Anchoring new approaches in the culture

care, and nurse attrition rates may create an impetus for change. However, appealing to the emotions and feelings of individuals tends to be more successful in changing behavior (Kotter & Cohen, 2012). The next step is to create a guiding coalition that agrees on the vision and communicates it to others. Enabling action is possible through empowerment and the removal of barriers that may hinder movement forward on this vision. This stage can be time-consuming and requires the buy-in of key stakeholders who are in positions of power. Small accomplishments or "wins" should be celebrated as the broader vision moves forward. In the last phase the focus turns to implementing and sustaining change while keeping the urgency fresh (Kotter, 1996).

Because there is a need to develop new models, here are two exemplars of nurses who have led bridge-building efforts and framed the learning, translation, and application of EBP in the global context.

■ Exemplar One: Clinical Nurse Leaders as Bridge-Builders

Gordana Dermody

Background

Although efforts are underway to transition the care of older adults from the hospital setting into the community, the average length of hospital stay in Japan (19 days) is much higher compared to the average length of hospital stay in Germany, United Kingdom, France, and the United States (6.45 days) (Motohashi, Hamada, Sekimoto, & Imanaka, 2013; OECD, 2009). The provision of evidence-based, efficient, and cost-effective health care is a complex challenge in health systems across the globe

(Lindberg, Nash, & Lindberg, 2008). Similarly to the United States, nursing leaders in Japan, as well as the Japanese healthcare system, are striving to better meet the demands of quality and cost-effective care for their aging society, while maintaining a strong nursing workforce at the bedside and in the community (Japanese Nurses Association, 2016; Poghosyan, Clarke, Finlayson, & Aiken, 2010; Statistics Bureau of Japan (SBJ) Ministry of International Affairs and Communication, 2014).

Care delivery models, supply and demand of human and fiscal resources, and population-specific healthcare needs within different sociocultural contexts are complicated issues that may result in nursing fatigue. This dilemma may in turn affect the integration of EBP, which could have an impact on patient outcomes (Poghosyan et al., 2010). For example, nurse burnout has been cited as a factor in the nursing shortage in Japan (Kanai-Pak, Aiken, Sloane, & Poghosyan, 2008). The literature suggests that links exist among patient outcomes, nurse satisfaction, and the nursing work environment (Poghosyan et al., 2010). As young nurses graduate and are confronted with the complexities of day-to-day clinical operations they soon feel overwhelmed by the demands placed upon them (Kanai-Pak et al., 2008). However, more knowledge about the association between the clinical nursing work environment and patient health outcomes in Japan is needed to mitigate this phenomenon. In addition, little is known about the use of evidence-based nursing practice and the autonomy of Japanese nurses to integrate EBP at the point of care (Delamaire & Lafortune, 2010; Kondo, 2013). Limitations in nursing autonomy also could be related to nursing fatigue because the integration of evidence-based nursing practice change may be inhibited.

The integration of evidence-based nursing practice requires creativity and the willingness of nurses and those with decision-making power to become innovators and take risks with the goal of bringing change to the nursing practice environment (Blakeny, Carleton, McCarthy, & Coakley, 2009). Taking nursing to the next level in Japan requires that Japanese nurses have a supportive work environment, that nurses with advanced degrees are given the opportunity to practice at a level that matches their credentials, and that nurses are empowered to be change-agents (Institute of Medicine, 2010).

The Introduction of the Clinical Nurse Leader Role in Japan

Clinical nurse leaders (CNLs) have unique microsystem expertise, are able to analyze gaps in care, and bring solutions for change in complex healthcare systems (Harris, Roussel, & Thomas, 2014). Integrating the CNL role into the Japanese healthcare system was first conceptualized as a bridge-building activity between US and Japanese nursing faculty, nursing managers, and nursing administrators, as well as bedside nurses and nursing students. A CNL project called: *The Development of a Nurse-Driven Mobility Protocol on a Certified Stroke Unit in a Magnet Designated Medical Center* was shared with Japanese nursing faculty and clinicians in Japan. Assumptions about the role of the CNL were introduced and discussed. The readiness for change among Japanese nurses and healthcare leaders was evident by their interest in the CNL as a new nursing role.

(continues)

The primary aim of the introduction of the CNL role into the Japanese health-care context was to contribute to the promotion of a better nursing work environment through the formation of teamwork, sharing of patient outcome data, and nursing empowerment at the point of care. Integrating the CNL role into the practice setting may have the potential to stave off nurse attrition and burnout. The secondary aim was to improve patient health outcomes through integrating evidence-based nursing practice and to promote efficient and cost-effective nursing care. A collaborative partnership was formed, and yearly educational sessions have been offered both in the United States and in Japan to disseminate how the CNL role could contribute to addressing nursing concerns in Japan. An immersion experience in a hospital setting with a mature CNL workforce and optimal model of CNL integration enhanced the learning about CNL role assumptions and bedside practices. The Japanese nurse-visitors had opportunity to shadow CNLs in the United States at the point of care. They observed how CNLs led daily huddles, rounded with physicians, and led quality improvement initiatives. Through this immersion experience, visiting Japanese nurses developed a more comprehensive understanding of how the CNL could contribute in Japanese hospitals. This collaboration between U.S. and Japanese nursing colleagues has fostered initiatives to promote nurse-faculty CNL certification, to develop a CNL curriculum, and to integrate the role of the CNL into some Japanese hospitals. These early efforts illustrate the developmental process of international partnerships in empowering nurses and promoting change in the clinical practice setting. In addition to laying the groundwork for integrating the role of CNL into the broader hospital settings, small-scale changes in nursing practice have occurred. One Japanese nurse manager from a large university hospital recognized the potential of the *Transforming Care at the Bedside* (TCAB) hourly rounding. This nurse manager aimed to decrease the call-lights on her 47-bed acute care unit. After this nurse-manager's visit to the United States, where she learned about TCAB, she utilized principles of EB nursing practice by implementing a TCAB hourly rounding protocol on the unit she was managing in Japan. This EB initiative reduced the call lights from approximately 1000 per day to 500 per day.

In another case, a Japanese nurse manager who had participated in the CNL immersion experience instituted interdisciplinary rounding on an acute-care internal medicine department, enhancing interdisciplinary collaboration. Bridges are built to allow crossing over from both sides. When U.S. nurse faculty and clinicians visited Japan they gained insight into the inner workings of the Japanese hospital system and nurse's work environment. The excellence in the disaster-preparedness of Japanese nurses and hospital systems is unmatched, and U.S. nurse faculty and clinicians learned much from their Japanese colleagues that could enable them to improve disaster-preparedness in the United States.

■ **Exemplar Two: Improving the Nursing Care of Older Adults: Building Bridges in Russia**

Catherine Van Son

Background

To improve the nursing care of older adults in Russia, a partnership was developed between the Dean of Nursing at a Russian school of nursing and an interdisciplinary team in the United States. Over the course of several years a series of annual professional development workshops for nursing faculty and administrators were planned and delivered. The aim of the workshops was to develop and deliver evidence-based geriatric content and teaching/learning principles, with the goal of integrating these principles into the nursing curriculum.

The geriatric nursing content was designed and delivered using best practices in teaching and learning, and incorporated healthcare administration/management and law, and nursing quality improvement. Each of the 5-week-long workshops focused on a different set of clinical topics including normal aging changes, mental health, prevention of falls and skin breakdown, end-of-life care (including pain management), interdisciplinary teams, and rehabilitation. The workshops were planned jointly by the American team members and the Russian school of nursing dean and were enhanced by conference participant input. The dean provided the team with an in-depth overview of the nursing curriculum and teaching methods utilized in Russia, providing a foundation for the workshop content and design. The Russian dean helped with the explanation of concepts, giving them a cultural context. Presentation slides and handouts were translated into Russian and the workshop was structured to match local customs and procedures.

Gerontological content was not previously part of the Russian nursing curriculum, thus clinical content began with fundamentals such as normal aging changes and physical and functional assessments. In addition to providing essential content, it was important to demonstrate active learning strategies during the workshops. The content presented was linguistically and culturally translated and the delivery of the workshops was tailored to the resources available in the host country. Show-and-tell of adaptive equipment and low-fidelity simulation are often utilized in the United States as a way to actively engage the learner; however, those resources may not be available in another country. Examples of resource tailoring in these workshops include the following. (a) In the United States, adaptive utensils for patients with arthritis can be readily purchased with built-up handles or can be made with thick foam tubing. In Russia, neither the specialized utensil nor foam is available, so participants were shown how to fold a washcloth in thirds, wrap it around the utensil handle and secure it with a rubber band. (b) Two sensory kits were brought for each participant, one to use during the workshop and one to take home to their schools and healthcare organizations. Presenters were careful to make the sensory

(continues)

kits practical so that they could be easily replicated with household materials that could be obtained locally in Russia. Learners experienced the sensory changes of older adults by using woolen gloves to experience peripheral neuropathy. Additional sensory changes are experienced by using needle and thread, plastic sandwich baggie, pieces of paper, a piece of sandpaper, etc. The presenters did not speak Russian; thus, their presentations required interpretation, which was one of the reasons for having workshop materials translated into Russian. Providing the workshop materials in Russian increased participants' understanding of the materials and made it easier to recall the content when sharing with their students and organizations back home.

To ground the learning strategies in theory, adult learning concepts were introduced. With permission, Kolb's (1993) learning style inventory was translated into Russian and completed by the participants as a classroom exercise. The participants were intrigued by the learning theory and explored the learning styles represented in the audience. This was followed by a discussion of different teaching strategies to address the four learning styles and how to incorporate all four phases of a learning cycle when teaching. Many of the teaching strategies used in the workshop were new to the participants, including experiential exercises, games, and role play. Participants soon found that learning through these teaching best-practices was effective and fun, and were eager to try these strategies when they returned home.

Each of the workshops was designed to be able to stand alone but also to build on the previous workshop content. This established continuity and enabled the presenter to "spiral up" the content by adding complexity, broadening the concepts, and allowing more independent learning. One example was the development of a case study, "Anna Petrovna," which evolved during each workshop. We began by introducing Anna in her home environment through a visit by the home health nurse. Anna Petrovna displayed symptoms of urinary tract infection and beginning dementia. The case contained home environment circumstances typical of Russian elders, such as living with family members in a high-rise apartment with a frequently nonfunctioning elevator and with minimal access to alternative living environments—for instance, assisted living. The case study highlighted issues of family caregiving and caregiver stress. In a subsequent workshop, Anna fell and broke her hip; she experienced issues of pain management and developed pressure ulcers. Eventually, Anna and her family dealt with issues regarding the end of life. The case study was supplemented through role play, giving participants the opportunity to discover unfolding issues in the case and to experience another form of interactive learning. This case study engaged the participants and provided an example of how to use case studies in teaching. Participants also received guidelines on how to develop and use case studies and role play as a classroom activity.

Russian literature was also accessed to illustrate another case study regarding the end of life (e.g., Tolstoy's [2003] short story *Death of Ivan Ilyich*). Using a case example from Russian literature allowed participants and instructors to have the same frame of reference for discussing end-of-life issues. To demonstrate how educators can integrate active learning methods into a lecture presentation, we included small groups, games, show and tell, and active demonstrations. Each of these teaching methods was used in the workshop, and handouts were provided to participants to guide them in facilitating these methods in their own teaching settings. Throughout the workshop the presenters were constantly assessing what the participants knew and adjusting their teaching methods to respond to the learning needs of the workshop participants. The necessity for this approach was made evident when discussing the teaching methods used by Russian nursing faculty when instructing on the reduction of pressure ulcers. For example, a bed was brought into the auditorium to observe the teaching methods used by Russian nursing faculty to address the reduction of pressure ulcers. This stimulated a lively conversation among participants regarding the different methods they used to turn and position patients. The workshop presenters then demonstrated evidenced-based methods for reducing the incidence of pressure ulcers and encouraged participants to practice methods of positioning patients that they had not used before (Melnyk, Fineout-Overholt, Feinstein, Sadler, & Green-Hernandez, 2008; Titler, 2008).

Historically, the Russian education paradigm includes didactic education delivery via a strict lecture methodology. As a result, the dialogue between educator and student was limited. Interaction among students was not a fundamental part of the education process, as it is in the United States. In this workshop series, through active learning strategies, the workshop presenter's demonstrated student-centered models of teaching and learning content that were new to the Russian colleagues. Because the participants were engaged in a learning dialogue with each other and their colleagues from the United States, these workshops encouraged professional collaboration and networking.

The Use of Culturally Appropriate Formats

Key to the success of these workshops was adapting to the cultural conventions of the country. Notions of hospitality, sharing a meal, and gift giving were important components of workshop gatherings in Russia. Cultural conventions dictated the length of each day, and time would be reserved on the last day of each workshop for a concluding ceremony, which entailed a formal presentation of certificates of attendance, refreshments, and gift exchanges. Ignoring these customs would have erected a barrier between the international faculty and the Russian participants. Setting aside time for and joining in these activities created bonds of friendship and opened the doors to understanding and shared learning.

Visiting faculty presenters must come to the workshops as learners. The purpose of the workshop was an exchange and valuing of each other's practices and ideas. Both faculty and participants have much to gain from open discussions and listening to each other for better understanding. For example, there is not a word for elder abuse in the Russian language. Instead, there are five different words/concepts in Russian that one can use to get at the issue of elder abuse. This example

(continues)

of linguistic differences suggests a move from pure lecture to active learning methods. Experiential exercises, games, simulations, role plays, and case studies rely on the active engagement of the learner and better mimic the situations in which learning will be applied. Participant learning is enhanced through modeling, discussing relevant theory, evaluating the merits of strategies, and planning and anticipating the use of these strategies in their home environment. Copyrighted materials should be kept to a minimum and should be identified with the copyright restriction. If possible, request permission from the copyright owner for one-time use at the workshop and for additional use by the workshop participants.

This series of workshops occurred over a period of several years. This is contrary to the format often employed in international work, in which an individual or group will have sustained contact with a community for 1–3 months, introduce a change, and then leave the area. Sustained (1 week) yet intermittent (over a period of years) contact allows participants to return to their home facilities and begin using workshop materials, gain experience with the methods and materials, and build on this knowledge at the next workshop session. As a result, participants were eager to return each year for the next installment of the program. Many brought additional members of their faculty and organizations to subsequent workshops. Because many of the participants returned year after year, they developed strong professional networks to share ideas and kept in touch with each other in between workshops, creating a network of support and innovation.

This exemplar describes a model for evidence-based teaching in an international arena. The series of workshops designed and offered by an international faculty focusing on the care of the older adult has influenced content and teaching strategies of Russian nursing curricula and healthcare facilities. Workshop materials have been shared with students, faculty, and practicing nurses and have served as the basis for additional nursing research and practice changes in both countries.

Discussion

Both exemplars demonstrate the successful development of ongoing collaboration. In addition, the exemplars show that evidence-based nursing practice can be promoted through sustained, cross-national partnerships. However, both authors are acutely aware that although the dissemination of EBP knowledge is important, knowledge alone is not sufficient for nurses and nursing leaders to have the power to integrate evidence-based nursing practices. The issue of empowering nurses is exceedingly important if evidence-based nursing practice is to be integrated into the model of nursing care delivery across the globe. Teaching EBP principles and concepts may need to be coupled with motivation and encouragement to overcome existing barriers. Other important aspects to consider are the readiness for change among nurses and healthcare settings and among those who may be empowered to remove the barriers that nurses' face in order to accelerate the building of cross-national bridges among nurse-educators nurse-clinicians and healthcare leaders worldwide (IHI, 2014; ICN, 2016).

REFERENCES

Abood, S. (2007). Influencing health care in the legislative arena. *OJIN: The Online Journal of Issues in Nursing, 12*(1), Manuscript 2. Retrieved from http://www.nursingworld.org/ojin/

American Nurses Association. (2001). *The code of ethics for nurses with interpretive statements.* Washington, DC: Nursesbooks.org.

American Nurses Association. (2010a). *Nursing's social policy statement: The essence of the profession* (3rd ed.). Silver Spring, MD: Nursebooks.org.

American Nurses Association. (2010b). *Nursing: Scope and standards of practice* (2nd ed.). Silver Spring, MD: Nursesbooks.org.

Berkowitz, B. (2012). The policy process. *Policy & Politics in Nursing and Health Care* (6th ed., pp. 49–64). St. Louis, MO: Saunders.

Blakeney, B., Carleton, P., McCarthy, C., & Coakley, E. (2009, May). Unlocking the power of innovation. *OJIN: The Online Journal of Issues in Nursing, 14*(2), Manuscript 1. doi:10.3912/OJINVol14No02Man01

Boström, A. M., Ehrenberg, A., Gustavsson, J. P., & Wallin, L. (2009). Registered nurses' application of evidence-based practice: A national survey. *International Journal of Public Health Services Research, 15,* 1159–1163.

Boström, A. M., Rudman, A., Gustavsson, J. P., & Wallin, L. (2013). Factors associated with evidence-based practice among registered nurses in Sweden: A national cross-sectional study. *BMC Health Service Research, 13,* 165.

Brown, C. E., Wickline, M. A., Ecoff, L., & Glaser, D. (2008). Nursing practice, knowledge, attitudes ad perceived barriers to evidence-based practice at an academic medical center. *Journal of Advanced Nursing, 65*(2), 371–381. doi:10.1111/j.1365-2648.2008.04878x

Campbell, R. J. (2008). Change management in healthcare. *Health Care Manager, 27*(1), 23–39.

Clark, C. (2010). From incivility to civility: Transforming the culture. *Reflections on Nursing Leadership, 36*(3), 2.

Delamaire, M., & Lafortune, G. (2010). Nurses in advanced roles: A description and evaluation of experiences in 12 developed countries. *OECD Health Working Papers* (No. 54). Paris, France: OECD Publishing. doi:10.1787/5kmbrcfms5g7-en

Ditlopo, P., Laauw, D., Penn-Kekana, L., & Rispel, L. C. (2014). Contestations and complexities of nurses' participation in policy-making in South Africa. *Global Health Action, 7,* 25237. Retrieved from http://dx.doi.org/10.3402/gha.v7.25327

Egerod, I., & Hansen, G. M. (2005). Evidence-based practice among Danish cardiac nurses: A national survey. *Journal of Advanced Nursing, 51*(5), 465–473.

Eizenberg, M. M. (2010). Implementation of evidence-based nursing practice: Nurses personal and professional factors? *Journal of Advanced Nursing, 67*(1), 33–42. doi:10.1111/j.1365-2648.2010.05488.x

Feetham, S., & Doering, J. (2015). Career cartography: A conceptualization of career development to advance health and policy. *Journal of Nursing Scholarship, 47*(1), 70–77.

Fineout-Overholt, E., Melnyk, B. M., & Schultz, A. (2005). Transforming health care form the inside out: Advancing evidence-based practice in the 21st century. *Journal of Professional Nursing, 21*(6), 335–344.

Green, L. W., Ottoson, J. M., Garcia, C., & Hiatt, R. A. (2009). Diffusion theory and knowledge dissemination, utilization, and integration in public health. *Annual Review of Public Health, 30,* 151–174.

Hall, H. R., & Roussel, L. A. (2014). *Evidence-based practice: An integrative approach to research, administration and practice.* Burlington, MA: Jones & Bartlett Learning.

Harris, J. L., Roussel, L., & Thomas, P. L. (2014). *Initiating and sustaining the clinical nurse leader role: A practical guide.* Burlington, MA: Jones & Bartlett Learning.

Hegge, M. J. (2011). The lingering presence of Florence Nightingale. *Nursing Science Quarterly, 24*(2), 152–162. doi:10.1177/0894318411399453

Hern, M. J., Vaughn, G., Mason, D., & Weitkamp, T. (2005). Creating an international nursing practice and education workplace. *Journal of Pediatric Nursing, 20*(1), 34–44.

Hinshaw, A. S., & Grady, P. A. (Eds.). (2011). *Shaping health policy through nursing research.* New York, NY: Springer.

Hudson, R. B. (2014). In R. B. Hudson (Ed.), *The new politics of old age policy.* (3rd ed.). Baltimore, MD: Johns Hopkins University Press.

Institute for Health Improvement (2014). *Improving health and healthcare worldwide.* Retrieved from http://www.ihi.org

Institute of Medicine. (2010). *The future of nursing: Leading change, advancing health.* Washington, DC: National Academy Press.

International Council of Nurses (2012). *Closing the gap: From evidence to action.* International Nurses Day (May 12, 2012), pp. 1–58. Geneva, Switzerland: Author. Retrieved from http://www.icn.ch/images/stories/documents/publications/ind/indkit2012.pdf

International Council of Nurses. (2016). *Education network fact sheet.* Retrieved from http://www.icn.ch/

Japanese Nurses Association. (2016). Nursing in Japan. Retrieved from: http://www.nurse.or.jp/jna/english/nursing/

Kanai-Pak, M., Aiken, L., Sloane, D. M., & Poghosyan, L. (2008). Poor working environments and nurse inexperience are associated with burnout, job dissatisfaction and quality deficits in Japanese hospitals. *Journal of Clinical Nursing, 17*, 3324–3329. doi:10.111/j.1365-2702.2008.02639

Keith, J. M. (1988). Florence Nightingale: Statistician and consultant epidemiologist. *International Nursing Review, 35*(5), 147–150.

Kolb, D. A. (1993). *Learning-style inventory: Self-scoring inventory and interpretation booklet—Revised scoring.* Boston, MA: Hay/McBer Training Resources Group.

Kondo, A. (2013). Advanced practice nurses in Japan: Education and related issues. *Journal of Nursing Care, S5*(4), 1–6. doi:10.4172/2167-1168.S5-004

Kopf, E. W. (1978). Florence Nightingale as statistician. *Research in Nursing and Health, 1*(3), 93–102.

Köpke, S., Koch, F., & Blazer, K. (2013). Einstellungen pflegender in Deutschen krankenhäusern zu einer evidenzbasierten pflegepraxis [German hospital nurses' attitudes concerning evidence-based nursing practice]. *Pflege, 26*(3), 163–175 [German].

Kotter, J. P. (1996). *Leading change.* Boston, MA: Harvard Business School.

Kotter, J. P., & Cohen, D. S. (2012). *The heart of change: Real life stories of how people change their organizations.* Boston, MA: Harvard Business School Press.

Levine, M. (2009). Transforming experiences: Nursing education and international immersion programs. *Journal of Professional Nursing, 25*(3), 156–169.

Lindberg, C., Nash, S., & Lindberg, C. (2008). *On the edge: Nursing in the age of complexity.* Bordentown, NJ: PlexusPress:

Matthews, J., (2012). Role of professional organizations in advocating for the nursing profession. *OJIN: The Online Journal of Issues in Nursing, 17*(1), Manuscript 3.

McAuliffe, M. S., & Cohen, M. Z. (2005). International nursing research and educational exchanges: A review of the literature. *Nursing Outlook, 53*(1), 21–25.

Melnyk, B. M., & Fineout-Overholt, E. (2015). *Evidence-based practice in nursing & healthcare: A guide to best practice* (3rd ed.). Philadelphia, PA: Wolters-Kluwer.

Melnyk, B. M., Fineout-Overholt, E., Feinstein, N. F., Sadler, L. S., & Green-Hernandez, C. (2008). Nurse practitioner educators' perceived knowledge, beliefs, and teaching strategies regarding evidence-based practice: Implications for accelerating the integration of evidence-based practice into graduate programs. *Journal of Professional Nursing, 24*(1), 7–13.

Moch, S. D., Cronje, R. J., & Branson, J. (2010). Part 1. Understanding nursing evidence-based practice education: Envisioning the role of students. *Journal of Professional Nursing, 26*(1), 5–13.

Moten, A., Schafer, D. F., & Montgomery, E. (2012). A prescription for health inequity: Building public health infrastructure I resources-poor settings. *Journal of Global Health, 2*(2), 1–4. doi:10.7189/jogh.02.020302

Motohashi, T., Hamada, H., Sekimoto, M., & Imanaka, Y. (2013). Factors associated with prolonged length of hospital stay of elderly patients in acute care hospitals in Japan: A multilevel analysis of patients with femoral neck fracture. *Health Policy, 111*, 60–67.

Nightingale, F. (1860). *Notes on nursing: What it is, and what it is not.* New York, NY: D. Appleton and Company.

Organisation for Economic Co-operation and Development. (2009). Average length of stay in hospitals. In *Health at a glance 2009*. Washington, DC: OECD.

Poghosyan, L., Clarke, S. P., Finlayson, M., & Aiken, L. H. (2010). Nurse burn-out and quality of care: Cross-national investigation in six countries. *Research in Nursing & Health, 33*(4), 288–298.

Poovey, M. (Ed.) (1992). *Florence Nightingale: Cassandra and other selections from Suggestions for Thought*. New York, NY: New York University Press.

Price, L. (2012). Research as a political tool and policy tool. *Policy and Politics in Nursing and Healthcare, 6*, 316–321.

Savage, C., & Kub, J. (2009). Public health and nursing: A natural partnership. *International Journal of Environmental Research Public Health, 6*, 2843–2848.doi:10.3390/ijerph6112843

Sherwood, G., & Liu, H. (2005). International collaboration for developing graduate education in China. *Nursing Outlook, 53*(1), 15–20.

Statistics Bureau of Japan (SBJ) Ministry of International Affairs and Communications. (2014). Population estimates by age (5 year age group) and sex: July 1, 2014 (final estimates), December 1, 2014 (provisional estimates). Retrieved from http://www.stat.go.jp

Stichler, J. F., Fields, W., Kim S. C., & Brown, C. E. (2011). Faculty knowledge, attitudes and perceived barriers to teaching evidence-based nursing. *Journal of Professional Nursing, 27*(2), 92–100.

Stokke, K., Olsen, N. R., Espehaug, B., & Nortvedt, M. W. (2014). Evidence based practice beliefs and implementation among nurses: a cross sectional study. *BMC Nursing 13*(8). Retrieved from http://www.biomedcentral.com

Thorsteinsson, H. S. (2013). Icelandic nurses' beliefs, skills, and resources associated with evidence-based practice and related factors: A national survey. *Worldviews on Evidence-Based Nursing, 10*(2), 116–126.

Titler, M. G. (2008). In R. G. Hughes (Ed.). *Patient safety and quality: An evidence-based handbook for nurses*. Rockville, MD: Agency for Healthcare Research and Quality.

Tolstoy, L. (2003). *Death of Ivan Ilych* (A. Maude, Trans.). New York, NY: Signet Classic. (Original work published 1886.)

Vikpeh-Lartey, B., Nkansah-Baidoo, M., & Furlane. (2016). Chiefs take active role in improving primary health care services in Western Ghana. Jhpiego: innovating to save lives, an Affiliate of Johns Hopkins University. Retrieved from https://www.jhpiego.org/success-story/chiefs-take-active-role-in-improving-primary-health-care-services-in-western-ghana/

Weston, M. J. (2008). Defining control over nursing practice and autonomy. *Journal of Nursing Administration, 38*, 404–408.

Weston, M. J. (2010) Strategies for enhancing autonomy and control over nursing practice. *OJIN: The Online Journal of Issues in Nursing, 15*(1). doi:10.3912/OJIN.Vol15No01Man02. Retrieved from http://www.nursingworld.org

World Health Organization. (2010). Wanted: 2.4 million nurses, and that's just in India (Bulletin), 88(5), 321–400.

World Health Organization. (2016). Global Health Observatory (GHO). Retrieved from http://www.who.int/gho/health_technologies/medical_devices/healthcare_infrastructure/en/

CHAPTER 19

Barriers to Evidence-Based Practice in Developing Countries

■ DUYGU HIÇDURMAZ, HANDAN BOZTEPE, AND LINDA ROUSSEL ■

■ Objectives:

- Recognize the importance of evidence-based practice (EBP) for developing countries.
- Identify the barriers to EBP in developing countries.
- Identify the strategies for overcoming barriers to EBP in developing countries.

■ Importance of Evidence-Based Practice for Developing Countries

Providing high-quality, cost-effective care, and improved patient outcomes necessitates specific guidance that healthcare providers can trust and act upon (Carlson & Plonczynski, 2008). EBP based on science involves the use of the most current and powerful research evidence in practice and suggests this proposition as the most successful and cost-effective approach to nursing care (Bartelt et al., 2011; Rudman, Gustavsson, Ehrenberg, Bostrom, & Wallin, 2012; Stetler, Ritchie, Rycroft-Malone, Schultz, & Charns, 2007). Results of high-quality research, evidence-based systematic reviews, and clinical guidelines are the tools that provide the guidance needed by healthcare professionals and nurses. However, today's healthcare literature is mainly based on evidence from developed countries such as the United States and Western Europe (Chinnock, Siegfried, & Clarke, 2005). This evidence may not be appropriate for developing countries with different socioeconomic, environmental, and cultural structures compared to developed countries.

The identity of "developing country" is based on an evaluation of socioeconomic variables. Developing countries are known as the countries that are poor or have limited resources; therefore, the policies managing the allocation of these resources require a rational, careful, and sensitive approach using scientifically sound evidence. On the other hand, the socioeconomic, political, environmental, and cultural characteristics of developing countries make production of evidence more difficult. Research-led practice seems to be irrelevant when systems are in disarray (Garner, Kale, Dickson, Dans, & Salinas, 1998). A circuitous path of strongly needed EBP and policies not allowing the implementation of these practices arises. In developing countries, this pathway needs to be addressed at different failure points that make EBP an important issue for developing countries.

■ Barriers to Evidence-Based Practice in Developing Countries

EBP necessitates integrating individual clinical expertise with the best available external clinical evidence from systematic research (Sackett, Rosenberg, Gray, Haynes, & Richardson, 1996). Nurses are expected to combine the best scientific evidence from nursing and other disciplines with their specialty clinical perspective during performance of the full range of care activities to conduct evidence-based nursing (McPheeters & Lohr, 1999). Attaining best practices through rigorous conduct of research evidence is problematic with multiple factors related to design, utilization, and critical appraisal of research characteristics of nursing professionals who will understand, interpret, and appropriately use this research and the system in which all of these phenomena occur. The complexity of the research and healthcare practice in developing countries makes the issue more complicated. On the other hand, it is necessary to look at the barriers to EBP in light of the literature published from developing countries. The international literature lacks high-level research evidence.

Barriers Related to Developing Country Realities

When EBP is viewed from a broader perspective, the policies of developing countries regarding research are the first to be seen. Research and policy-making are strongly interlinked. However, there are some misconceptions about this interlinkage. Policy-making is conceptualized as a linear and logical process. Policy-makers identify a problem, conduct research, take note of the results, and make sensible policies that are implemented. Clearly, this is not the case in policy-making relevant to EBP and setting care standards (Young, 2005). Policy-making is a dynamic, complex, and chaotic process, especially in developing countries. Research-policy links are dramatically shaped by the political context (Young, 2005). In workshops organized by the Overseas Development Institute with participants from developing countries, the most crucial challenges in the process of informing policy with evidence-based research in developing countries include instability and high turnover of key positions, authoritarianism as a virtue, favoritism, empirical policy-making, and lack of transparency (Young, 2005). Additionally, lack of high-quality credible research, limited awareness of the dramatic influence of donors and grant institutions on research and policy processes, poor recognition of civil society organizations by policy-makers, and lower involvement of these organizations in policy-making are but a few of the factors that have an impact on EBP in developing countries (Young, 2005).

Most research addresses health conditions and nursing issues that are priorities in the developed world (Swingler, Volmink, & Ioannidis, 2003) and focuses on the discussion of the results in the United States and Western Europe (Chinnock et al., 2005). Although nurses and other healthcare professionals in developing countries use relatively older and cheaper technology, the authors assessed the evidence for more recent and expensive technologies (Chinnock et al., 2005). Because of a lack of research conducted in developing countries and difficulties in publishing research in a journal or in an indexed journal (Horton, 2003), most of the research published is conducted in developed countries (Chinnock et al., 2005). Also, difficulties of conducting randomized controlled trials that reveal the type of evidence to have the greatest credibility in resource-poor countries result in the exclusion of many developing country studies from the literature. The differences in patient populations and in the delivery of health care between developed and developing countries make the transferability of the evidence derived in developing countries into developed countries problematic at best (Chinnock et al., 2005).

Evidence-based nursing cannot be isolated from other political, organizational, and social factors that affect nurses and healthcare environments (Estabrooks, Floyd, Scott-Findlay, O'Leary, & Gushta, 2003). Rapid alterations are present in developing countries with regard to political, organizational, and social factors, and this slippery ground mostly influence counterparts in negative ways. Accessibility of research findings, anticipated outcomes, administration, and organizational support are challenges that developing countries struggle with on a daily basis. Garnering support from others to use the evidence, financial support, and nurses' understanding of evidence-based nursing and its clinical relevance are requisite best practices. Logistical issues such as the availability of journals, knowledge, and skills in searching for and evaluating research evidence and authority to change practice are factors hindering evidence and practice-based nursing (Brown, Wickline, Ecoff, & Glaser, 2009; Chau, Lopez, & Thompson, 2008; DiCenso et al., 2004; Funk, Champagne, Wiese, & Tornquist, 1991; Funk, Tornquist, & Champagne, 1995; Glacken & Chaney, 2004; Hannes et al, 2007; Hutchinson & Johnston, 2004; Kajermo et al., 2010; Kajermo, Nordstrom, Krusebrant, & Bjorvell, 1998; Koehn & Lehman, 2008; Melnyk et al., 2004; Melnyk, Fineout-Overholt, Gallagher-Ford, & Kaplan, 2012; Nagy, Lumby, McKinley, & Macfarlane, 2001). When conditions of evidence-based nursing are assessed in light of disadvantages in developing countries, the magnitude and variety of barriers to EBP may be better understood. In several studies conducted in Turkey, the most important factors hindering utilization of research findings in practice were reported as (a) inappropriate environments to implement research findings; (b) difficulty in understanding the literature because it is not presented in one resource; (c) lack of awareness of EBP (Sarı, Turgay, Genç, & Bozkurt, 2012); (d) difficult identifying time to read the research (Öztürk, Kaya, Ayık, Uygur, & Cengiz, 2010; Tan, Akgün Sahin, & Kardas Özdemir, 2012); and (e) lack of time, collaboration, and autonomy (Demir et al., 2012).

Barriers Related to Theory-Practice Gap and Professional Realities

The gap between theory and practice in nursing and reflection of EBPs in clinical practices have been discussed in the literature. Different strategies have been suggested to close the gap (Carlson & Plonczynski, 2008; Champion & Leach, 1989; Rosswurm & Larrabee, 1999). This theory-practice gap remains a major issue hindering evidence-based nursing in developing countries, as well. In a study focused on knowledge and perceptions of medical, nursing, and allied health practitioners in Malaysia, 61% of nurses and other health practitioners agreed that there is an exaggeration of the importance of EBP in patient care whereas only 33% of physicians agreed with this finding. In the same study, 46% of nurses and other health practitioners reported that "evidence-based practice is too tedious and impractical"; 21% of physicians reported the same (Lai, Teng, & Lee, 2010).

Wide gaps between evidence and practice make it increasingly important to influence change in health professionals' clinical practice in developing countries. Use of clinical guidelines and policies to inform and reinforce good practice is desirable (Siddiqi, Newell, & Robinson, 2005). However, in the majority of healthcare settings in developing countries, clinical policies do not exist or lack consistent adherence to standards of care (Heiby, 1998; Oranta, Routasalo, & Hupli, 2002).

Educational Barriers

In developing countries, nursing education is another problem area relative to EBP. In some developing countries the title "nurse" may be given equally to all nurses despite different levels of educational background, including vocational high school degree, associate degree, and baccalaureate of science or graduate degrees. Legal authorities such as ministries of health entitle all nurses with the same "nurse" title with little expectation for understanding and using research evidence. In a qualitative study conducted in Iran, nurses were asked "what is the meaning of evidence-based nursing" and for many, it was the first time that they had encountered the idiom of evidence-based nursing (Adib-Hajbaghery, 2007). In the same study, participants defined evidence-based nursing as nurses using their knowledge obtained professionally to care for and respond to patients' needs. These nurses were seeing professional knowledge as basic evidence for nursing care and report paying little attention to research evidence to change practice. This was likely due to no or limited research knowledge or skills (Adib-Hajbaghery, 2007; Retsas, 2000).

Another barrier to EBP relates to nurses' having limited awareness of what constitutes evidence and how evidence is translated into practice (Özdemir & Akdemir, 2009). In developing countries, the expectation is that entry into the nursing profession is at the bachelor's level. Undergraduate nursing education programs do provide content in research and EBP for the beginning generalist in nursing. Most of the research education in developing countries is provided in graduate programs. Yet, graduates of these programs prefer to work in administrative nursing roles or in academic positions (Bahçecik & Ecevit, 2009). Highly research-qualified nurses generally are not working in clinical practice, thus further widening the gap between theory, research, and practice.

Organizational Barriers

Utilization of research findings in practice depends on individual and organizational factors (Forsman, Rudman, Gustavsson, Ehrenberg, & Wallin, 2010). Organizational characteristics, including structure and functioning of healthcare organizations, were determined as the most substantial factors affecting EBP uptake (Cummings, Hutchinson, Scott, Norton, & Estabrooks, 2010). Leadership, workload, staffing, and organizational culture are factors in healthcare organizations influencing EBP. Adib-Hajbaghery (2007) determined lack of professional knowledge and experience, limited time and opportunity for evidence-based care, and increased number of patients, were reasons Iranian nurses did not readily embrace research evidence. Heavy workload, inadequate staffing, traditional task-oriented work, lack of self-confidence affected by role ambiguity, and physician centered structure of the health system are also themes identified in this qualitative study. Educational barriers such as low quality of nursing education, inexperienced and task-oriented nurse educators, inefficient management and supervision, senior managers devaluing EBP were also described as problematic for EBP as a professional mandate. In a study conducted in Turkey, Özdemir and Akdemir (2009) reported factors ranging from issues related to basic nursing education to more complex topics involving politics of health care, organizational support, and context as the most important factors influencing EBP. In the same study, they determined a positive relationship between research utilization and organizational support (Özdemir & Akdemir, 2009). Similarly, Parahoo (2000) reported management style, listening to staff, particularly their successes as factors enabling utilization of research. For overcoming identified barriers, Munroe, Duffy, and Fisher (2008) organized an education program to develop knowledge, skills, and attitudes of nurses toward research and EBP reporting an increase in nurses' knowledge and skills after program implementation. In a similar study aiming to develop research utilization in practice via an education program, findings suggested the program was helpful in improving nurses' attitudes toward using research findings (Tsai, 2003). Programs targeting development of EBPs are found to be more successful if organizational support exists (Royle & Blythe, 1998). In similar studies, organization support was reported as one of the most essential facilitators of EBP (Kajermo et al., 1998; Parahoo, 2000; Chau et al., 2008; Ghada, Shereen, & Reda, 2012; Solomons, & Spross, 2011).

Individual Barriers

Self-perception and self-confidence play an essential role in governing an individual's motivation to learn, practice, and maintain skills (Bandura, 1994). Self-confidence of healthcare professionals in their application of EBPs plays an important role in their attitudes and activities. However, nurses of developing countries show poor self-confidence in the translating EBP. This phenomenon may be related to factors such as educational background, culture, and organization of healthcare systems that prioritize physicians' education and practice. In a study on knowledge and perceptions of medical, nursing, and allied health practitioners toward EBP in Malaysia (Lai et al., 2010), physicians were found more confident and more positive in their perception of EBP than nurses and other allied healthcare professions. When searching for evidence, the majority of the physicians were more satisfied with their search results. On the other hand, over half of the nurses and other allied health professions either hardly performed any search or were seldom satisfied with their searches (Lai et al., 2010). In another study conducted with nurses working in the Eastern Anatolian Region of Turkey, the rate of the nurses participating in scientific research activities as well as keeping up with the professional journals was found to be low (Tan et al., 2012). This study reported that although nurses considered research important to their nursing practice, they continued their profession practice using traditional methods and rituals, with limited acknowledgment of utilizing research findings in care delivery (Tan et al., 2012).

Barriers Related With Access to Evidence

Supply and utilization of information technologies are generally poor in developing countries, forming a barrier to EBP. In a study on the barriers to EBP, the largest proportions of the medical, nursing, and allied health practitioners reported a lack of good information technology support in delivering care (Lai et al., 2010).

Another dimension of access in developing countries is related to access to knowledge and resources. In a study on awareness, use, and barriers of EBPs in reproductive health, lack of awareness, and lack of supplies and materials were determined as the major barriers to EBP (Tita, Selwyn, Waller, Kapadia, & Dongmo, 2005).

Not knowing a foreign language—mainly English—may be listed among the factors hindering access to research findings in developing countries because most of the research has been published in international journals are English-centric. In their study, conducted in Turkey, Kelleci, Gölbaşı, Yılmaz, and Doğan (2008) reported the rate of nurses who regularly followed professional publications as low as 11%.

■ Strategies for Overcoming Barriers to Evidence-Based Practice in Developing Countries

Work environments are the main variables affecting implementation of evidence-based nursing. For EBP uptake, decreasing the barriers to access of information, and educational readiness, creating opportunities for a research-friendly environment, can go far to influence care delivery using best practices. Organizations require a supportive and powerful management and supervisory system by providing adequate staff, encouraging teamwork, and creating user-friendly work environment that empower nurses to seek out and use evidence in their practice. Although senior nurse managers of developing countries report awareness of barriers to evidence-based nursing, it was noted that lowering expectations for the use of research evidence rather than removing barriers was the preferred option. Essentially, the researcher found that carrying out traditional, task-oriented roles was the overall expectation of senior nurse leadership for staff nurses (Adib-Hajbaghery, 2007). It is difficult for evidence-based nursing to flourish in environments that support ritualistic practices. Manager and supervisor inexperience, insecurity, lack of self-confidence, or being overly concern for self-promotion were found to negatively contribute to this environment (Adib-Hajbaghery, 2007). A patient-centered focus is required throughout an organization, where managers are not intent on doing more work with fewer nurses, and nurses are therefore not encouraged to adopt EBP, preferring routine-oriented, task-based methods of working (Adib-Hajbaghery, 2007). Time and opportunity are other important factors affecting implementation of evidence-based nursing, and that lack of time, caused by unbalanced ratio of nurses to patients, is an important barrier to EBP. It is essential that managers take responsibility for overcoming these barriers and redesign care delivery systems that include time and opportunity for nurses to implement evidence-based nursing (Adib-Hajbaghery, 2007). Nurses who have time and participate in research projects use EBPs more than other nurses (Royle & Blythe, 1998; Fink, Thompson, & Bonnes, 2005).

For creating a research-friendly work environment, the institutions can organize educational programs, conferences, interactive meetings to create and strengthen a positive attitude toward EBPs. The importance of teaching evidence-based processes and learning how to access online resources can accelerate and ease the access to research findings. Also, developing clinical guidelines to inform and reinforce good practice are necessary to inform clinical care (Siddiqi et al., 2005).

Nursing education plays a critical role in preparing nurses for EBP. For enabling utilization of EBP, nurses should have a sound educational base, have the power to make a change and have appropriate role models. Nurses who discover the value and importance of EBP can be a role model for others. Hence, some organizations have developed programs to generalize EBPs and support nurses' utilization of research findings in practice, revealing successful efforts (Schulman 2008; Straka, Brandt, & Brytus, 2013). Senior healthcare professionals may be role models for junior healthcare professionals, as well. Dedicated EBP programs for senior clinicians and policy-makers may be the key to changing practice culture (Lai et al., 2010).

Differentiating good-quality from poorer quality evidence requires critical appraisal skills. The foundations of critical appraisal skills should be laid during undergraduate education of nurses and other healthcare professionals in developing countries. These appraisal skills can be improved with continuing education programs during their professional working lives (Lai et al., 2010).

Negative attitudes toward EBP may arise from lower self-confidence in EBP. Greater efforts to promote EBP in undergraduate curriculum are needed.

Incorporating multidisciplinary evidence-based approach into this curriculum will make the efforts more successful as a multidisciplinary evidence-based culture (Lai et al., 2010).

Nurses and other healthcare professionals report poor access to evidence and poor information technologies as barriers to EBP. Efforts to provide reliable access to clinical evidence at the point of care provide user-friendly and preappraised evidence-based resources, and journals should be made available (Lai et al., 2010). A lack of systematic reviews relevant to the priorities of developing countries has been reported. Preparing and publishing systematic reviews considering the needs of developing countries will be instrumental in EBP uptake for these countries.

Better use of research-based evidence in policy-production and practice can help save lives, reduce poverty, and improve the quality of life in developing countries. Delivering academically credible research-based evidence and advice to policy-makers in the right format at the right time can be a very helpful strategy. This strategy is referred to as "Think Tanks" and considered to be relatively low in developing countries (Young, 2005). Another strategy in developing evidence-based policy-making can be using networks (Young, 2005). National, regional, and global networks play a remarkable role in development policy (Stone & Maxwell, 2005) and many national and international networks were cited as influential during the workshops organized by the Overseas Development Institute (Young, 2005).

Finally, a more systematic understanding of the external context, the political context, the evidence, and the links between them will help researchers, policy-makers, practitioners, and civil society organizations decide how they can best promote evidence-based policy. Particular attention needs to be given in developing countries to the factors that shape local policy and political processes. The capacity to generate and use research-based evidence effectively, donor and grant institution influence on research and policy processes, and empowerment of civil society can go far in promoting evidence-based policy-making (Young, 2005).

■ **Exemplar One: Overcoming Barriers to Evidence-Based Culture: The Formation Story of the Turkish Psychiatric Nurses Association**

The idea of formation of the Turkish Psychiatric Nurses Association goes back to the early 1990s. A group of academician psychiatric nurses from Istanbul, Turkey came together to discuss issues in psychiatric nursing, including the barriers to adopting EBP, the status of psychiatric nurses in education, practice, and society, and the necessity of standards for psychiatric nursing practice, education, and research. They were aware of the gaps between research and practice and expressed a need for talking the same language that could be based on evidence. The first meeting was organized in March 17, 1991 with the desire to share problems with more psychiatric nurses. Participants of this meeting were limited and included psychiatric nursing faculty from major universities of Istanbul. This first formal meeting became the beginning of the Turkish Psychiatric Nurses Association. This first meeting launched a small group of academician and clinical psychiatric nurses passionate to keep the association alive and ultimately developing an infrastructure for the group. They stressed the collaboration between psychiatric nurses from the academia and clinical practice. They organized another meeting on April 17, 1996 to share their work with a larger audience and increase participation and membership. Many academic and clinical psychiatric nurses all over the country joined this meeting and adopted the course of action on formation of the association and writing its charter. The association was formally founded on May 15, 2000. Since its foundation, the association has worked to fill in gaps between research and practice and develop evidence-based psychiatric nursing practice guidelines. The Turkish Psychiatric Nursing Journal was born from this initiative, as well an International and National Psychiatric Nursing Conference hosted every year (the 4th International and 8th National Psychiatric Nursing conference will be held in 2016). Committees have been formed and are working on issues related to psychiatric nursing (evidence-based psychiatric nursing, psychiatric nursing education). The association has participated in several levels of policy-making related to psychiatric nursing in Turkey (Turkish Psychiatric Nurses Association, 2016).

■ Exemplar Two: Efforts to Improve Evidence-Based Practices in Hacettepe University Hospitals: By Narration of Nursing Services Directorate Fusun Terzioglu

Hacettepe University comprises adult, child, oncology, and physical therapy hospitals and outpatient clinics. Directorate of Nursing Services in Hacettepe University Hospitals was established in 2012 as a result of adjustments on the hospital organizational chart. In the context of these adjustments, Administrative Affairs Coordinator, Treatment and Clinical Services Coordinator, Financial Affairs Coordinator, and Directorate of Nursing Services were connected to the Hospitals General Director with a horizontal arrangement. Since its formation, the aims of Nursing Services Directorate are planning, organizing, managing, supervising, evaluating, and coordinating the services to provide high-quality nursing services in accordance with Joint Commission International quality policies. It is responsible for working in coordination with other disciplines, managing nursing resources, and appointing appropriate staff to fulfill functions of improving implementation, management, education, research, and quality in care. Ensuring the implementation of

(continues)

professional nursing care standards is included in its function. It is also responsible for monitoring quality improvement trends in nursing across the world, adapting improvements to Hacettepe University Hospitals, and announcing innovations made in Hacettepe University Hospitals to national and international platforms. The Directorate has recognized an urgent need to improve EBPs and made considerable effort to develop these practices in all of the embodied hospitals and clinics since 2012.

One of the most important determinants of nursing service quality was EBPs. Studies were conducted with more than 1200 nurses working at the hospitals to determine factors affecting nurses' performance and productivity, the people and behaviors causing the bullying at work environment, and the professional attitudes of nurses. Study findings propelled action including establishing quality-improvement teams and identifying problem-solving techniques to address barriers. These efforts have been conducted to make nursing services visible, one of the most important issues for nursing in influencing current nurse workforce productivity. Nurses' scientific knowledge could be improved through research. Practice-oriented research topics and preparation of proposals to ensure the development and cost-effectiveness of patient care have been extremely important. Twenty-five certificate programs in different fields such as operating room nursing, emergency room and intensive care unit nursing, stoma and wound care nursing, palliative care nursing, and home care nursing were created. These programs developed competencies of nurses, aligning the future mission and vision of the Directorate of the Nursing Services. The Directorate has made contribution to the development of nurses' individual competencies and improvement of their professional motivation with activities, including regular education programs, opportunities to participate in graduate training, and conferences. The Directorate now believes that mentor nurse education conducted by the Directorate will improve nursing students' practices and knowledge. Projects proposed by the Directorate for international training of nurses and nursing students provided opportunities for making Hacettepe University Hospitals a preferred institution by graduate nurses. These driving forces are substantial elements for improving EBPs in their hospitals (F. Terzioglu, personal narration, February 18, 2016).

■ **Exemplar Three: Developing New Evidence-Based Practice Insights: Our Visiting Scholarship Process in the University of Alabama at Birmingham School of Nursing (UABSON), USA**

UABSON in the United States, and Hacettepe University Faculty of Nursing, Turkey, started an international partnership allowing mutual exchange of academic staff and students in 2013. Within the scope of this partnership we—the authors of this chapter—visited UABSON in 2015–2016. During our visit, we had the opportunity to work with Dr. Linda Roussel and participated in various EBP activities in UABSON and UAB Medicine Hospitals ranging from critical appraisal classes to meetings on developing clinical guidelines. During our EBP journey, we met with other academicians working on EBPs, Doctor of Nursing Practice (DNP) students from UABSON, and nurses from the UAB hospitals. We have had valuable discussions on production and utilization of evidence, types and credibility of evidence, contribution of systematic reviews and clinical guidelines to EBP, differences between the United State and Turkey in terms of evidence-based culture, and how to develop an EBP culture. Each of these activities has broadened our vision and provided insight about developing EBPs in our university and in our country.

■ Conclusion

EBP is still a developing area for the world. Considering sociological, economic, policy-based, environmental, cultural structure of developing countries, the quantity and density of problems in utilization of EBP in these countries are higher. Overcoming these problems and barriers in front of EBP is possible by understanding them better and developing comprehensive strategies to solve them.

REFLECTIVE ACTIVITIES

1. In light of the information provided in this chapter regarding barriers to EBP in developing countries, compare the conditions of your country with those of developing countries.
2. Propose new strategies for overcoming barriers to EBP in developing countries and how evidence would inform your strategies.

REFERENCES

Adib-Hajbaghery, M. (2007). Factors facilitating and inhibiting evidence-based nursing in Iran. *Journal of Advanced Nursing, 58*(6), 566–575.

Bahçecik, N., & Ecevit, A. S. (2009). Nursing education in Turkey: From past to present. *Nurse Education Today, 29*(7), 698–703.

Bandura, A. (1994). Self-efficacy. In V. Ramachaudran (Ed.), *Encyclopedia of human behavior* (Vol. 4, pp. 71–81). San Diego, CA: Academic Press.

Bartelt, T. C., Ziebert, C., Sawin, K. J., Malin, S., Nugent, M., & Simpson, P. (2011). Evidence-based practice: Perceptions, skills, and activities of pediatric health care professionals. *Journal of Pediatric Nursing, 26*(2), 114–121.

Brown, C. E., Wickline, M. A., Ecoff, L., & Glaser, D. (2009). Nursing practice, knowledge, attitudes and perceived barriers to evidence-based practice at an academic medical center. *Journal of Advanced Nursing, 65*(2), 371–381.

Carlson, C. L., & Plonczynski, D. J. (2008). Has the BARRIERS Scale changed nursing practice? An integrative review. *Journal of Advanced Nursing, 63*(4), 322–333.

Champion, V. L., & Leach, A. (1989). Variables related to research utilization in nursing: An empirical investigation. *Journal of Advanced Nursing, 14*(9), 705–710.

Chau, J. P. C., Lopez, V., & Thompson, D. R. (2008). A survey of Hong Kong nurses' perceptions of barriers to and facilitators of research utilization. *Research in Nursing and Health, 31,* 640–649.

Chinnock, P., Siegfried, N., & Clarke, M. (2005). Is evidence-based medicine relevant to the developing world? *PLoS Med, 2*(5), e107.

Cummings, G. G., Hutchinson, A. M., Scott, S. D., Norton, P. G., & Estabrooks, C. A. (2010). The relationship between characteristics of context and research utilization in a pediatric setting. *BMC Health Services Research, 10,* 168.

Demir, Y., Ak, B., Bilgin, N. Ç., Efe, H., Albayrak, E., Çelikpençe, Z., & Nurgülay, G. (2012). Barriers and facilitating factors to research utilization in nursing practice. *Journal of Contemporary Medicine, 2*(2), 94–101.

DiCenso, A., Prevost, S., Benefield, L., Bingle, J., Ciliska, D., Driever, M., ... Titler, M. (2004). Evidence-based nursing: Rationale and resources. *Worldviews on Evidence-based Nursing, 1*(1), 69–75.

Estabrooks, C. A., Floyd, J. A., Scott-Findlay, S., O'Leary, K. A., & Gushta, M. (2003). Individual determinants of research utilization: A systematic review. *Journal of Advanced Nursing, 43*(5), 506–520.

Fink, R., Thompson, C., & Bonnes, D. (2005). Overcoming barriers and promoting the use of research in practice. *Journal of Nursing Administration, 35*(3), 121–129.

Forsman, H., Rudman, A., Gustavsson P., Ehrenberg A., & Wallin L. (2010). Use of research by nurses during their first two years after graduating. *Journal of Advanced Nursing, 66*(4), 878–890.

Funk, S. G., Champagne, M. T., Wiese, R. A., & Tornquist, E. M. (1991). Barriers to using research findings in practice: The clinician's perspective. *Applied Nursing Research, 4*(2), 90–95.

Funk, S. G., Tornquist, E. M., & Champagne, M. T. (1995). Barriers and facilitators of research utilization: An integrative review. *Nursing Clinics of North America, 30*(3), 395–407.

Garner, P., Kale, R., Dickson, R., Dans, T., & Salinas, R. (1998). Implementing research findings in developing countries. *British Medical Journal, 317,* 531–535.

Ghada, A. E. B., Shereen, R. D., & Reda, A. E. S. (2012). Barriers to research utilization in clinical practice. *Journal of American Science, 8*(4), 392–403.

Glacken, M., & Chaney, D. (2004). Perceived barriers and facilitators to implementing research findings in the Irish practice setting. *Journal of Clinical Nursing, 13*(6), 731–740.

Hannes, K., Vandersmissen, J., De Blaeser, L., Peeters, G., Goedhuys J., & Aertgeerts, B. (2007). Barriers to evidence-based nursing: A focus group study. *Journal of Advanced Nursing, 60*(2), 162–171.

Heiby, J. R. (1998). Quality improvement and the integrated management of childhood illness: Lessons from developed countries. *The Joint Commission Journal on Quality Improvement, 24,* 264–279.

Horton, R. (2003). Medical journals: Evidence of bias against the diseases of poverty. *Lancet, 361,* 712–713.

Hutchinson, A. M., & Johnston, L. (2004). Bridging the divide: A survey of nurses' opinions regarding barriers to, and facilitators of, research utilization in the practice setting. *Journal of Clinical Nursing, 13,* 304–315.

Kajermo, K. N., Boström, A. M., Thompson, D. S., Hutchinson, A. M., Estabrooks, C. A., & Wallin, L. (2010). The BARRIERS scale: The barriers to research utilization scale—A systematic review. *Implementation Science, 5,* 32. doi:10.1186/1748-5908-5-32

Kajermo, K. N., Nordstrom, G., Krusebrant, A., & Bjorvell, H. (1998). Barriers to and facilitators of research utilization, as perceived by a group of registered nurses in Sweden. *Journal of Advanced Nursing, 27*(4), 798–807.

Kelleci, M., Gölbaşı, Z., Yılmaz, M., & Doğan, S. (2008). The views of nurses, about carrying out research and utilization of research results in nursing care in a university hospital. *Journal of Research and Development in Nursing, 2,* 3–16.

Koehn, M. L., & Lehman, K. (2008). Nurses' perceptions of evidence-based nursing practice. *Journal of Advanced Nursing, 62*(2), 209–215.

Lai, N. M., Teng, C. L., & Lee, M. L. (2010). The place and barriers of evidence based practice: Knowledge and perceptions of medical, nursing and allied health practitioners in Malaysia. *BMC Research Notes, 3,* 279.

McPheeters, M., & Lohr, K. N. (1999). Evidence-based practice and nursing: Commentary. *Outcomes Management for Nursing Practice, 3*(3), 99–101.

Melnyk, B. M., Fineout-Overholt, E., Feinstein, N. F., Li, H., Small, L., Wilcox, L., & Kraus, R. (2004). Nurses' perceived knowledge, beliefs, skills and needs regarding evidence-based practice: Implication for accelerating the paradigm shift. *Worldview on Evidence Based Nursing, 1*(3), 185–192.

Melnyk, B. M., Fineout-Overholt, E., Gallagher-Ford, L., & Kaplan, L. (2012). The state of evidence-based practice in US nurses. *The Journal of Nursing Administration, 42*(9), 410–417.

Munroe, D., Duffy P., & Fisher, C. (2008). Nurse knowledge, skills, and attitudes related to evidence-based practice: Before and after organizational supports. *Medical Surgical Nursing, 17*(1), 55–60.

Nagy, S., Lumby, J., McKinley, S., & Macfarlane, C. (2001). Nurses' beliefs about the conditions that hinder or support evidence-based nursing. *International Journal of Nursing Practice, 7*(5), 314–321.

Oranta, O., Routasalo, P., & Hupli, M. (2002). Barriers to and facilitators of research utilization among Finnish Registered Nurses. *Journal of Clinical Nursing, 11*(2), 205–213.

Özdemir, L., & Akdemir, N. (2009). Turkish nurses' utilization of research evidence in clinical practice and influencing factors. *International Nursing Review, 56,* 319–325.

Öztürk, A., Kaya, N., Ayık, S., Uygur, E., & Cengiz, A. (2010). Barriers to research utilization in nursing practice. *Florence Nightingale Journal of Nursing, 18*(3), 144–155.

Parahoo, K. (2000). Barriers to, and facilitators of, research utilization among nurses in Northern Ireland. *Journal of Advanced Nursing, 31,* 89–98.

Retsas, A. (2000). Barriers to using research evidence in nursing practice. *Journal of Advanced Nursing, 31*(3), 599–606.

Rosswurm, M. A., & Larrabee, J. H. (1999). A model for change to evidence-based practice. *Image: Journal of Nursing Scholarship, 31*(4), 317–322.

Royle, J., & Blythe, J. (1998). Promoting research utilization in nursing: The role of the individual, organization, and environment. *Evidence-Based Nursing, 1,* 71–72.

Rudman, A., Gustavsson, P., Ehrenberg, A., Bostrom, A. M., & Wallin, L. (2012). Registered nurses' evidence-based practice: A longitudinal study of the first five years after graduation. *International Journal Nursing Studies, 49,* 1494–1504.

Sackett, D. L., Rosenberg, W. M., Gray, J. A., Haynes, R. B., & Richardson, W. S. (1996). Evidence based medicine: What it is and what it isn't. *British Medical Journal, 312*(7023), 71–72.

Sarı, D., Turgay, A. S., Genç, E. R., & Bozkurt, D. O. (2012). Research activities and perceptions of barriers to research utilization among Turkish nurses. *Journal Continuing Education Nursing, 43*(6), 251–258.

Schulman, C. S. (2008). Strategies for starting a successful evidence-based practice program. *AACN Advanced Critical Care, 19*(3), 301-311. doi:10.1097/01.AACN.0000330381.41766.2a

Siddiqi, K., Newell, J., & Robinson, M. (2005). Getting evidence into practice: What works in developing countries? *International Journal for Quality in Health Care, 17*(2), 447–453.

Solomons, N. M., & Spross, J. A. (2011). Evidence-based practice barriers and facilitators from a continuous quality improvement perspective: An integrative review. *Journal of Nursing Management, 19,* 109–120

Stetler, C. B., Ritchie, J., & Rycroft-Malone J., Schultz, A., & Charns, M. (2007). Improving quality of care through routine, successful implementation of evidence-based practice at the bedside: An organizational case study protocol using the Pettigrew and Whipp model of strategic change. *Implementation Science, 2*(3), 1–13.

Stone, D., & Maxwell, M. (2005). *Global knowledge networks and international development: Bridges across boundaries.* Oxford, UK: Routledge.

Straka, K. L., Brandt, P., Brytus, J. (2013). Brief report: Creating a culture of evidence-based practice and nursing research in a pediatric hospital. *Journal of Pediatric Nursing, 28*(4), 374–378.

Swingler, G. H., Volmink, J., & Ioannidis, J. P. A. (2003). Number of published systematic reviews and global burden of disease: Database analysis. *British Medical Journal, 327,* 1083–1084.

Tan, M., Akgün Sahin, Z., & Kardas Özdemir, F. (2012). Barriers of research utilization from the perspective of nurses in Eastern Turkey. *Nursing Outlook, 60*(1), 44–50.

Tita, A. T. N., Selwyn, B. J., Waller, D. K., Kapadia, A. S., & Dongmo, S. (2005). Evidence-based reproductive health care in Cameroon: Population-based study of awareness, use and barriers. *Bulletin of the World Health Organization, 83*(12), 895–903.

Tsai, S. (2003). The effects of a research utilization in-service program on nurses. *International Journal of Nursing Studies, 40,*105–113.

Turkish Psychiatric Nurses Association. (2016). *History of Turkish Psychiatric Nurses Association.* Retrieved from http://phdernegi.org/hakkimizda/psikiyatri-hemsireleri-dernegi-kisa-tarihce/

Young, J. (2005). Research, policy and practice: Why developing countries are different. *Journal of International Development, 17,* 727–734.

CHAPTER 20

Dissemination of the Evidence

■Heather R. Hall and Linda A. Roussel■

■ Objectives:

- Explain the importance of publishing the results of your work.
- Identify the processes of disseminating findings from evidence-based practice (EBP).
- Communicate the structure of academic papers, presentations, and posters.

The dissemination of the evidence is the final and most important step in the research process (Lyder & Fain, 2009). Disseminating the evidence is vital to the application of research in practice. It is the communication of research findings that allows for meaningful critique, evolution of new clinical questions, and application of research-based evidence in practice. Research is of no value if the findings are not shared (Fain, 2009). This chapter provides information related to disseminating evidence, which includes peer-reviewed journal publishing, poster and podium presentations, and journal club presentations.

■ Publishing in Peer-Reviewed Journals

The improvement of EBP relies on the efforts of researchers to publish the findings of their research. Publishing in a professional journal guarantees broad distribution of research-based evidence. It is an advantage for professionals to publish their work; perhaps it should be a requirement for researchers to do so as well (Polit & Beck, 2012).

Tappen (2011) gave researchers advice concerning the difficult process of producing a manuscript worthy of being published in a professional journal. Tappen stated that a researcher who strives for publication must be able to endure criticism, to maintain staying power, and to tolerate the requirement of revising submitted manuscripts. In addition to this advice, Tappen listed other essential characteristics of a manuscript worthy of publication, which include (a) choosing to send the written article to a journal that publishes corresponding studies; (b) reading the journal requirements that are listed for authors; (c) compiling proper literature review for research conducted; (d) including the proper headings in the submitted article, which are specified in the author requirements; (e) proofreading the article from beginning to end and revising if necessary; (f) requesting another professional to proof the document and provide feedback; (g) double-checking the format to be certain it follows all guidelines stated in the author's requirements; (h) changing the manuscript as per reviewers' comments and resubmitting as soon as possible; and (i) refusing to concede defeat if one journal rejects the manuscript; simply revise the manuscript and submit it to another journal (Tappen, 2011).

■ Presentations

Researchers or clinical scholars may apply for the opportunity to present their findings as either a poster presentation or a podium presentation. An outline, abstract, or summation of data concerning an issue is appropriate for a poster presentation and can provide significant information (Brown, 2012). Attendees at conferences are given opportunities to examine posters as carefully as they choose. Conference sponsors expect poster presenters to stand beside their posters so conference attendees may ask questions (Brown, 2012). Posters give presenters an opportunity to showcase their work and themselves.

Podium presentations are talks normally given within a specified time frame as a part of a panel related to a particular topic. A podium presentation includes visual (e.g., slides) and oral components (Shepherd & Plichta, 2013). Conveying confidence with and knowledge of the subject matter is important to a successful presentation. Knowledge of the subject matter and the ability to share this information with credibility can be facilitated by planning ahead with a short presentation and handouts for participants. This affords presenters the opportunity to organize their thinking by preparing for possible questions in advance (Zaccagnini & White, 2011).

Poster Presentations

A poster is usually organized by following the *introduction, methods, results, and discussion* (IMRAD) format (University of Tampere, 2012). However, consideration should be given to the graphics and the simplicity of the poster. IMRAD is a format used for posters with a scientific focus (Day & Gastel, 2006; University of Tampere, 2012). A well-designed poster does not include a large amount of text. The illustrations should constitute the majority of the space (Day & Gastel, 2006).

The introduction should briefly present the problem statement. The purpose statement should be at the beginning of the poster. The methods component of the poster should be to the point; one or two sentences is appropriate to explain the method used. The results are typically the main component of a well-designed poster (in contrast, the results section is frequently the shortest section of a paper). The results should be illustrated using the largest part of the poster's available space. The discussion must be concise. The discussion heading is not used in the best posters. Instead, a conclusions section consisting of a heading and short sentences is placed on the far right. It is important to keep the reference citations to a minimum (Day & Gastel, 2006). In addition, include an acknowledgments section to thank specific individuals for their contribution to the success of the project (Shepherd & Plichta, 2013).

The poster should conform to the guidelines of the program meeting (Shepherd & Plichta, 2013). The title of the poster should be short and capture attention. If the title is lengthy, it might not fit the available space. The title should be clear from a distance of 10 feet (about 3 meters; Day & Gastel, 2006). Make the typeface bold and dark, and the type at least approximately 1 inch (about 250 mm). The authors' names should be a size or two smaller. Avoid big blocks of type, and use bulleted lists if possible (Day & Gastel, 2006). White space is important all over the poster; disorder is confusing and unattractive. Visual impact is critical in a poster session. If necessary, consider asking a graphic artist in a publications department for assistance (Day & Gastel, 2006). Exemplar posters have been presented at conferences (see **Figure 20-1**). Bad posters have been presented as well. Attempting to present too much information is one characteristic of a bad poster. People will congregate around posters that are straightforward and well illustrated. Disorganized and wordy posters will be disregarded (Day & Gastel, 2006).

Preparing a poster may be considered an easier task than preparing an oral presentation. However, presenters are cautioned about becoming complacent concerning poster presentations. When preparing a poster, the developer should be discerning about content because too much or too little data can cause people to become uninterested quickly (Brown, 2012). The main idea of a poster should be easy to find and read. If the idea is interesting to someone, he or she will ask questions or read further from the poster. The poster developer provides the interested person with additional information. The poster serves to attract the readers. Poster presentations assist professionals with their growth; therefore, professionals are encouraged to prepare posters to display their findings and make proper requests to exhibit their posters at appropriate conferences (Brown, 2012).

Podium Presentations

Professional podium presentations are normally given at conferences. In some cases, an individual might be invited to present his or work. However, if someone is interested in presenting at a major conference, he or she must take the initiative by submitting an abstract of the paper to be presented. All submitted abstracts go through a peer review process. It is important to follow all guidelines and word the abstract succinctly so that it is informative and to the point. Submitters of the strongest abstracts may be asked to give podium presentations (Day & Gastel, 2006).

Polit and Beck (2012) described podium presentations as usually having a specific time allotment, with an additional few minutes for questions from the audience.

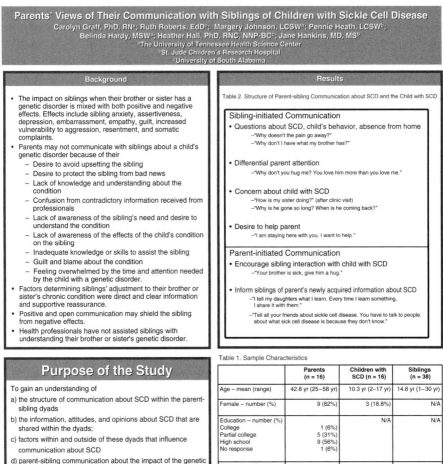

Parents' Views of Their Communication with Siblings of Children with Sickle Cell Disease

Carolyn Graff, PhD, RN[a]; Ruth Roberts, EdD[b]; Margery Johnson, LCSW[b]; Pennie Heath, LCSW[b]; Belinda Hardy, MSW[a]; Heather Hall, PhD, RNC, NNP-BC[c]; Jane Hankins, MD, MS[b]

[a]The University of Tennessee Health Science Center
[b]St. Jude Children's Research Hospital
[c]University of South Alabama

Background

- The impact on siblings when their brother or sister has a genetic disorder is mixed with both positive and negative effects. Effects include sibling anxiety, assertiveness, depression, embarrassment, empathy, guilt, increased vulnerability to aggression, resentment, and somatic complaints.
- Parents may not communicate with siblings about a child's genetic disorder because of their
  - Desire to avoid upsetting the sibling
  - Desire to protect the sibling from bad news
  - Lack of knowledge and understanding about the condition
  - Confusion from contradictory information received from professionals
  - Lack of awareness of the sibling's need and desire to understand the condition
  - Lack of awareness of the effects of the child's condition on the sibling
  - Inadequate knowledge or skills to assist the sibling
  - Guilt and blame about the condition
  - Feeling overwhelmed by the time and attention needed by the child with a genetic disorder.
- Factors determining siblings' adjustment to their brother or sister's chronic condition were direct and clear information and supportive reassurance.
- Positive and open communication may shield the sibling from negative effects.
- Health professionals have not assisted siblings with understanding their brother or sister's genetic disorder.

Results

Table 2. Structure of Parent-sibling Communication about SCD and the Child with SCD

Sibling-initiated Communication
- Questions about SCD, child's behavior, absence from home
  - –"Why doesn't the pain go away?"
  - –"Why don't I have what my brother has?"
- Differential parent attention
  - –"Why don't you hug me? You love him more than you love me."
- Concern about child with SCD
  - –"How is my sister doing?" (after clinic visit)
  - –"Why is he gone so long? When is he coming back?"
- Desire to help parent
  - –"I am staying here with you. I want to help."

Parent-initiated Communication
- Encourage sibling interaction with child with SCD
  - –"Your brother is sick, give him a hug."
- Inform siblings of parent's newly acquired information about SCD
  - –"I tell my daughters what I learn. Every time I learn something, I share it with them."
  - –"Tell all your friends about sickle cell disease. You have to talk to people about what sick cell disease is because they don't know."

Purpose of the Study

To gain an understanding of
a) the structure of communication about SCD within the parent-sibling dyads
b) the information, attitudes, and opinions about SCD that are shared within the dyads;
c) factors within and outside of these dyads that influence communication about SCD
d) parent-sibling communication about the impact of the genetic disorder stigma on the sibling and relationships within the family.

Methods

- Parents recruited through St. Jude Comprehensive Sickle Cell Center
- Semi-structured focus group interviews with parents of children sickle cell disease
- Transcribed interview data imported into NVivo7 and coded
- Emerging categories analyzed to identify themes

Table 1. Sample Characteristics

	Parents (n = 16)	Children with SCD (n = 16)	Siblings (n = 38)
Age – mean (range)	42.8 yr (25–58 yr)	10.3 yr (2–17 yr)	14.8 yr (1–30 yr)
Female – number (%)	9 (82%)	3 (18.8%)	N/A
Education – number (%)		N/A	N/A
College	1 (6%)		
Partial college	5 (31%)		
High school	9 (56%)		
No response	1 (6%)		
Race – number (%)			
Black or African American	16 (100%)	16 (100%)	38 (100%)
Birth order– number (%)			
First-born		7 (43.8%)	
Second-born		2 (12.5%)	
Third-born		2 (12.5%)	
Fourth-born		3 (18.8%)	
Fifth-born		1 (6.2%)	
Seventh-born		1 (6.2%)	
Health of child with SCD – number (%)			
Poor		3 (18.8%)	
Fair		4 (25%)	
Good		7 (43.8%)	
Very Good		2 (12.5%)	

■ **Figure 20-1** Parents' Views of Their Communication With Siblings of Children With Sickle Cell Disease

Parents' Views of Their Communication with Siblings of Children with Sickle Cell Disease

Carolyn Graff, PhD, RN[a]; Ruth Roberts, EdD[a]; Margery Johnson, LCSW[b]; Pennie Heath, LCSW[b];
Belinda Hardy, MSW[a]; Heather Hall, PhD, RNC, NNP-BC[c]; Jane Hankins, MD, MS[b]
[a]The University of Tennessee Health Science Center
[b]St. Jude Children's Research Hospital
[c]University of South Alabama

Results

Table 3. Information, Attitudes, and Opinions about SCD Shared between Parents and Siblings

Explanation of child's behaviors
–"If I say he is having a bone crisis, then I have to go on and on about what a bone crisis is."
Genetics of SCD
–"It's a blood disease. She got it from me and your father. I did not know I had it."
–"I told my daughter who has the trait that if she gets a boyfriend with the trait, she will likely have a child with it. I told my son that he does not have the trait."
Impact of SCD on child with SCD
–"It's the cell you have in your body. It's like when you have candy and it gets stuck. You have to break it away. You have to wash it with hot water until it comes loose. Sometimes you have to take medicine and once the medicine starts working, you feel better."

Table 4. Factors Influencing Parent-sibling Communication about SCD

- Behavior of child with SCD
- Family and friends (attitudes, support)
- Health of child with SCD (clinic visits, hospitalizations)
- Parent awareness of sibling needs
- Parent concerns about future of child with SCD
- School problems for child with SCD
- Sibling age
- Sibling behavior problems
- Sibling-child with SCD relationship
- Strategies to prevent SCD crisis and complications

Conclusion

Parents of children with SCD engaged in communication with siblings on topics similar to parents of children with other chronic conditions. Factors related to parents, siblings, the child with SCD, extended family, friends, and the school influenced parent sibling communication about SCD. Parents reported that clinic visits or hospitalizations of the child with SCD resulted in parent-sibling discussion about SCD and the child with SCD. Several parents reported open discussion with siblings about the pattern of inheritance of SCD. Their decision to discuss the genetics of SCD with siblings was related to sibling age, the questions asked by questions, and parents' understanding of the genetics of SCD. Parents engaged in practical, unique, and creative ways of sharing information about SCD with siblings.

References

- Ashley-Koch, A., Yang, Q., & Olney, R.S. (2000). Sickle hemoglobin (HbS) allele and sickle cell disease. American Journal of Genetics, 151, 839–845.
- Gallo, A., Breitmayer, B., Knafl, K., & Zoeller, L. (1993). Mother's perceptions of sibling adjustment and family life in childhood chronic illness. Journal of Pediatric Nursing, 8, 318–324.
- QSR International. (2006). NVivo7. Victoria, Australia: QSR International, Pty Ltd.
- Stein, R.E.K., & Jessop, D.J. (1989). What diagnosis does not tell: The case for a noncategorical approach to illness in childhood. Social Science and Medicine, 29, 769–778.
- Tesch, R. (1990). Qualitative research: Analysis types and software tools. New York: Falmer Press.
- Williams, P.D. (1997). Siblings and pediatric chronic illness: A review of the literature. International Journal of Nursing Studies, 34, 312–323.

Recommendations

- Talk with parents about sharing information about SCD with siblings
- Consider offering informational sessions on SCD for siblings
- Generate informational materials about SCD that are geared for siblings of varying developmental ages
- Recognize that some parents may have extra responsibilities and stressors that prevent them from recognizing sibling needs or acting when they recognize sibling needs

Acknowledgments

- Society of Pediatric Nurses, Corrine Barnes Research Grant Award
- St. Jude Children's Research Hospital Comprehensive Sickle Cell Center and Department of Hematology
- Susan Neely-Barnes, PhD, College of Social Work, University of Tennessee
- Connie Burgess, College of Nursing, University of Tennessee Health Science Center

■ **Figure 20-1** *(Continued)*

The presentation should consist of important information related to the study, and the presenter should be certain to highlight results of the study. A qualitative research report can be difficult to shorten to a time-limited oral presentation, because there is a risk for eliminating rich data. It takes approximately 2.5 to 3 minutes to read one page of double-spaced typescript; however, a podium presentation is more effective if it is given informally rather than read to the audience (Polit & Beck, 2012). To maintain the audience's attention, provide smart visuals and maintain an enthusiastic tone of voice (Shepherd & Plichta, 2013). It is best to rehearse the presentation multiple times to gain confidence with the text and stay within time constraints (Polit & Beck, 2012).

Scholarly podium presentations, for the most part, follow a similar format (Shepherd & Plichta, 2013). The title should communicate the topic in a few words (one slide). The coauthors and institutional affiliations, and, if they are not too long, the acknowledgments, should appear on the same slide. An abstract is not included in a presentation. However, the presenter may consider a one-page summary of the findings as a handout for interested members of the audience. Address the problem first in the introduction. Then, present a succinct literature review (three to four slides). The methods should be explained concisely using applicable tables and figures if possible. The presentation methods section does not have the same level of detail as a manuscript methods section. The slides should be neat (five to six slides). The first slide of the results section should include the key finding. The remaining results slides may include tables and graphs (five to eight slides). The initial slide of the conclusions should describe the successfulness of the project using qualitative and quantitative results. Interesting results should be discussed. Describe the importance to policy, practice implications, and potential research (five to eight slides). Individuals who contributed to the project should be acknowledged for their efforts. The disclosure of conflicts of commitment should be included unless addressed on the first slide. End the presentation with a closing slide that includes an email address and additional contact information. The literature cited throughout the presentation should be the last slide shown to the audience, but it is not discussed. However, members of the audience might find a reference slide to be useful (Shepherd & Plichta, 2013). The value of a scientific presentation is significantly increased with slides that are thoughtfully designed, well organized, and proficiently used (Day & Gastel, 2006).

■ Journal Club Presentations

A journal club consists of a group of people who meet for educational purposes to discuss current publications. These meetings provide an environment that assists people in their efforts to keep up with recent literature. The purpose of a journal club is to facilitate the evaluation of a particular research study and discuss study implications for clinical practice. Taking part in a journal club has advantages, including keeping up with new knowledge, supporting research findings, being able to critique and critically appraise research-based evidence, recognizing the best research evidence in a journal, and promoting the use of research evidence. Specific steps to establishing a journal club in an academic or clinical setting include the following (Kleinpell, 2002):

1. Establishing a clinical question that will direct the research study article choice.
2. Send to all interested individuals a copy of the article and the discussion questions developed for the journal club.
3. Schedule an appropriate time and place for everyone to meet.
4. Name a meeting facilitator; "Initially this could be a clinical educator, clinical nurse specialist, clinical nurse leader, nurse manager, or senior staff members with journal club members taking turns to lead subsequent journal club sessions" (Kleinpell, 2002, p. 412).
5. The journal club should meet regularly and use discussion questions to maintain active participant involvement.
6. Assess the journal club, including comments from participants related to the meeting. Make a decision on how the next journal club gathering could be more valuable—for example, promoting more attendance, having more than one journal club meeting, and recording the meeting for participants unable to attend.
7. Plan the next journal club meeting.

Multiple factors are key in the success of maintaining a journal club, including promoting awareness, presence, and participation (Kleinpell, 2002). See **Table 20-1** for an outline of a journal club.

■ Executive Summary

An executive summary is a clear and concise document that reviews the important points of a lengthier document or article. This document is for an individual that does not have the time to read the full report. An actual executive summary examines and reviews the key points in the report and will frequently make a recommendation dependent on the analysis. Executive summaries are documents that do not need additional documents as a supplement. These summaries are mostly read individually of the documents they review (University of Maryland University College, 2016).

There are questions to consider when developing an executive summary, including the following:

■ Does the executive summary have a projected audience? It is important to remember that the individual reading the summary needs to know all of the significant information in the chief document without having to read the document.
■ Does the chief document have a key theme? The theme should be included in the summary.

Table 20-1 Online Journal Club

Outline of the Journal Club

1. A specific clinical question is chosen.

2. All evidence-based literature related to the question is derived from online databases.

3. A reference list of all literature for review is generated.

4. High-level-evidence randomized controlled trials and systematic reviews are critiqued and given more weight than quasi-experimental case studies and opinions.

5. Participants critically appraise the relevant literature before attending the journal club.

6. Journal club discussions center on the critical appraisal of evidence found for clinical interventions.

7. Implications for practice and further research are discussed, with key findings recorded in minutes.

8. A resource folder that includes a reference list of resource critiques, guidelines for practice, treatment resources, standardized assessments, disease management strategies, and gaps in evidence is created.

9. A system for ongoing evaluation of outcomes and changes in practice is developed and communicated.

Source: Adapted from McQueen, J., Miller, C., Nivison, C., & Husband, V. (2006). An investigation into the use of a journal club for evidence-based practice. *International Journal of Therapy and Rehabilitation, 13*(7), p. 313.

- Does the chief document have a purpose? The purpose should be summarized in a few sentences.
- Does the document have sections? The sections should be included that are crucial to understanding the issue. Some of the sections could be left out if necessary.
- Does the document recommend a specific action? The course of action recommended should be included in the summary. If no recommendation is discussed, the data should be analyzed and an action will be recommended in the summary.
- Are there benefits or penalties of the specific action? A discussion should be included related to the recommendation being a worthy idea. The benefits should be stated to support the recommendation. The positive benefits should be highlighted; however, the consequences should be stated as well (University of Maryland University College, 2016).

■ Digital Repository

A reliable digital repository provides dependable, long-term access to digital resources to its community. Digital repositories may be diverse in format. Some institutions may develop local repositories, whereas others may elect to manage the intellectual characteristics of a repository and contract the storage and maintenance with a third-party provider. The overall structure should meet expectations of the community. All reliable digital repositories must take responsibility for the continued preservation of digital resources. Methods should be established to evaluate the system to meet the expectations of the community (Research Libraries Group, 2002).

■ Redundant Publications

When an author publishes an article that is much like another article or main portions of an article that he or she has previously published (online or print) without giving notice to the editors or citing the other article, this is known as a redundant publication. Another term for redundant publication is "self-plagiarism"; it is considered unethical and is a type of scientific misconduct (Burns & Grove, 2009; Shepherd & Plichta, 2013). Duplicate publications can be avoided by educating authors on how to become mindful about this issue, how to keep it from occurring, what transpires when it takes place, and the penalties associated with it (Shepherd & Plichta, 2013).

Guidelines focused on duplicate publications have been published by the International Committee of Medical Journal Editors (2009) and the International Academy of Nursing Editors (Yarbro, 1995). Authors should read the portion related to redundant publications if they have thought about publishing in multiple journals (Shepherd & Plichta, 2013). Because it is unethical, publishing duplicate articles can lead to many problems. Publishing duplicate articles could cause other authors to consider the result of one study multiple times if the data are used for a meta-analysis or review of the literature. In addition, an editor must devote time to investigating whether duplicate publishing occurred (Burns & Grove, 2009; Hegyvary, 2005; Shepherd & Plichta, 2013). The manuscript will be rejected if the duplication is noticed before it is published. If the duplication is discovered after the work has been published, multiple actions could be taken to rectify the situation (Hegyvary, 2005; Shepherd & Plichta, 2013).

There are many steps an author can take to avoid duplicate publication—for example, (a) citing all papers (e.g., those published and those submitted for publication) related to the manuscript; (b) ensuring that new information is apparent when submitting a manuscript; and (c) choosing to publish a manuscript with the potential of being a classic and comprehensive article rather than dividing the results into multiple manuscripts (Shepherd & Plichta, 2013).

■ Conclusion

One's research findings may be presented through several mediums, including peer-reviewed journals, poster presentations, podium presentations, and journal club meetings. Generally, an outline, abstract, or summation of data concerning a clinical issue is appropriate for poster and podium presentations, and a solo talk (or a talk as part of a panel) on a particular topic is required for a podium presentation. This is done within a specified time frame. Being part of a journal club can be advantageous from a professional development perspective because it allows one to keep up with new knowledge, support research findings, and garner the ability to critique and critically appraise research-based evidence. Redundant publications should be avoided, sparing the research future problems related to ethical concerns. If data are being used for a meta-analysis or a literature review, redundant publications could cause other authors to factor in the result of one study multiple times.

REFLECTIVE ACTIVITIES

1. Select a peer-reviewed journal that reflects your research interest or area of practice. Using the journal's manuscript guidelines, develop an outline with the topical areas that would be included in your manuscript.
2. Select a conference, seminar, or workshop that has recently disseminated a call for abstracts. Using the guidelines outlined in the call, write the abstract and discuss it with peers.

REFERENCES

Brown, S. J. (2012). *Evidence-based nursing: The research-practice connection* (2nd ed.). Burlington, MA: Jones & Bartlett Learning.

Burns, N., & Grove, S. K. (2009). *The practice of nursing research: Appraisal, synthesis, and generation of evidence* (6th ed.). St. Louis, MO: Saunders.

Day, R. A., & Gastel, B. (2006). *How to write and publish a scientific paper* (6th ed.). Westport, CT: Greenwood Press.

Fain, J. A. (2009). *Reading, understanding, and applying nursing research* (3rd ed.). Philadelphia, PA: F. A. Davis.

Hegyvary, S. (2005). What every author should know about redundant and duplicate publications. *Journal of Nursing Scholarship, 37*(4), 295–297.

International Committee of Medical Journal Editors. (2009). *Publishing and editorial issues related to publication in biomedical journals: Overlapping publications.* Retrieved from http://www.icmje.org/recommendations/browse/publishing-and-editorial-issues/overlapping-publications.html

Kleinpell, R. M. (2002). Rediscovering the value of the journal club. *American Journal of Critical Care, 11*(5), 412–414. Retrieved from http://ajcc.aacnjournals.org/content/11/5/412.full

Lyder, C., & Fain, J. A. (2009). Interpreting and reporting research findings. In J. A. Fain (Ed.), *Reading, understanding, and applying nursing research* (3rd ed., pp. 233–250). Philadelphia, PA: F. A. Davis.

Polit, D. F., & Beck, C. T. (2012). *Nursing research: Generating and assessing evidence for nursing practice* (9th ed.). Philadelphia, PA: Lippincott Williams & Wilkins.

Research Libraries Group. (2002, May). *Trusted digital repositories: Attributes and responsibilities.* An RLG-OCLC Report. Retrieved from http://www.oclc.org/content/dam/research/activities/trustedrep/repositories.pdf

Shepherd, L. G., & Plichta, S. B. (2013). Writing and presenting for publication. In S. B. Plichta and E. A. Kelvin (Eds.), *Munro's statistical methods for health care research* (6th ed., pp. 445–453). Philadelphia, PA: Lippincott Williams & Wilkins.

Tappen, R. M. (2011). *Advanced nursing research: From theory to practice.* Burlington, MA: Jones & Bartlett Learning.

University of Maryland University College. (2016). Writing executive summaries. Retrieved from http://www.umuc.edu/writingcenter/writingresources/exec_summaries.cfm

University of Tampere, Department of Translation Studies. (2012). *The IMRAD research paper format.* Retrieved from http://www.uta.fi/FAST/FIN/RESEARCH/imrad.html

Yarbro, C. H. (1995). Duplicate publication: Guidelines for nurse authors and editors. *Image: The Journal of Nursing Scholarship, 27*(1), 57.

Zaccagnini, M. E., & White, K. W. (2011). *Doctor of nursing practice essentials: A new model for advanced practice nursing.* Burlington, MA: Jones & Bartlett Learning.

Collaborating for Clinical Scholarship through Integration of Evidence-Based Practice

■ LINDA A. ROUSSEL AND HEATHER R. HALL ■

This chapter highlights the synthesis of scientific research within an administrative context and clinical practice that supports an infrastructure for patient care improvement. Focusing on safe patient care delivery, quality, and accountability within learning organization requires the integration of evidence in support of best practices. This involves knowing what questions to ask as well as having an understanding of how good science is structured. Knowing how administrative and clinical practices provide contextual relevance for translational research is a process that guides the work of healthcare providers. Advanced leadership skills, team science, the ability to understand complex adaptive systems (CASs), high-reliability organizations, and clinical scholarship enhance this process. Each chapter outlines critical aspects of integrative collaboration.

Clinical scholarship requires identification of desired outcomes and systematic observations that are scientifically based. Gonzales and Esperat (2010) stated that to improve outcomes, "clinical decisions must be grounded in clinical inquiry where nurses who practice in a scholarly manner work directly and collegially with other health care providers in other settings, both in the discovery and the application of new knowledge" (p. 199). The conclusion focuses on integration of best science, translation into evidence-based practice (EBP), and collaboration to achieve patient-centered care. It is because of the integration and collaboration of scholars that healthcare providers are able to achieve quality patient outcomes, facilitate team science, and create a culture of safety. It is within this integrative work that clinical scholars come together to reach beyond each individual expert knowledge for the greater aim of safe, quality, and patient-centered care.

To better understand integrative collaboration, it is important to describe integration and collaboration and how best to accomplish these goals through enhanced clinical scholarship. Our second edition provides ample tools, methods, and examples to achieve this end, integrating research principles for translation and the best administrative and clinical practices.

Integrative collaboration necessitates a deliberate process of bringing together individual professionals and their requisite skills as a scientific team. Providing a process that is reliable and understandable is essential to integrative collaboration of clinical scholars. Finding what works in health care is multifaceted, as illustrated by our second edition text. For example, from a research perspective, systematic reviews, meta-analyses, meta-synthesis, and clinical practice guidelines are intended to provide organized and systematic aids in making complex healthcare decisions (Eden, Levit, Berg, & Morton, 2011; Graham, Mancher, Wolman Miller, Greenfield, & Steinberg, 2011).

Technology and informatics enhance clinical decision-making and decision-support. The use of big data and data repositories further support standardization, a shared language, and ways to best talk about translation in the "doing" of improvement work (Lloyd, 2011). Evidence-based decision-making provides standardization, reducing variation and improving consistency of shared solutions, and care delivery. Examples include clinical decisions related to preventive and monitoring tasks, the prescribing of drugs, and diagnosis and management (Briere, 2001). "Carefully designed, evidence-based processes, supported by automated clinical information and decision support systems, offer the greatest promise of achieving the best outcomes for care for chronic conditions" (Briere, 2001, p. 10). Integrating research, administrative leadership, systems, and clinical practice maximizes our best single efforts at improvement science.

Foundational to the concept of integrative collaboration is understanding that it involves combining or coordinating separate elements to create a harmonious, interrelated whole. Through a complexity lens, the whole is greater than the sum of its parts, as in CASs. Nonlinear, interactive systems that adapt to changing environments are known as CASs. These systems are self-organizing and composed of many independent agents that interact at all levels. The interaction is a true maxim of our healthcare systems today, which will only become more complicated and stretched to their limits. Relationships in CASs create new ideas, structures, and patterns (Crowell, 2011). In complex systems, positive deviance provides another lens to experience outliers who are making a difference despite overwhelming challenges of resource constraints, limited access to experts, and a dismal future (Marsh, Schroeder, Dearden, Sternin, & Sternin (2004). Disruptive innovation also provides insights into strategies that may have limited research evidence and are steeped in strong principles supporting more nimble and informed ways to lead and innovate (Yu & Hang, 2010).

Today's healthcare system requires an intense look at relationships and patterns created through sense-making, networking, and making connections (Guiette & Vandenbempt, 2016). These organizational and structural components are organized or structured so that units function cooperatively. Integration means bringing together or incorporating (parts) into a whole. Integrating systems can be challenging;

the rewards far outweigh the costs, thus necessitating a new lens through which to view the healthcare world (Capra, 2002; Crowell, 2011; Lindberg, Nash, & Lindberg, 2008). High-reliability organizations provide an example of ongoing work needed to ensure a culture of safety with minimal to zero error rates (Chassin & Loeb, 2013).

An integrated delivery system (IDS) can be defined as a network of healthcare providers and organizations that provides or arranges a coordinated continuum of services to a defined population. An IDS is willing to be held clinically and fiscally accountable for the clinical outcomes and health status of the population served (Crosson, 2009). IDSs have a number of objectives, including quality improvement and cost savings that serve to reduce administrative and overhead costs, share risks, and eliminate cost shifting. Outcomes management, continuous quality improvement, reduction of inappropriate and unnecessary resource use, value-based care, and efficient use of capital and technology also can be achieved with an IDS (Crosson, 2009). Economies of scale are encouraged through providers' motives and the mission of organizations involved. An example might include, at the hospital level, varying degrees of organizational consolidation that lead to improved utilization of resources, both capital and operating.

Through coordinated activities, integration can enable the system to meet the same level of demand with less capacity than that required for individual systems. Having a larger scale of operations affords increased productivity, lower staffing requirements, and reduced unit costs through joint activities. An integrative collaboration approach is not only the right thing to do, but also good business practice (Crosson, 2009)!

Collaborating in an integrative way centers on working together as a team to achieve goals and to think big about improvement. It is a process whereby two or more people (e.g., organizations, programs, and systems) work together to realize a shared vision created by a shared mental model (Senge, 1990). Considering a shared vision, collaboration is more than the intersection of common aims, as in a cooperative venture. Collaboration is a deep, collective determination of a shared connection, a "sacred covenant" (DePree, 1990); it is the sharing of knowledge, team learning, and consensus building. Collaboration requires transformational and servant leadership. Humility for the greater good is the backdrop of all sustained excellence. Collaboration calls on courageous teams working collectively to obtain greater resources and recognition. In particular, teams that work collaboratively can increase capacity building and rewards when facing competition for finite resources (Senge, 1990). Being fluid, nimble, and "good enough," requires mindful reflection of our daily work and its relationship to the larger vision. It is being present and intentional and giving voice to our observations, along with deep learning of our systems, communication, and organizing structure. This provides real time (just in time) strategies that have the background of thoughtfulness and using tools such as appreciative inquiry, storytelling, and creative teaming.

Collaboration embraces introspection, appreciative inquiry, and crucial conversations (Cooperrider, 1990; Patterson, Grenny, McMillan, & Switzler, 2002). Aims of collaboration include increasing the success of teams as they engage in collabora-tive problem-solving and decision-making. Gardner (2005) described 10 lessons in collaboration that are helpful to the integrative collaboration process:

1. Know thyself.
2. Learn to value and manage diversity.
3. Develop constructive conflict resolution skills.
4. Use your power to create win-win situations.
5. Master interpersonal and process skills.
6. Recognize that collaboration is a journey.
7. Leverage all multidisciplinary forums.
8. Appreciate that collaboration can occur spontaneously.
9. Balance autonomy and unity in collaborative relationships.
10. Remember that collaboration is not required for all decisions.

Collaboration may necessitate letting go and loss. Loss of face, status, and ego may thwart collaboration. Collaborative partners face difficulties such as poor listening and new languages, conflicts over goals, and methods to achieve them (Gardner, 2005).

In Part I, Critical Appraisal of Research to Support Scholarship, foundational research tools and methods were described and the authors explored the best ways to conduct the research process through the use of quantitative, qualitative, and mixed methods approaches. The data analysis process of research was discussed, as well as understanding how to determine sound research evidence translatable to practice. In navigating the institutional review board process, the authors described the his-torical perspective on current practice mandates regarding human subject protection for implementing quality improvement and research studies. Part I further defined critical appraisal of the research design methods evaluating the evidence for its ap-propriateness in relation to better patient outcomes. Understanding critiquing skills that enhance the ability to critically appraise is also discussed. The link between critiquing, critical appraisal, and critical thinking is underscored and establishes the foundation for sound clinical decision-making. Exemplars of strategies to enhance critical appraisal skills were described.

In Part II, Scholarship of Administrative Practice, evidence supporting the need for evidence-based leadership practices was discussed within the context of under-standing sound organizational systems. Leadership is a complex phenomenon; it in-volves the ability to be persuasive with research evidence in response to the demand for large-scale transformation and cost containment, the result of chaos, complexity, rapid change, and a shrinking of the world through global communication. It involves going beyond quantitative evaluations to "see" the big picture and "hear" the voice through storytelling to convey our true purpose, providing context for quality im-provement systems change. Lloyd (2011) claimed that "aggregated data presented in tabular formats or with summary statistics will not help you measure the impact of process improvement/redesign efforts. Aggregated data can only lead to judgment, not to improvement" (Slide 42). He stressed the need to understand the variation, noting that if we do not understand the variation that lives in the data, we will be misguided from the beginning. For example, we may be blinded and deny that data presented fit our view of reality; see trends where there are no trends; try to explain natural variation as special events; blame and give credit to people for things over which they have no control; distort the process that produced the data; and kill the messenger (Lloyd, 2011, Slide 44). An understanding of the politics and financial implications enables the evidence-based policy changes necessary for widespread adoption of innovation. Part II provides an excellent backdrop for understanding the translation process and the importance of leadership, systems dynamics, and the political context.

Part III, Scholarship of Clinical Practice, identifies critical issues in clinical practice. For example, philosophical and theoretical perspectives to guide inquiry delineate processes of making sense of real-time, relevant issues. The theoretical underpinnings that support evidence-based clinical practice described the frameworks, theories, and models necessary to guide sound practice and systems improvement.

EBP research and the technology supporting the search for sound science are guided by an intensive step-by-step process of search strategies, best databases for efficient location, and rich resources that promote clinical scholarship.

Collaborating for clinical scholarship through integration of EBP is a relationship-centered holistic approach to safe, quality practice. Collaborative models, collaborative modeling, and integrative delivery systems are not new to interprofessional work. The Institute for Healthcare Improvement (IHI) offers a series on collaborative modeling for achieving breakthrough improvement. This initiative supports healthcare change improvement. Collaborative learning, as a vehicle for breakthrough improvement offered through the IHI, has been developed to assist organizations in closing the gap by supporting an infrastructure in which interested organizations can easily learn from each other. Recognized experts in topic areas are brought together for this purpose.

According to the IHI, the Breakthrough Series Collaborative is a short-term (6–15 months) learning system that brings together a large number of teams from hospitals and clinics to seek improvement in a specific area (IHI, 2003). Since 1995, the IHI has sponsored more than 50 such collaborative projects on several dozen topics involving more than 2000 teams from 1000 healthcare organizations. Examples include reduction of cesarean rates by 30% or more within 12 months, the asthma care collaborative, and reduction of delays and wait times.

REFERENCES

Briere, R. (2001). *Crossing the quality chasm*. Washington, DC: National Academies Press.
Capra, F. (2002). *The hidden connection*. New York, NY: Doubleday.
Chassin, M. R., & Loeb, J. M. (2013). High-reliability health care: getting there from here. *The Milbank Quarterly, 91*(3), 459–490.

Cooperrider, D. L. (1990). Positive image, positive action: The affirmative basis of organizing. In S. Srivastva & D. L. Cooperrider (Eds.), *Appreciative management and leadership: The power of positive thought and action in organizations* (pp. 91–125). San Francisco, CA: Jossey-Bass.

Crosson, F. (2009). 21st-century health care: The case for integrated delivery systems. *New England Journal of Medicine, 361,* 1324–1325. Retrieved from http://healthpolicyandreform.nejm.org/?p=1887

Crowell, D. M. (2011). *Complexity leadership.* Philadelphia, PA: F. A. Davis.

DePree, M. (1990). *Leadership is an art.* New York, NY: Random House.

Eden, J., Levit, L., Berg, A., & Morton, S. (2011). *Finding what works in health care: Standards for systematic reviews.* Washington, DC: National Academies Press.

Gardner, D. (2005). Ten lessons in collaboration. *Online Journal of Issues in Nursing, 10*(1). Retrieved from http://www.nursingworld.org/ojin

Gonzales, E. W., & Esperat, M. C. (2010). The clinical scholar role in doctoral advanced nursing practice. In H. Michael Dreher & M. W. Smith Glasgow (Eds.), *Role development for doctoral advanced nursing practice* (pp. 199–212). New York, NY: Springer.

Graham, R., Mancher, M., Wolman Miller, D., Greenfield, S., & Steinberg, E. (2011). *Clinical practice guidelines we can trust.* Washington, DC: National Academies Press.

Guiette, A., & Vandenbempt, K. (2016). Learning in times of dynamic complexity through balancing phenomenal qualities of sensemaking. *Management Learning, 47*(1), 83–99.

Institute for Healthcare Improvement. (2003). *The breakthrough series: IHI's collaborative model for achieving breakthrough improvement* (IHI Innovation Series White Paper). Boston, MA: Author. Retrieved from http://www.IHI.org

Lindberg, C., Nash, S., & Lindberg, C. (2008). *On the edge: Nursing in the age of complexity.* Bordentown, NJ: Plexus Institute.

Lloyd, R. (2011, June). *Quality improvement: Building basic competencies.* Podium presentation, University of Texas Health Science Center at San Antonio, Academic Center for Evidence Based Practice.

Marsh, D. R., Schroeder, D. G., Dearden, K. A., Sternin, J., & Sternin, M. (2004). The power of positive deviance. *British Medical Journal, 329,* 1177–1179.

Patterson, K., Grenny, J., McMillan, R., & Switzler, A. (2002). *Crucial conversations: Tools for talking when stakes are high.* New York, NY: McGraw-Hill.

Senge, P. (1990). *The fifth discipline: The art and practice of the learning organization.* New York, NY: Random House.

Yu, D., & Hang, C. C. (2010). A reflective review of disruptive innovation theory. *International Journal of Management Reviews, 12*(4), 435–452.

Index

Note: Page numbers followed by *b*, *f*, or *t* indicate material in boxes, figures, or tables, respectively.

6S hierarchy of pre-appraised evidence, 293, 294*f*, 301, 302
six Sigma process, for quality improvement, 220–221
small troubles, adaptive responses (STAR-2), 201
SMART, 217
Snow, John, 268, 269
snowball sampling, 8*t*, 26
social structure, empiricism and, 269
software programs
　for qualitative data analysis, 61–62
　for qualitative research, 28
Solomon four-group design, 15–16, 16*t*
solutions, to problems, 203
　grand schemes, 203
　rapid *vs.* slow, 203
　tried and true, 203
SORT, 346
space, cause and effect and, 203
special variation, 204
staff education, 338
staff engagement surveys, 208
staff knowledge, increasing, 339–340, 341*f*
standard deviation (SD), 81
standards of care, variations in, 204
statistical processes, in quality improvement plan, 223
statistics, 69
stratified purposive sampling, 58
stratified random sampling, 7*t*
stressors
　in double ABCX model of family behavior, 274, 275*f*
　perception of, in double ABCX model of family behavior, 274, 275*f*, 276
structure, quality improvement and, 215–216
SUMARI (System for the Unified Management, Assessment and Review of Information), 311
summary, 133–134
summary statistics, generation, 92
supplies/equipment, failure, 204
supportiveness of the larger system, as microsystem characteristic, 199
surgical site infection prevention, 242–243
survey sampling, 71
SWAT team approach, for quality improvement, 220
SWOT, 335
synopsis of studies, 310
synthesis, 93
systematic random sampling, 7*t*
systematic reviews
　in 6S hierarchy of pre-appraised evidence, 293, 294*f*
　critique, 129–133
　description of, 19
　in evidence pyramid, 290–291, 291*f*
　as knowledge synthesis method, 296
systems. *See also specific types of systems*
　change
　　leadership and, 204–205, 205*f*
　　management, 224–225
　　organizational frameworks, evaluation of, 167–185
　　readiness for, 333
　　small tests, as microsystem growth/development stage, 195
　　transformational, exemplar of, 159–160
　characteristics of, 170–171, 198–199
　properties, 204
　qualities, definition of, 193–194
systems approach, to human error, 233, 234
systems theory, complexity science and chaos theory, 279
systems thinking
　description of, 170–171
　organizational learning and, 202–203
　theory of profound knowledge and, 232

T

target population, 69
Taylor, Frederick, 214
TCAB. *See* Transforming Care at the Bedside (TCAB)
team members, collaboration among, 236, 237
TeamSTEPPS training program, 237, 238*f*, 279
teamwork training programs, 236
test-retest reliability, 9*b*
Texas Nurses Association (TNA), 174–175
text, examination methods, 92
thematic content analysis, 61
theme clusters, 94–95, 94*t*
theme, definition of, 91
theoretical sampling, 26
theorizing, 68–69
theory-guided practice, 271
theory/theories
　conceptual frameworks/models and, 270–271
　definition of, 68, 267, 270, 273
　grand, 271
　ladder of abstraction and, 242*f*, 272–273
　middle-range, 271–272
　practice, 272
　of profound knowledge, 232
　in quantitative research, 270, 271